VETERINARY EMBRYOLOGY

VETERINARY EMBRYOLOGY

T. A. McGeady, MV[
Former Senior Lectu[
Department of Veteri[
Faculty of Veterinary[
University College D[

P. J. Quinn, MVB, P[
Professor Emeritus,[
Former Professor of [
Faculty of Veterinary[
University College D[

E. S. FitzPatrick, FI[
Department of Veteri[
Faculty of Veterinary[
University College D[

M. T. Ryan, MSc, Ph[
Molecular Biology L[
Faculty of Veterinary[
University College D[

Illustrations by
S. Cahalan, MVB
Faculty of Veterinary[
University College D[

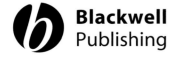
Blackwell
Publishing

© 2006 TA McGeady, PJ Quinn, ES FitzPatrick, MT Ryan and S Cahalan

Editorial Offices:
Blackwell Publishing Ltd, 9600 Garsington Road, Oxford OX4 2DQ, UK
 Tel: +44 (0)1865 776868
Blackwell Publishing Professional, 2121 State Avenue, Ames, Iowa 50014-8300, USA
 Tel: +1 515 292 0140
Blackwell Publishing Asia, 550 Swanston Street, Carlton, Victoria 3053, Australia
 Tel: +61 (0)3 8359 1011

First published 2006 by Blackwell Publishing Ltd

ISBN-10: 1-4051-1147-X
ISBN-13: 978-1-4051-1147-8

Library of Congress Cataloging-in-Publication Data

Veterinary embryology / T.A. McGeady . . . [et al.].; illustrations by S. Cahalan.— 1st ed.
   p. cm.
  Includes bibliographical references and index.
  ISBN-13: 978-1-4051-1147-8 (pbk. : alk. paper)
  ISBN-10: 1-4051-1147-X (pbk. : alk. paper)
  1. Veterinary embryology.   I. McGeady, T. A. (Thomas A.)

  SF767.5.V48 2006
  636.089′264—dc22

                                                2005022781

A catalogue record for this title is available from the British Library

Set in 10/12.5pt Times
by Graphicraft Limited, Hong Kong
Printed and bound in Great Britain
by TJ International Ltd, Padstow, Cornwall

The publisher's policy is to use permanent paper from mills that operate a sustainable forestry policy, and which has been manufactured from pulp processed using acid-free and elementary chlorine-free practices. Furthermore, the publisher ensures that the text paper and cover board used have met acceptable environmental accreditation standards.

For further information on Blackwell Publishing, visit our website:
www.blackwellpublishing.com

Contents

Preface

An understanding of the origin, development and maturation of cells in the developing embryo and, later, in the foetus provides veterinary students with information relevant to organ primordia and development of body systems. A study of embryology offers the student an understanding of the development, structure, final form and relationships of tissues and organs. Developmental defects and the clinical conditions to which they give rise can be more completely understood through a knowledge of the factors which control developmental processes and the deleterious affects of environmental teratogens on normal embryological development.

This book is primarily concerned with developmental aspects of cells, tissues, organs and body systems of animals. Where feasible, comparative aspects of human embryology are included. Drawings of cells, tissues and organs, along with flow diagrams and tables, are used to provide a clear understanding of information contained in the text.

There are 24 chapters in this book, each dealing with topics which are fundamental to an understanding of the sequential stages of embryological and foetal development. Cell division, gametogenesis, fertilisation, cleavage and gastrulation are presented in sequential chapters. Succeeding chapters are concerned with cell signalling, establishment of a body plan, formation of foetal membranes and placentation. Body systems are considered in separate chapters and the embryological aspects of structures associated with special senses are reviewed. Age determination and aspects of mutagenesis and teratogenesis are briefly reviewed in final chapters.

Although this book is intended primarily as a textbook for undergraduate veterinary students, it may be of value to colleagues engaged in teaching embryology, either as part of a veterinary curriculum or in courses relating to animal science or developmental biology. Research workers engaged in projects on animal reproduction and allied topics may find particular chapters relevant to their fields of investigation.

Throughout the book, emphasis is placed on the origin and differentiation of tissues and organs and their relationships to each other. This approach provides a logical foundation for acquiring an understanding of the form and relationships of cells, tissues, organs and structures in defined regions of the body. Such knowledge is a fundamental requirement for the appreciation of topographical anatomy, a cornerstone in the acquisition of clinical skills, interpretation of diagnostic imaging and the implementation of surgical procedures. Molecular aspects of embryology provide an introduction to genes and the transcription factors which promote or regulate orderly development of the embryo and foetus. Developmental defects of clinical significance are also included. The classification used throughout the book generally conforms to the *Nomina Embryologica Veterinaria* system proposed in 1994. Selected review articles and textbooks are listed in each chapter as sources of additional information.

1 Division, Growth and Differentiation of Cells

The mammalian body is composed of an array of organs, tissues and individual cells which function in a specialised and highly coordinated manner. Although these cells, tissues and organs exhibit considerable diversity in both structure and function, they all derive from a single cell, a fertilised ovum. The fertilised ovum is a product of the fusion of two specialised reproductive cells, gametes, of male and female origin. Following fertilisation, the ovum undergoes a series of divisions which ultimately lead to the formation of pluripotent stem cells, from which all cells, tissues and organs of the body arise. The study of this process of growth and differentiation, beginning with the fertilisation of an ovum and progressing to a fully formed individual animal, is termed embryology.

Cells associated with tissue formation and regeneration are described as somatic cells. Specialised reproductive cells, referred to as germ cells, include gametes of male and female origin and their precursors.

Coordinated and regulated cell division is essential for embryological development. Somatic cell division consists of nuclear division, mitosis, followed by cytoplasmic division, cytokinesis. In mitotic division of somatic cells, the daughter cells produced are genetically identical. A form of cell division distinctly different from mitosis occurs in germ cells. In this form of cell division, referred to as meiosis, the cells produced contain half the number of chromosomes of the progenitor germ cell and are not genetically identical. Somatic cell division combined with other cellular processes such as progressive differentiation, migration, adhesion, hypertrophy and apoptosis are prerequisites for embryological development.

The cell cycle

Somatic cells undergo a series of molecular and morphological changes as part of the cell cycle. These changes occur in four sequential phases, namely G_1, S, G_2 and M, and also a quiescent phase, termed G_0 (Fig. 1.1). The G_1 and G_2 phases are termed resting phases. In these phases, the cell is metabolically active, fulfilling its specialised function preparatory to the next phase of the cycle, but DNA replication does not take place. During the S phase, DNA synthesis occurs prior to chromosomal replication. This is followed by mitosis which occurs during the M phase. Collectively, the G_1, S and G_2 phases constitute the interphase (Fig. 1.1). Cells which enter a G_0 state may remain transiently or permanently in that state. Certain fully differentiated cells, such as neurons, do not divide, and continue to function permanently in a G_0 state. Other cell types, such as epithelial cells and hepatocytes, can re-enter the cell cycle from G_0 and proceed to mitotic division in response to appropriate stimuli.

A number of stimuli such as growth factors, mitogens and signals from other cells and from the extra-cellular matrix can induce cells in a G_0 state to re-enter the cell cycle near the end of the G_1 phase. Growth factors which bind to cell surface receptors activate intra-cellular signalling pathways. In most mammalian cells, the activation of genes encoding cyclins and cyclin-dependent kinases (Cdks) specific to the G_1 phase regulate the cell cycle and commit the cell to enter the S phase. This process is initiated at the restriction point, a stage at which mammalian cells become committed to entering the S phase and are then capable of completing the cell cycle independent of extra-cellular influences.

The rate of cell division varies in different cell types and at different stages of differentiation. Variations in cell cycle length are largely attributed to differences in the length of the G_1 phase, which can range from six hours to several days. Early embryonic development is characterised by rapid cell division, but as cells become more differentiated during organ development, the rate of cell division generally decreases.

Mitosis

The nuclei of somatic cells of each mammalian species have a defined number of chromosomes (Table 1.1). A somatic cell with a full complement of chromosomes

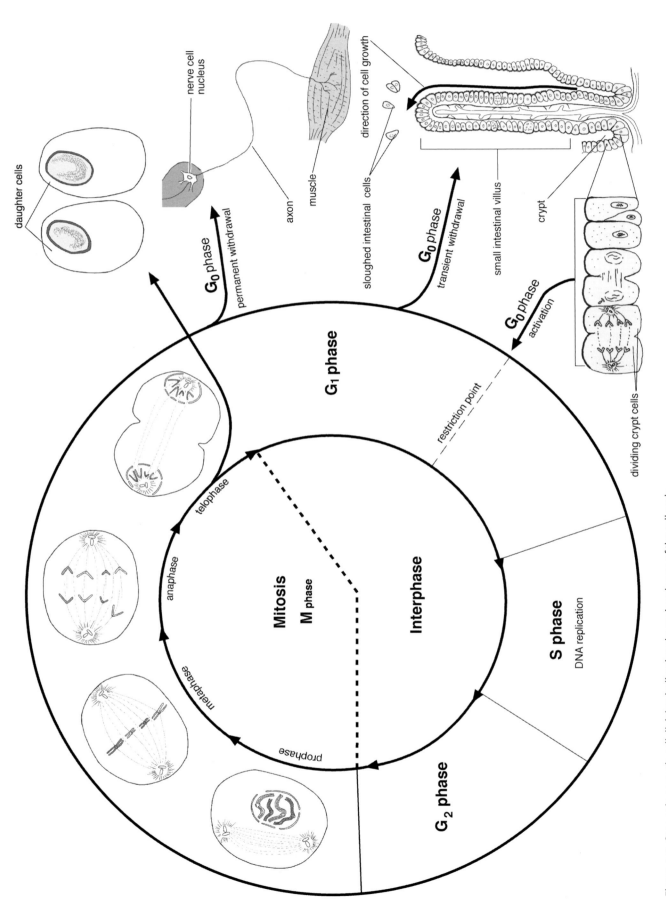

Figure 1.1 Stages in somatic cell division indicating the major phases of the cell cycle.

Table 1.1 The number of chromosomes in diploid human and animal cells.

Species	Number of chromosomes (2n)
Humans	46
Cats	38
Cattle	60
Chickens	78
Dogs	78
Donkeys	62
Goats	60
Horses	64
Pigs	38
Rabbits	44
Rats	42
Sheep	54

is referred to as diploid and given the designation 2n. The term mitosis is used to describe nuclear division of somatic cells, a process which usually results in the production of two cells, with the same chromosome complement as the progenitor cell from which they derived. Mitosis is essential for embryonic growth and development and for repair and replacement of tissue throughout life. The stages of mitosis occur as a distinct sequence of cytological events, which are part of the cell cycle.

Stages of mitosis

Preparatory to mitosis, the chromosomes are replicated in the S phase of the cell cycle forming sister chromatids. Within the nuclear envelope sister chromatids remain attached at a constricted region of the chromosome called a centromere. Following the G_2 phase, mitosis, which can be divided into four stages, prophase (Fig. 1.2B), metaphase (Fig. 1.2C), anaphase (Fig. 1.2D) and finally telophase (Fig. 1.2E), begins. The stages of mitosis are usually followed by cytoplasmic division or cytokinesis (Fig. 1.2F).

Prophase

The first stage of mitosis is prophase (Fig. 1.2B). During this period, the chromosomes, consisting of closely associated sister chromatids, condense. Outside the nucleus, the centrosomes, composed of paired centrioles previously replicated during interphase, begin to form

microtubule spindles or asters. The spindles are responsible for the movement of the centrosomes to opposite poles of the dividing cell.

Microtubules, an essential part of the mitotic apparatus, are visible microscopically only during the M phase. Individual microtubules are cylindrical structures, composed of 13 parallel protofilaments consisting of alternating α-tubulin and β-tubulin subunits. An individual microtubule may grow or shrink by a process of polymerisation of α-tubulin and β-tubulin. A growing microtubule has a structure referred to as a guanidine-triphosphate (GTP) cap. The β-subunit of a microtubule contains GTP capable of being hydrolysed to guanidine-diphosphate (GDP). This, in turn, alters the conformation of the subunits, resulting in shrinking of the microtubules. If GTP hydrolysis occurs more rapidly than subunit addition, the cap is lost and the microtubule shrinks. Shrinking and growing are a dynamic process and these changes enable the microtubules to actively orientate and move chromosomes during mitosis and meiosis.

Metaphase

Events during the metaphase stage of mitosis can be divided into two phases, pro-metaphase and metaphase. Disintegration of the nuclear envelope marks the beginning of pro-metaphase. A kinetochore, a protein complex which forms on the centromeres during late prophase, acts as a platform for attachment to microtubules. Chromosomes attach to the microtubules via their kinetochores and the combination of these two latter structures is termed a kinetochore microtubule. The formation of the kinetochore microtubule enables the movement of chromosomes to take place. During metaphase, the chromosomes are positioned midway between the poles of the cell at a region termed the metaphase plate. Each sister chromatid is attached to the centrosome by its kinetochore microtubule (Fig. 1.2C).

Anaphase

During the anaphase stage, the pairs of conjoined sister chromatids synchronously separate as the centromeres split and the attached kinetochore microtubules shorten. The newly separated chromatid sets are drawn towards opposite poles of the cell (Fig. 1.2D).

Telophase

The two groups of identical chromosomes (former chromatids) clustered at their respective poles, de-condense and a nuclear envelope forms around each set. The formation of nuclear envelopes marks the end of mitosis, a process which results in equal and symmetrical division of the nucleus (Fig. 1.2E).

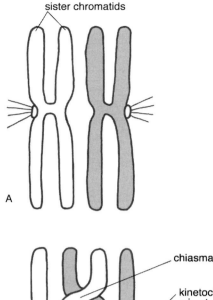

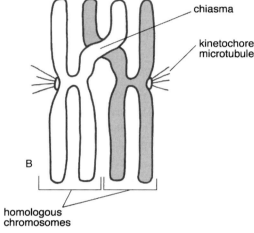

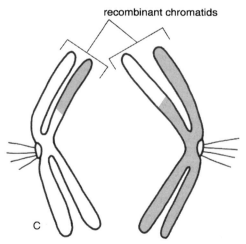

Figure 1.3 Chiasma formation and reciprocal exchange of genetic material between non-sister homologous chromatids during meiosis I.

Metaphase I

As in mitosis, homologous chromosome pairs attach via their kinetochores to the microtubules arising from the centrosomes which are located at opposite poles of the cell. During metaphase, the homologous chromosome pairs are positioned at the metaphase plate by the kinetochore microtubules (Fig. 1.4D).

Anaphase I

During anaphase I, the tetrad splits into two dyads (half a tetrad), which move to opposite poles of the cell. Unlike the anaphase stage of mitosis, splitting of the centromeres does not occur because in this instance only one kinetochore forms on each dyad. The distribution of paternally derived and maternally derived homologous chromosomes at this point is random, and it is this variable arrangement which underlies the Mendelian principle of random assortment (Fig. 1.4E).

Telophase I

In telophase I, nuclear envelopes develop around the separate chromosome sets and cytokinesis follows (Figs. 1.4F and G). In the formation of primary spermatocytes, progenitors of male gametes, the cytoplasm is divided equally between the two cells. However, during the formation of oocytes, female gametes, one of the two resulting cells retains the greater portion of cytoplasm. The smaller of the two cells is termed a polar body. A short resting phase, termed interkinesis, follows telophase I and replication of DNA does not occur during this phase.

The second meiotic division

Prophase II

The events of prophase II are similar to prophase I. The nucleus contains a set of dyads each composed of a pair of chromatids connected by a shared centromere (Fig. 1.5A).

Metaphase II

The phase termed metaphase II is similar to metaphase I in that the chromosomes are positioned at the metaphase plate by the kinetochore microtubules. In this instance, however, kinetochores form on each of the individual chromatids. This allows the microtubules to attach separately to each chromatid (Fig. 1.5B).

Anaphase II

During anaphase II, the dyads are separated into individual chromatids by the kinetochore microtubules and the sets of chromatids are drawn towards opposite poles of the dividing cell (Fig. 1.5C).

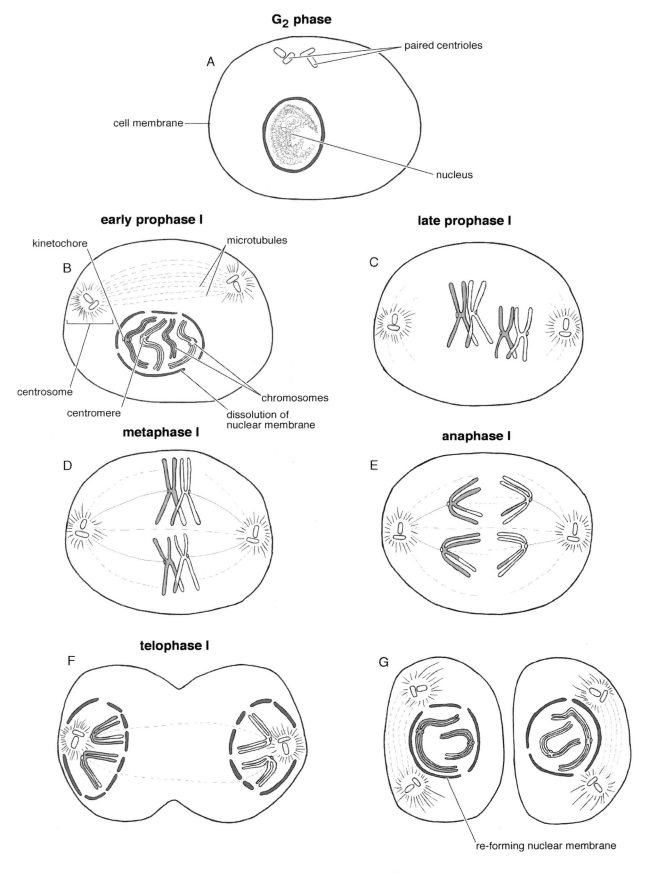

Figure 1.4 An outline of the sequential stages of the first meiotic division (A to G). After the G_2 phase, prophase I commences followed by metaphase I, anaphase I and telophase I.

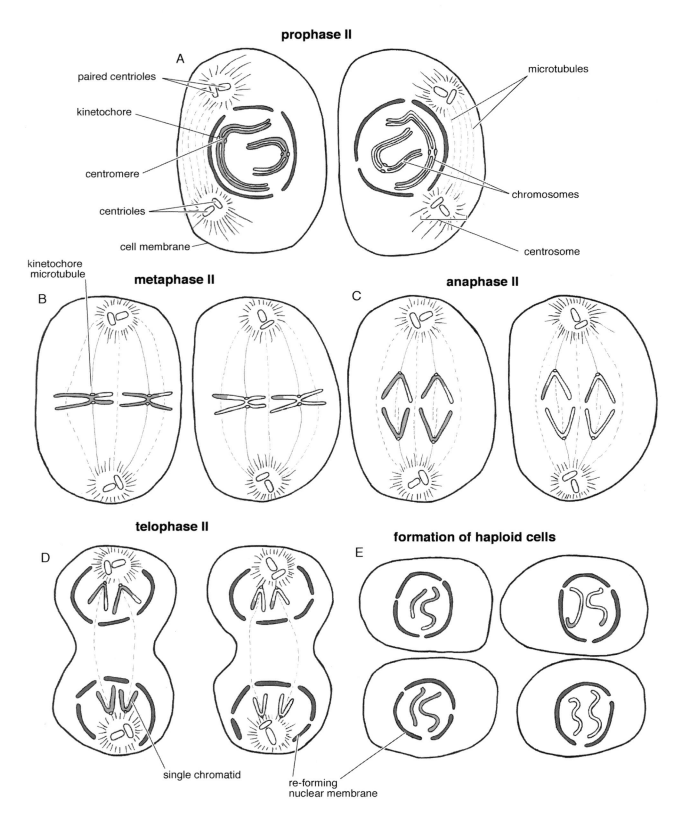

Figure 1.5 An outline of the sequential stages of the second meiotic division (A to G). After meiosis I, prophase II commences, followed by metaphase II, anaphase II, and telophase II, leading to the formation of four haploid gametes. Only two pairs of chromosomes are represented for clarity.

Telophase II

At the end of telophase II, nuclear envelopes form around each set of chromatids and the cytoplasm divides again (Fig. 1.5D). As a consequence of meiosis I and II, four haploid cells are formed from a single diploid germ cell (Fig. 1.5E).

Consequences of non-dysjunction of chromosomes during meiosis

The term non-dysjunction describes the failure of two homologous chromosomes in meiosis I, or sister chromatids in meiosis II, to separate properly and to move correctly to opposite poles. Meiosis depends on the establishment of specialised interactions between chromosomes along with specific modifications to the mitotic cell cycle regulatory processes. Errors in these processes, which usually occur during meiosis I, can result in defective segregation. Abnormalities arising from this include numerical alteration and structural defects in chromosomes. While chromosomal defects associated with germ cells generally lead to embryonic death, in some instances offspring may survive and exhibit developmental defects. Alterations of chromosome numbers may involve either autosomes or sex chromosomes.

Further reading

Alberts, B., Johnson, A., Lewis, J., Raff, M., Roberts, K. and Walter, P. (2002) *Molecular Biology of the Cell*, 4th edn. Garland Science, New York.

Klug, W.S. and Cummins, M.R. (1999) *Essentials of Genetics*. Prentice-Hall, Upper Saddle River, New Jersey.

Levine, E.M. (2004) Cell cycling through development. *Development* **131**, 2241–2246.

Marston, A.L. and Amon, A. (2004) Meiosis: cell-cycle controls shuffle and deal. *Nature Reviews: Molecular and Cell Biology* **5**, 983–997.

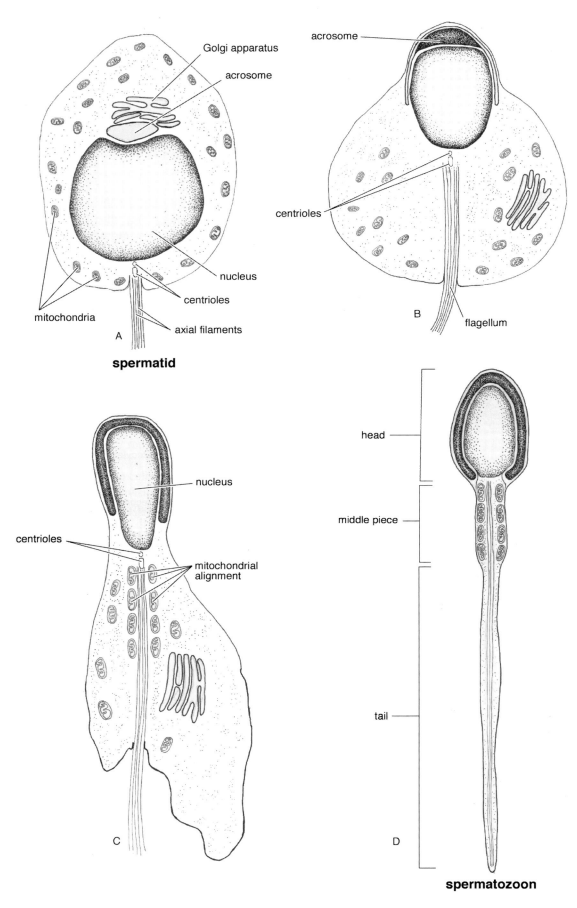

Figure 2.2 The morphological changes whereby a mammalian spermatid is converted into a spermatozoon.

the epididymis for only a few days before losing their viability. Most of the unejaculated spermatozoa are gradually discharged into the urinary system; a small percentage which remain in the epididymis undergo degenerative change and are phagocytosed. The transport of spermatozoa through the epididymis, due to contractions of the smooth muscle of the epididymal duct wall, takes up to 12 days in the bull and ram and up to 14 days in the boar and stallion. With increased frequency of ejaculation, transport time may be reduced.

Oogenesis

Oogonia, which arise from primordial germ cells in the endoderm, undergo repeated mitotic divisions in the foetal ovary. The duration of this period of mitosis varies in individual species. Irrespective of species, the mitotic phase of oogenesis ceases in mammals soon after birth. When they have completed their cycles of mitosis, oogonia enter the prophase of the first of two meiotic divisions and become primary oocytes which are diploid. Such diploid cells are given the designation 2n to indicate that they contain a full complement of chromosomes. All primary oocytes are formed before puberty (Fig. 2.3).

A primary oocyte surrounded by a single layer of squamous epithelial cells is known as a primordial follicle (Fig. 2.4). Primary oocytes do not complete the prophase of the first meiotic division but enter a prolonged resting or dictyate stage until activated by gonadotrophic hormones which induce further development. During both the proliferative and resting phases, a high proportion of primordial follicles undergo atresia. Completion of the initial stage of the first meiotic division follows hormonal stimulation. During puberty, the oocyte increases in size and the surrounding epithelial follicular cells form a stratified layer around the oocyte. This structure is now known as a primary follicle. Glycoproteins, secreted primarily by the oocyte, condense forming a prominent translucent acellular layer, the zona pellucida, located between the vitelline membrane of the oocyte and the follicular cells. As the follicle enlarges, the thickness of the zona pellucida increases. The oocyte and the follicular cells maintain contact by means of microvillous cytoplasmic processes which penetrate the zona. Gap junctions between the oocyte and the cytoplasmic processes of follicular cells allow intercellular communication. As the follicle continues to increase in size, small fluid-filled spaces appear between the follicular cells which gradually coalesce forming a fluid-filled cavity known as the antrum. The squamous follicular cells, which become cuboidal, form stratified layers and are referred to as granulosa cells. The oocyte remains attached to the follicular wall by an accumulation of granulosa cells termed the cumulus oophorus (Fig. 2.4). Those granulosa cells which surround the

oocyte in a radial fashion are referred to as the corona radiata. The mature follicle is now referred to as a vesicular or Graafian follicle. The completion of the first meiotic division results in the production of two haploid cells of unequal size. The cell which receives most of the cytoplasm is referred to as the secondary oocyte and the other, which receives a minimal amount of cytoplasm, is the first polar body (Fig. 2.3). Following formation of the first polar body, the secondary oocyte commences the second meiotic division.

Ovulation

Release of the ovum from the follicle is referred to as ovulation (Fig. 2.4). Prior to ovulation, the oocyte and corona radiata detach from the cumulus oophorus and float in the follicular fluid. Rupture of the follicle is attributed to the formation of a blister-like area, the stigma, on the ovarian surface directly above the follicle. While it is accepted that the stigma arises from constriction of blood vessels as a result of hormonal or enzymatic activity, the exact details of follicular rupture are poorly understood.

Although ovulation generally occurs near the end of oestrus, the precise time at which it occurs differs among domestic species (Table 2.1). Ovulation occurs spontaneously in most species (spontaneous ovulation). In cats, rabbits, ferrets and camels, however, ovulation is induced by coitus (induced ovulation). The number of ova released, which is characteristic for a given species, is strongly influenced by genetic factors. In most mammals, ovulation occurs during the metaphase of the second meiotic stage of oogenesis. Exceptions include dogs and foxes, where ovulation usually occurs during the metaphase of the first meiotic division. Completion of the second meiotic division and formation of the second polar body occur after fertilisation.

Transport of ova in the uterine tube

After ovulation, the ovum enters the uterine tube, the site of fertilisation in mammals. Tubal wall contractions aided by the ciliary beat of the epithelium of the tube are responsible for the transportation of ova along the tube. Whether or not they are fertilised, ova normally reach the uterus within three to four days after ovulation. However, in domestic carnivores it may take up to seven days for ova to reach the uterus. Fertilised ova of horses and bats enter the uterus, whereas non-fertilised ova are retained at the isthmus of the uterine tube. In rabbits, opossums and dogs, a mucopolysaccharide coat forms around the zona pellucida while the ovum is in the uterine tube. As the uterus provides a favourable environment for the survival of spermatozoa but not for the blastocyst, it is essential that fertilised ova be transported

Table 2.1 Features of the oestrous cycle in domestic animals.

Animal	Length of oestrous cycle in days	Duration of oestrus	Number of ova usually released from ovary	Time at which ovulation occurs
Bitch	140	9 days	2 to 10	2 to 3 days after commencement of oestrus
Cow	18 to 24	18 hours	1	14 hours after end of oestrus
Ewe	15 to 17	36 hours	1 to 3	24 to 30 hours after onset of oestrus
Goat	18 to 22	24 to 48 hours	2 to 3	24 to 36 hours after onset of oestrus
Mare	18 to 24	4 to 8 days	1	1 to 2 days before end of oestrus
Queen	17	3 to 6 days	2 to 8	24 hours after coitus
Sow	19 to 22	48 hours	10 to 25	36 to 48 hours after onset of oestrus

from one uterine horn to the other up to 14 times per day. While intrauterine migration can occur in cattle and sheep, the frequency is low in sheep (4%) and rare in cattle (0.3%). Embryo migration and spacing within the uterus appear to be regulated by peristaltic contractions of the myometrium, influenced by hormones released from the conceptus.

Optimal time for fertilisation of the ovum

In individual species, there is a maximum period during which an ovum remains capable of being fertilised. Loss of viability is gradual and although ageing ova may be fertilised, the resulting embryos are usually not viable. Senescence appears to predispose to polyspermy, the entry of more than one spermatozoon into the ovum. Fertilisation involving aged gametes is considered to contribute to the occurrence of some congenital abnormalities, particularly in the human population. Unfertilised ova undergo fragmentation and are phagocytosed in the female reproductive tract.

Retention of fertilising capacity of spermatozoa

In the female reproductive tracts of domestic animals, spermatozoa retain their ability to fertilise ova for at least 24 hours. It has been suggested that there is a correlation between the duration of oestrus and the retention of viability of spermatozoa and their ability to fertilise ova after deposition in the female reproductive tract. Motile spermatozoa have been observed in the reproductive tracts of mares for up to six days after mating, and for up to 11 days in bitches. In domesticated fowl, spermatozoa, which are stored in special sperm nests in the female tract, may remain capable of fertilising ova for up to 21 days. In some species of bats in which coitus takes place in the autumn, spermatozoa remain viable in the female reproductive tract until ovulation occurs in the spring.

Semen used for artificial insemination retains its viability at 4°C for several hours. When stored at −196°C in liquid nitrogen, viability is retained indefinitely.

Further reading

Bracket, B.J. (2004) Male reproduction in mammals. In *Duke's Physiology of Domestic Animals.* Ed. W.O. Reece. Comstock Publishing Association, Cornell University Press, Ithaca, NY, pp. 670–691.

Eddy, E.M. and O'Brien, D.A. (1994) The spermatozoon. In *Physiology of Reproduction*, Vol. 1, 2nd edn. Eds. E. Knobil and J.D. Neill. Raven Press, NY, pp. 29–77.

Hafez, E.S.E. and Hafez, B. (2000) Folliculogenesis, egg maturation, and ovulation. In *Reproduction of Farm Animals*, 7th edn. Eds. E.S.E. Hafez and B. Hafez. Lippincott, Williams, and Wilkins, Philadelphia, pp. 68–82.

Robl, J.M. and Fissore, R.A. (1999) Gametes, an overview. In *Encyclopedia of Reproduction*, Vol. 2. Eds. E. Knobil and J.D. Neill. Academic Press, San Diego, pp. 430–434.

Senger, P.L. (2003) Endocrinology of the male and spermatogenesis. In *Pathways to Pregnancy and Parturition.* Current Conceptions Inc., Pullman, Washington, pp. 214–240.

Thompson, T.N. (2004) Female reproduction in mammals. In *Duke's Physiology of Domestic Animals*, Ed. W.O. Reece. Comstock Publishing Association, Cornell University Press, Ithaca, NY, pp. 692–719.

Wassarman, P.M. and Albertini, D.F. (1994) The mammalian ovum. In *Physiology of Reproduction*, Vol. 1, 2nd edn. Eds. E. Knobil and J.D. Neill. Raven Press, NY, pp. 79–122.

3 Fertilisation

The process whereby a spermatozoon and an ovum fuse to form a single-celled zygote is termed fertilisation. Following penetration of the vitelline membrane by the spermatozoon, the activated ovum completes meiosis and extrudes the second polar body. The chromosomes contained in the haploid male pronucleus align with their corresponding chromosomes in the female pronucleus. The paternal and maternal chromosomes condense, become attached to mitotic spindles and align themselves centrally. The first mitotic division of cleavage follows. The integration of the paternal and maternal genetic material, which occurs during these processes, is referred to as syngamy. As a consequence of fertilisation, the diploid number of chromosomes is restored, the sex of the individual is determined and biological variation results from the integration of paternal and maternal hereditary characteristics.

Many aquatic animals release ova and spermatozoa into the water and fertilisation takes place in this aqueous environment. The fact that gametes are released at approximately the same time and in close proximity to each other, usually as a consequence of courtship, contributes to the likelihood of fertilisation taking place. In addition, mutual chemical attraction between male and female gametes increases the probability of fertilisation. This selective attraction is considered to be important in the attachment of the spermatozoon to the ovum and in the inhibition of cross-fertilisation between unrelated species. Relative to mammalian species, aquatic animals and amphibians produce large quantities of zygotes; however, the parental energy invested per zygote (PEI/Z) is low. In contrast, birds and mammals produce relatively fewer zygotes, but the PEI/Z involved is much greater. This investment can take many forms and in mammalian species it encompasses the parental investment provided both during gestation and post-natally.

When ova are retained within the female reproductive tract and are fertilised by spermatozoa deposited there, this type of fertilisation is referred to as internal fertilisation. Factors which increase the probability of fertilisation taking place are the high numbers of spermatozoa released at copulation and the relatively large size of the ovum. Despite the fact that millions of spermatozoa are deposited in the female tract, only hundreds of spermatozoa reach the site of fertilisation. Involvement of more than one spermatozoon in fertilisation (polyspermy) is an abnormal occurrence in mammals and invariably leads to early embryonic death. Accordingly, the female tract controls the transport of spermatozoa so that the number reaching the site of fertilisation is sufficient to fertilise ova released from the ovary without the likelihood of polyspermy.

In mammals, millions of spermatozoa are deposited in the female reproductive tract at coitus (Table 3.1). Depending on the species, the spermatozoa may be deposited in either the vagina or the uterus. From this location, they are transported to the uterine tube which is arbitrarily divided on a functional basis into three regions, infundibulum, ampulla and isthmus. The infundibulum, the region closest to the ovary, is funnel shaped and its free edge possesses regular processes known as fimbriae which play an important role in the capture of ova (ova pickup). The infundibulum is continuous with a tubular portion which is divided into two regions of comparable length. The proximal region where fertilisation takes place is the ampulla, and the narrower terminal segment, which opens into the uterus, is the isthmus. Despite past uncertainty about the rate of transportation of spermatozoa within the female

Table 3.1 Volume of ejaculate, number of spermatozoa per ml, and site of deposition of spermatozoa in the female reproductive tract of domestic animals.

Species	Approximate volume of ejaculate (ml)	Number of spermatozoa per ml ($\times 10^6$)	Site of deposition of spermatozoa in the female reproductive tract
Cats	0.5	60	Vagina
Cattle	4.0	800 to 1,500	Vagina
Dogs	10	250	Uterus
Horses	70	150 to 300	Uterus
Pigs	250	200 to 300	Uterus
Sheep	1.0	2,000 to 3,000	Vagina

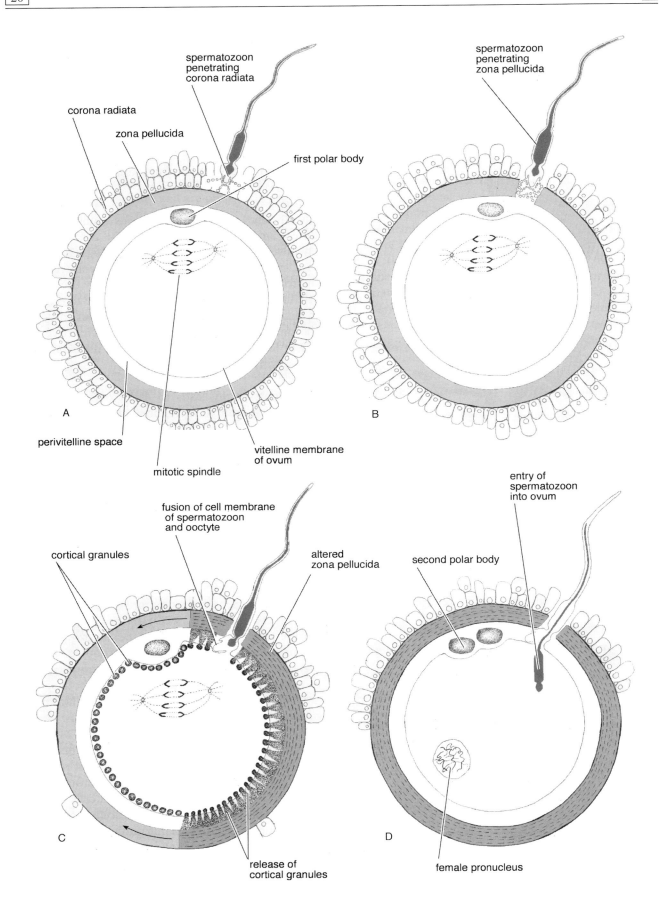

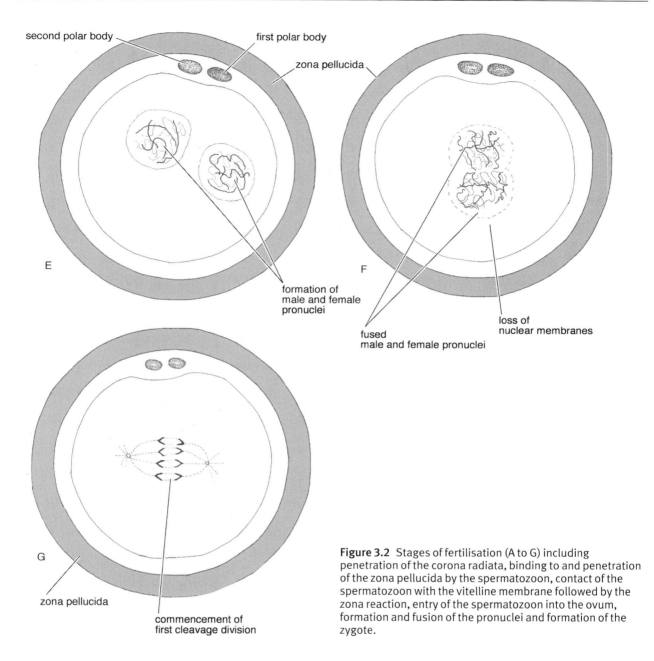

Figure 3.2 Stages of fertilisation (A to G) including penetration of the corona radiata, binding to and penetration of the zona pellucida by the spermatozoon, contact of the spermatozoon with the vitelline membrane followed by the zona reaction, entry of the spermatozoon into the ovum, formation and fusion of the pronuclei and formation of the zygote.

in calcium concentrations is reported to facilitate escape from meiotic arrest and to promote embryonic mitosis. At a later stage, ovum activation responses include recruitment of maternal mRNA for translation, changes in protein synthesis and activation of the zygotic genome. The factors which promote ovum activation are reported to be associated with the pronucleus of the spermatozoon but the mechanisms involved are ill-defined.

In vitro fertilisation

The process whereby secondary oocytes are fertilised with capacitated spermatozoa outside the body is termed *in vitro* fertilisation (IVF). In this procedure, under appropriate laboratory conditions, spermatozoa fertilise oocytes and the resulting embryos can be cultured to the cleavage stage prior to transfer to a female of the same species. The recipient's oestrous cycle is hormonally regulated to the appropriate stage for implantation. In cattle, sheep, pigs and humans, IVF has been employed successfully. Its success rate, however, is currently low. Applications of IVF include increased production of offspring of genetically superior breeding stock and the enhancement of the breeding rate of endangered species.

Comparative fertilisation rates

Fertilisation rate refers to the percentage of ova released at ovulation which are fertilised following natural or artificial insemination. In polytocous species such as pigs, dogs and cats, the fertilisation rate following natural mating ranges from 85% to 100%, while in monotocous species such as cattle and sheep, the range is from 85% to 95%. The fertilisation rate in horses is reported to be approximately 60%.

Sex determination

Every normal nucleated cell in the animal body contains a fixed number of chromosomes which is constant for a given species (Table 1.1). The chromosome complement is composed of paired autosomes and one pair of sex chromosomes. In normal mammalian female animals, the sex chromosomes, which are morphologically identical, are given the designation XX. The sex chromosomes of normal mammalian male animals, which are different from each other, are given the designation XY. Thus, female mammals are homogametic whereas male mammals are heterogametic.

In mammals, half of the spermatozoa contain an X chromosome and half contain a Y chromosome. Unlike spermatozoa, ova contain only X chromosomes. An ovum which is fertilised by an X-bearing spermatozoon is destined to become a female (XX) animal, while an ovum which is fertilised by a Y-bearing spermatozoon is destined to become a male (XY) animal (Fig. 3.3).

Sex determination in avian species is different from that in mammals as the male is homogametic and the female is heterogametic. Avian spermatozoa contain Z chromosomes only, while ova contain either Z or W chromosomes (Fig. 3.4). The designation XY in mammals and

the designation ZW in birds is conventional to facilitate genetic distinction. The ZZ/ZW designation is also used in fish, amphibians and reptiles.

The process of chromosomal determination of sex is referred to as genotypic sex determination as the sex of an individual is determined by genes on the sex chromosomes. Although, in the majority of reptiles, the sex of an individual is determined by sex chromosomes, the sex of most turtles and all crocodiles is determined by the incubation temperature of the fertilised ovum. Tortoise ova produce only male offspring at incubation temperatures from 16°C to 28°C. At a temperature of 32°C, only female offspring are produced. Reptiles lacking heteromorphic sex chromosomes therefore depend on incubation temperatures for determination of the sex of offspring. Incubation temperature has no effect on the sex ratio of reptiles which have heteromorphic sex chromosomes.

Parthenogenesis

Parthenogenesis is the development of an embryo from an ovum that has been activated by means other than a spermatozoon. The process occurs naturally in insects and lower animals. Experimentally, parthenogenesis can be induced in amphibians, birds and mammals by different techniques. Imprinting, which results in selective gene repression, follows a different pattern in male and female gametes. As a consequence of this differential gene expression, fusion of homologous gametes does not produce viable offspring. However, experimental interruption of the normal process of imprinting has succeeded in producing viable offspring in mice

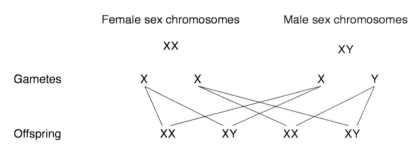

Figure 3.3 The chromosomal basis of sex determination in mammals.

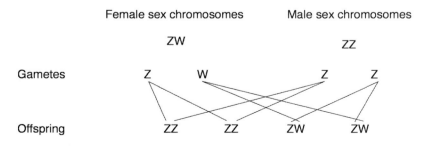

Figure 3.4 The chromosomal basis of sex determination in avian species.

from the fusion of two female gametes. These findings indicate that it is possible to overcome the barrier to parthenogenesis by circumventing the normal process of imprinting.

Natural parthenogenesis occurs infrequently in turkeys and rarely in chickens. In most cases, the embryos degenerate early in development. However, viable offspring have hatched in turkeys and chickens as a result of parthenogenesis. The sex of turkeys and chickens produced by parthenogenesis is always male (ZZ) and they have a diploid number of chromosomes due either to the suppression of the second stage of meiosis, or to the recombination of the second polar body with the nucleus of the ovum. For natural embryological development in mammals, a contribution from both the maternal and paternal genomes is a requirement. However, using experimental methods, viable offspring can be produced in mammals by parthenogenesis.

Sex ratio

The primary sex ratio is the proportion of male to female zygotes which result from fertilisation in mammals. The proportion of male animals to female animals at birth is referred to as the secondary sex ratio (Table 3.2).

Chromosomes of domestic animals

During metaphase, when the chromatids condense, their number, size and morphology can be observed by light microscopy. At this time, chromosomes of different species have recognisable characteristics. Two sets of chromosomes, present in somatic cells, constitute the diploid or 2n number. The classification of chromosomes is based on the length of their arms and the position of the centromere, which is observed as a constriction. At metaphase, each arm consists of two

Table 3.2 Primary and secondary sex ratios per 100 individuals in humans and domestic animals.

Species	Primary sex ratio		Secondary sex ratio	
	Male	Female	Male	Female
Humans	50	50	51	49
Cattle	50	50	52	48
Dogs	50	50	54	46
Horses	50	50	52	48
Pigs	50	50	52	48
Sheep	50	50	50	50

chromatids side by side. When the two arms are approximately equal in length, the chromosome is termed metacentric. When one arm is only one-half to one-third as long as the other, the chromosome is termed submetacentric. If the centromere is close to or at the end of the chromosome, such a chromosome is referred to as acrocentric.

The chromosomal complement of a cell, individual or species is known as the karyotype. Normally, the karyotype is constant for somatic cells of individuals within a species. Karyotyping, whereby chromosomes at metaphase can be drawn or photographed and arranged in homologous pairs in a systematic manner, is undertaken to determine the number and morphology of chromosomes in somatic cells. This technique is used to identify abnormalities such as the presence of additional chromosomes (trisomy), missing chromosomes (monosomy), the relocation of segments of chromosomes (translocation) and the loss of segments (deletion). Alteration of chromosome numbers may be associated with either the autosomes or the sex chromosomes. In humans an additional autosome gives rise to conditions such as Down Syndrome (47 chromosomes), while alterations in the number of sex chromosomes can lead to Klinefelter Syndrome (XXY) or Turner Syndrome (XO).

Further reading

Bedford, J.M. and Cross, N.L. (1999) Sperm capacitation. In *Encyclopedia of Reproduction*, Vol. 4. Eds. E. Knobil and J.D. Neill. Academic Press, San Diego, pp. 597–601.
Dunbar, B.S. and O'Rand, M.G. (Eds.) (1991) *A Comparative Overview of Mammalian Fertilization.* Plenum Press, New York.
Eisenbach, M. (1995) Sperm changes enabling fertilization in mammals. *Current Opinion in Endocrinology and Diabetes* **2**, 468–475.
Evans, J.P. and Florman, H.M. (2002) The state of the union: the cell biology of fertilization. *Nature Cell Biology, Suppl.* **4**, 57–63.
Hunter, R.H.F. (1991) Fertilization in pig and horse. In *A Comparative Overview of Mammalian Fertilization.* Eds. B.S. Dunbar and M.G. O'Rand. Plenum Press, New York, pp. 329–350.
Hunter, R.H.F. (2002) Vital aspects of fallopian tube physiology in pigs. *Reproduction in Domestic Animals* **37**, 186–190.
Hunter, R.H.F. (2003) Reflections upon sperm–endosalpingeal and sperm–zona pellucida interactions *in vivo* and *in vitro*. *Reproduction in Domestic Animals* **38**, 147–154.
Hyttel, P., Greve, T. and Callesen, H. (1989) Ultrastructural aspects of oocyte maturation and fertilization in

cattle. *Journal of Reproduction and Fertility* **39**, Suppl., 35–47.

Kono, T., Obata, Y., Wu, Q., Niwa, K., Ono, Y., Yamamoto, Y., Park, E.S., Soe, J. and Ogawa, H. (2004) Birth of parthenogenic mice that can develop into adulthood. *Nature* **428**, 860–864.

Longo, T.J. (1997) *Fertilization*, 2nd edn. Chapman and Hall, London.

Mahi-Brown, C.A. (1991) Fertilization in dogs. In *A Comparative Overview of Mammalian Fertilization.* Eds. B.S. Dunbar and M.G. O'Rand. Plenum Press, New York, pp. 281–298.

Moore, H.D.M. (2001) Molecular biology of fertilization. *Journal of Reproduction and Fertility* **57**, Suppl., 105–110.

Nomina Embryologica Veterinaria (1994) Published by the International Committees on Veterinary Gross Anatomical Nomenclature, Veterinary Histological Nomenclature and Veterinary Embryological Nomenclature. Zürich, pp. 1–59.

Primakoff, P. and Myles, D.G. (2002) Penetration, adhesion, and fusion in mammalian sperm–egg interaction. *Science* **296**, 2183–2185.

Rothchild, I. (2003) The yolkless egg and the evolution of eutherian viviparity. *Biology of Reproduction* **68**, 337–357.

Runft, L.L., Jaffe, L.A. and Mehlmann, L.M. (2002) Egg activation at fertilization: where it all begins. *Developmental Biology* **245**, 237–254.

Schatten, G. (1999) Fertilization. In *Encyclopedia of Reproduction*, Vol. 1. Eds. E. Knobil and J.D. Neill. Academic Press, San Diego, pp. 256–264.

Smith, T.T. (1998) The modulation of sperm function by the oviductal epithelium. *Biology of Reproduction* **58**, 1102–1104.

Suarez, S.S. (2002) Formation of a reservoir of sperm in the oviduct. *Reproduction in Domestic Animals* **37**, 140–143.

Wassarman, P.M. (1999) Mammalian fertilization: molecular aspect of gamete adhesion, exocytosis, and fusion. *Cell* **96**, 175–183.

Wasserman, P.M., Jovine, L. and Litscher, E.S. (2001) A profile of fertilization in mammals. *Nature Cell Biology* **3**, E59–E64.

Yanagimachi, R. (1994) Mammalian fertilization. In *The Physiology of Reproduction*, 2nd edn. Eds. E. Knobil and J.D. Neill. Raven Press, New York, pp. 189–318.

4 Cleavage

The fertilised ovum, with a diameter of 80–120 μm, is one of the largest mammalian cells and has a large amount of cytoplasm relative to the size of its nucleus. For structural development to take place, the zygote must divide. This series of mitotic divisions is referred to as cleavage or segmentation. A distinguishing feature of cleavage over the usual form of mitosis is that daughter cells become progressively smaller with each division, hence the term segmentation. As cleavage proceeds, division of the cytoplasm follows nuclear division and the two daughter cells produced are referred to as blastomeres. The two blastomeres divide repeatedly, producing four, eight, 16 and 32 cells, and division continues until a spherical mass of cells, termed a morula, is formed. The first cell divisions tend to occur synchronously in all blastomeres. Later, synchronous division is lost and blastomeres divide independently.

Division of the fertilised ovum is usually regular with the plane of the first division orientated vertically, passing through the main axis of the ovum from the animal pole at the top to the vegetal pole below. The succeeding division, which is also vertical and passes through the main axis at a right angle to the first division, results in four blastomeres (Fig. 4.1A). The third division takes place in the equatorial plane. As a consequence of the planes in which division takes place, eight blastomeres are formed, four in the animal hemisphere and four in the vegetal hemisphere.

The yolk content of the fertilised ovum determines the pattern of cleavage in individual species; retardation of the completion of cytokinesis correlates with increased yolk content. Accordingly, the relative amount of yolk and its distribution throughout the ovum has a profound influence on how cleavage proceeds and, subsequently, on germ layer formation. Ova with a small amount of evenly distributed yolk are referred to as miolecithal (isolecithal) ova. When the amount of yolk present displaces the embryo-forming cytoplasm into a small area at the animal pole, such ova are referred to as megalecithal (telolecithal). The term medialecithal (mesolecithal) is applied to ova with a moderate amount of yolk. Based on the abundance and distribution of the yolk, cleavage can be classified in a number of ways. The term total or holoblastic cleavage is used to describe divisions in which the entire ovum divides and the blastomeres produced are of either equal or unequal size. In miolecithal ova, such as those produced by some primitive chordates and placental mammals, blastomeres are of approximately equal size. In medialecithal ova, yolk accumulation at the vegetal pole retards mitosis, and blastomeres of unequal size are produced. This latter form of cleavage occurs in amphibians. In megalecithal ova, mitosis is restricted to the animal pole where the cytoplasm is devoid of yolk. The inert yolk mass at the vegetal pole does not divide. This type of division, referred to as partial or meroblastic cleavage, applies to fish, reptiles and birds. Because the site of cleavage is confined to a disc-shaped area at the animal pole, this type of cleavage is also known as discoidal. The final stage of cleavage is marked by the formation of a blastula which consists of a single layer of cells lining a central cavity known as the blastocoele.

Cleavage in primitive chordates, amphibians, avian species and mammals

Primitive chordates

Cleavage in *Amphioxus lanceolatum*, a primitive chordate, is holoblastic and the blastomeres produced are of almost equal size. As cleavage proceeds, surface depressions between dividing cells are referred to as cleavage furrows (Fig. 4.1). The first cleavage spindle forms near the centre of the ovum. The second division also produces cells of equal size, but after the third division the four cells at the animal pole are slightly smaller than those at the vegetal pole. As divisions proceed and a morula is formed, differences in cell size become more pronounced, with cells at the animal pole smaller than those at the vegetal pole. At the end of cleavage, the developing *Amphioxus* embryo is referred to as a blastula (Fig. 4.1A). This structure consists of a single layer of cells surrounding a central cavity, the blastocoele.

Amphibians

As ova of amphibians are medialecithal, cleavage is holoblastic and unequal. The first two cleavage divisions result in four equally-sized blastomeres but the third

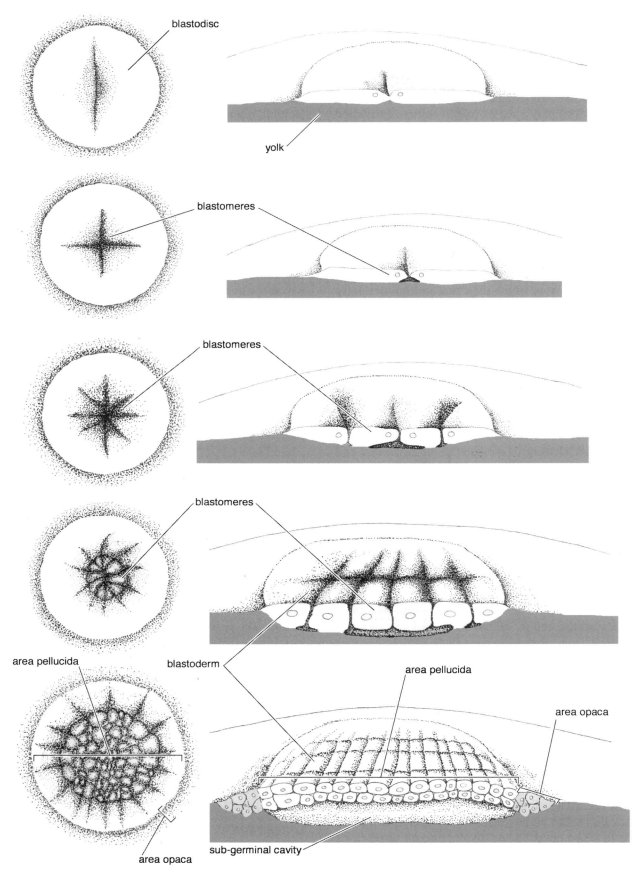

Figure 4.2 Stages of cleavage in the avian zygote from the first cleavage division to the formation of a blastoderm. Blastodisc viewed from above (left), and in cross-section (right).

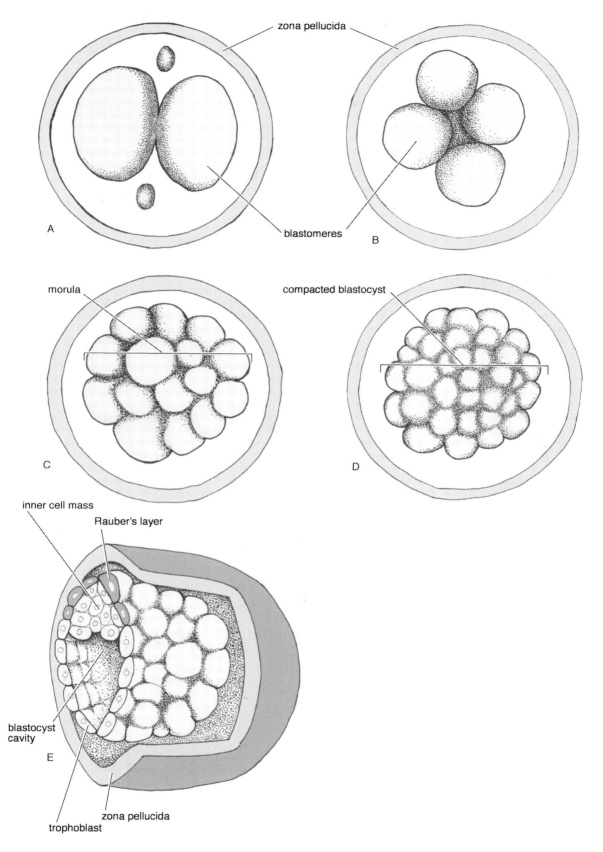

Figure 4.3 Stages of cleavage in a mammalian zygote from the two-cell stage to the formation of a blastocyst, A to D. The section through the blastocyst in E shows the inner cell mass and blastocyst cavity.

This process, which is termed compaction, gives the blastomeres a defined orientation for the first time, as each cell has a fixed contact area with adjacent cells and a free outer surface. Compaction occurs in humans and mice at the eight-cell stage, at the 16-cell stage in sheep, and at the 32-cell stage in cattle. After several cleavage divisions, the resultant group of blastomeres constitutes a compact sphere of cells, the morula, consisting of a superficial layer around a central core of cells. The superficial layer of cells ultimately gives rise to an epithelial layer known as the trophoblast, or trophoectoderm, which forms the outer surface of the extra-embryonic membranes and attaches the developing embryo to the uterine wall. From the central core of cells, the inner cell mass, the embryo develops (Fig. 4.3). Secretions from the blastomeres cause fluid-filled intercellular spaces to form which later coalesce into a single cavity, the blastocyst cavity. As fluid accumulates, the inner cell mass remains attached to an area of the trophoblast. At this stage of development, the mammalian embryo is called a blastocyst. The progressive development of those cells which constitute the inner cell mass is determined by their immediate environment. The tight junctions which exist between the trophoblastic cells are believed to form a barrier between the immediate environment of the cells of the inner cell mass and the external environment. The cellular arrangement whereby trophoblastic cells are exposed to an external environment and cells of the inner cell mass are in an enclosed environment is known as the 'inside–outside' hypothesis of embryological development. The functional fate of trophoblastic cells becomes determined more quickly than cells of the inner cell mass. The cavitation and fluid accumulation in the blastocyst cavity is an active process involving sodium and potassium pump activity across the outer cells of the compact morula which occurs at the 16-cell stage in pigs and at the 64-cell stage in humans, cattle and sheep. In the 11- to 12-day-old bovine blastocyst, the cells of the inner cell mass account for about 25% of the 1000-cell structure. Up to 10% of blastomeres may undergo programmed cell death (apoptosis). In marsupial embryos, no inner cell mass forms and the blastocyst appears as a hollow sphere of cells, all of a similar type.

Species variation is observed in the fate of the trophoblastic cells overlying the inner cell mass, Rauber's layer (Fig. 4.3E). In primates, bats and some rodents, Rauber's layer persists while in other species, including domestic mammals, it disappears prior to implantation. The inner cell mass forms a disc of cells, the embryonic disc, which becomes incorporated into the wall of the blastocyst and corresponds to the blastoderm in avian species (Fig. 4.4).

It is probable that autocrine factors, together with paracrine and endocrine factors of maternal origin and of embryonic origin, regulate growth and development of the early embryo.

Blastocyst elongation

Although the blastocyst commences expansion within the zona pellucida, it must emerge from the zona before it can undergo further development. In some species such as rodents and horses, the zona disintegrates, while in other species such as cattle, sheep and pigs, the blastocyst 'hatches' from a cracked zona.

Species variation is evident in the growth and expansion of the blastocyst prior to its attachment to the endometrium. In primates, rodents and guinea-pigs, because the blastocyst invades the endometrium, little expansion can occur. Associated with superficial or central attachment as observed in horses, dogs, cats and rabbits, there is marked round to oval expansion of the blastocyst. Marked thread-like expansion occurs in cattle, sheep and pigs. The porcine blastocyst undergoes exceptional morphological change from a 10 mm diameter sphere at 9 days of gestation to an elongated, filamentous structure of up to 100 cm in length by day 13. These changes occur through cellular remodelling and restructuring rather than by an increase in mitotic activity. Uterine secretions probably influence this form of blastocyst expansion.

Stem cells

Cells in the embryo which have the inherent ability to differentiate into all the cell types required for the formation of tissues, organs and systems are referred to as embryonic stem cells. In contrast, stem cells present in tissues or organs of mature animals are generally considered to be more lineage-restricted in their ability to differentiate than embryonic stem cells. Diversification of cell types is usually complete at or shortly after birth.

Embryogenesis is characterised by a gradual restriction in the developmental potential of cells which constitute the embryo. From the zygote, successive divisions of blastomeres give rise to cells with totipotential capability. However, as blastomeres continue to divide, they lose the potential to differentiate into all cell lineages of the embryo. With the formation of the blastocyst, lineage restriction becomes apparent. At this stage, cells located on the surface of the blastocyst form the trophoblast, from which the embryonic component of the placenta derives. Cells located inside the developing embryo, the inner cell mass, give rise to all cell lineages of the embryo itself but they do not have the ability to contribute to trophoblast formation. Expression of the transcription factor Oct-4 is required for the maintenance of pluripotency. At high levels, Oct-4

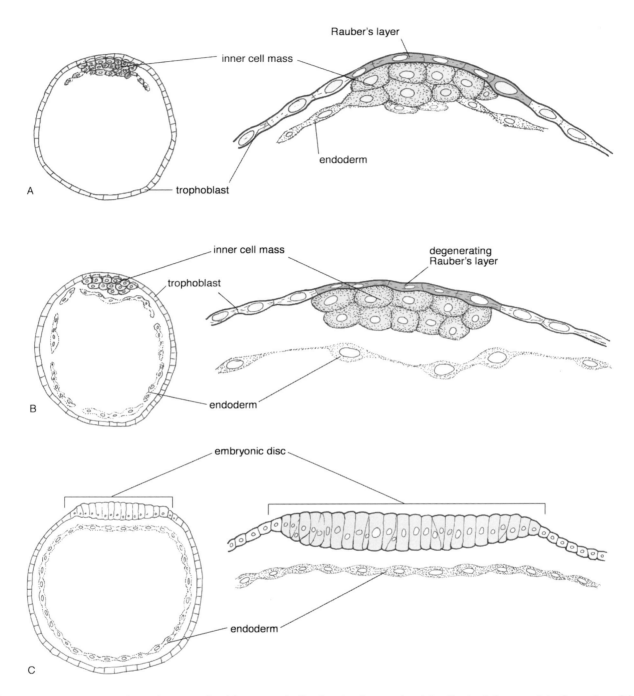

Figure 4.4 Cross-sections through mammalian blastocysts indicating the changes involving Rauber's layer and the formation of the embryonic disc and endoderm.

promotes pluripotency; lower concentrations can promote lineage differentiation, such as trophoblast formation.

Many tissues in the body of a mature animal have the inherent capability of self-renewal. Epidermal cells shed from the surface of the body are replaced at intervals of 3–4 weeks. Likewise, red blood cells and white blood cells have defined life spans in the circulation and are constantly being replaced by cells which originate in the bone marrow and develop in a lineage-restricted pattern. Stem cells are required to replace ageing tissues or cells as they reach the end of their normal life span. Although it was formerly considered unlikely that some specialised tissues such as neural tissue contained stem cells, that view is being questioned. It seems probable that most body tissues contain cells which are capable of self-renewal and which have the ability to differentiate into specialised cells in response to stimulatory signals from depleted tissues or organs, or as a consequence of environmental factors activating tissue responses.

Undifferentiated stem cells, present in the embryo at an early stage of development, can give rise to multipotential stem cells with the ability to form a wide range of tissues and organs ranging from muscle and bone to blood cells and neural cells. When suitably activated, these embryonic stem cells are ultimately responsible for the formation of all the tissues, structures and organs present in the embryo. Stem cells, which persist past the embryonic and foetal stages of development, can produce either more stem cells or more differentiated cells in the mature animal in response to appropriate cell signals or tissue injury. Following stimulation or injury, skeletal muscle fibres can be repaired or undergo proliferation. The cells responsible for repair are quiescent satellite myoblasts which become reactivated, proliferate and fuse, forming differentiated myotubules which interact with and repair muscle fibres. In mature animals, stem cells are reported to be slow-cycling cells capable of responding to specific microenvironmental signals and either generating new stem cells or differentiating into a particular cell lineage. Prior to differentiation, stem cells in mature animals undergo a transient state of rapid proliferation followed by differentiation along a defined pathway.

The epidermis, cells of hair follicles, and cells of the small intestine and of the haematopoietic system are examples of cells or tissues in mature animals with the ability to give rise to new cells with a defined life span which can divide and terminally differentiate. Because the epidermis and hair follicles of mammals are naturally exposed to ultraviolet irradiation, dehydration and physical contact with abrasive surfaces, a means of replacing sloughed cells is required. The basal layer of the epidermis is a single layer of cells which previously withdrew from the cell cycle. Following activation, these specialised cells can divide and differentiate terminally and move towards the surface of the epidermis, replacing surface cells which have been sloughed.

The precursors of haematopoietic stem cells are mesodermally-derived cells which migrate to an environment supportive of haematopoiesis in the aorta–gonad–mesonephros region of the embryo. The first blood cells, called embryonic nucleated erythrocytes, are produced in the yolk sac and express special transcription factors which determine their haematopoietic role. In murine models, vascular endothelial growth factor or its tyrosine-kinase receptor-Flk1 signal transduction pathway are reported to be essential for regulating the migration of embryonic blood cells and endothelial progenitor cells to the aorta–gonad–mesonephros region. Subsequently, migration of haematopoietic stem cells to the foetal liver relies on $\beta 1$ integrin and associated molecules. These molecules on the surfaces of haematopoietic stem cells respond to environmental factors which promote expression of new intrinsic factors. While in the environment of the foetal liver, haematopoietic stem cells differentiate and give rise to progenitor cells restricted to the myeloid and lymphoid lineages. Late in the foetal period, haematopoietic stem cells migrate to the bone marrow, the site of blood cell formation for the animal's post-natal life.

During embryogenesis, neural progenitor cells develop in the neural crest. These cells detach from the dorso-lateral margins of the neural tube and migrate to particular sites throughout the developing embryo where they differentiate into neurons and glial cells of the peripheral nervous system. They also give rise to melanocytes, smooth muscle cells, facial bones and cartilage. The cells or structures formed by neural crest cells are determined in part by the migratory pathway taken by these cells and also by factors secreted locally by cells in their immediate vicinity when they arrive in a defined site. Recent experimental data indicate that multipotential cells in the brains of mature mice may be either ependymal cells or astrocytes, and in culture these multipotential cells gave rise to both neurons and glial cells. In olfactory epithelium, basal cells can differentiate into olfactory neurons to replace these specialised cells which have a life span of approximately 30 days.

A distinguishing feature of stem cells which sets them apart from other cells is their ability to undergo self-renewal while still retaining their multipotency. Maintenance of the unique characteristics of stem cells has at least three distinct requirements: inhibition of differentiation, sustained proliferative capacity and retention of multipotency. Although it was formerly considered that the properties of stem cells present in a given tissue or system were fixed and immutable, experimental evidence suggests that stem cells from sites such as the bone marrow may be 'plastic' in the types of lineages to which they can give rise. Because it is highly probable that stem cells have the capability to respond to multiple instructive signals *in vivo*, their derivatives may be determined in part by the microenvironment in which these multipotent cells are normally located or the sites into which they are experimentally transplanted. In the course of stem cell self-renewal, symmetrical cell division gives rise to two stem cells, whereas asymmetrical cell division results in one stem cell and either one differentiated daughter cell or a stem cell with restricted capacity for differentiation. Self-renewal by asymmetrical cell division may occur in stem cells in embryos or foetuses late in development and also in animals post-natally as a means of ensuring homeostasis of the established body plan.

Murine embryonic stem cell research

Murine embryonic stem cells have been used extensively as models to elucidate the unique characteristics of mammalian stem cells. Pluripotent stem cells have unique properties which include unlimited self-renewal capability, a stable karyotype and resistance to senescence. These cells possess a highly efficient and reproducible differentiation potential: they can give rise to cell types which would normally derive from the three embryonic germ layers both *in vivo* and *in vitro*. In addition, these cells can be grown as separate colonies which can be expanded as independent subclones following genetic manipulation.

Murine embryonic stem cells were first recovered from embryos cultured on a layer of mitotically inactivated mouse fibroblasts. Currently, it is recognised that a number of growth factors, including leukaemia inhibitory factor, basic fibroblast growth factor and stem cell factor, are essential for retention of embryonic stem cell pluripotency, self-renewal capability and suppression of differentiation. Fibroblasts maintain pluripotency of embryonic stem cells by secreting leukaemia inhibitory factor, a member of the interleukin-6 family of cytokines. Along with leukaemia inhibitory factor, this family contains interleukin-6, oncostatin M, ciliary neurotrophic factor and cardiotrophin-1. Members of the interleukin-6 family of cytokines, which are functionally related, can mediate proliferation or differentiation of target cell types. It has been suggested that leukaemia inhibitory factor may influence the rate of embryonic stem cell proliferation or cell cycle progression. This factor may also act on the stem cell phenotype by activating a signalling cascade which operates on the up-regulation of genes expressed exclusively in pluripotent cells and on the down-regulation of genes expressed in differentiated cells. The receptors involved in the interleukin-6 family signalling cascade belong to the cytokine receptor class I family.

Because of their therapeutic potential in the treatment of degenerative diseases in humans, studies on the innate properties of stem cells have been intensified in recent years. A central objective is the generation of immortalised unipotential progenitor cells which do not have an increased risk of becoming neoplastic. Telomerase, an enzyme crucial for the maintenance of chromosome integrity, is expressed at high levels in mitotically-active pluripotent stem cells. Experimentally-induced overexpression of this enzyme in mitotically-inactive progenitor cells has been shown to immortalise them and to restore their replicative potential. The use of telomerase-immortalised progenitor cells as therapeutic agents is currently being clinically evaluated.

Further reading

Albert, B., Johnson, A., Lewis, J., Raff, M., Roberts, L.S. and Walter, P. (2004) Development of multicellular organisms. In *Molecular Biology of the Cell*, 4th edn. Garland Science, New York, pp. 1157–1258.

Carlson, B.M. (2004) Cleavage and implantation. In *Human Embryology and Developmental Biology*, 3rd edn. Mosby, Philadelphia, PA, pp. 44–63.

Cavaleri, F. and Schöler, H. (2004) Molecular facets of pluripotency. In *Handbook of Stem Cells*, Vol. 1. Ed. R. Lanza. Academic Press, San Diego, pp. 27–44.

Daley, G.Q. (2004) Hematopoietic stem cells. In *Handbook of Stem Cells*, Vol. 1. Ed. R. Lanza. Academic Press, San Diego, pp. 279–283.

Fuchs, E. and Segre, J.A. (2000) Stem cells: a new lease of life. *Cell* **100**, 143–155.

Gardner, R.L. (2004) Pluripotential stem cells from vertebrate embryos: present perspective and future challenges. *Handbook of Stem Cells*, Vol. 1. Ed. R. Lanza. Academic Press, San Diego, pp. 15–26.

Hafez, E.S.E. and Hafez, B. (2000) Fertilization and cleavage. In *Reproduction in Farm Animals*, 7th edn. Eds. E.S.E. Hafez and B. Hafez. Lippincott, Williams, and Wilkins, Philadelphia, pp. 110–125.

Körbling, M. and Estrov, Z. (2003) Adult stem cells for tissue repair – a new therapeutic concept? *New England Journal of Medicine* **349**, 570–582.

Lanza, R. and Rosenthal, N. (2004) The stem cell challenge. *Scientific American* **290**, 60–67.

Noden, D.M. and de Lahunta, A. (1985) Early stages of development in birds and mammals. In *Embryology of Domestic Animals, Developmental Mechanisms and Malformations.* Williams and Wilkins, Baltimore, pp. 23–45.

Pedersen, R.A. and Burdsal, G.A. (1994) Mammalian embryogenesis. In *The Physiology of Reproduction*, 2nd edn. Eds. E. Knobil and J.D. Neill. Raven Press, New York, pp. 319–390.

Trounson, A. (2005) Derivation characteristics and perspectives for mammalian pluripotential stem cells. *Reproduction, Fertility and Development* **17**, 135–141.

Twyman, R.M. (2001) Cleavage and gastrulation. In *Instant Notes: Developmental Biology*. Bioscientific Publishers, Hong Kong, pp. 161–186.

Wilt, F.H. and Hake, S. (2004) Oogenesis and early development of birds. In *Principles of Developmental Biology*. W.W. Norton and Co., New York, pp. 80–83.

Wolpert, L. (1998) Morphogenesis: change in form in the early embryo. In *Principles of Development*. Oxford University Press, Oxford, pp. 231–268.

5 | Gastrulation

Gastrulation, or germ layer formation, is a stage of embryological development during which the single-layered blastula is converted into a trilaminar structure consisting of an outer ectodermal, a middle mesodermal, and an inner endodermal layer. These changes occur through a series of orderly cell migrations from the surface of the blastula into its interior. Cells arising from each germ layer ultimately give rise to specific tissues and organs. Ectoderm differentiates into the epidermis of the skin and into neural tissue, endoderm forms the lining of the gastrointestinal and respiratory tracts, and from the middle mesodermal layer the urogenital, circulatory and supportive muscular and skeletal systems are formed. Using labelling techniques, it is possible to identify the cells in the blastula from which the germ layers arise and from which specific organ primordia develop. Data compiled in this manner can be used to construct a diagrammatic illustration of the migration of cells from their origin within the blastula to specific tissues or organs in later stages of development. Such diagrammatic illustrations are termed fate maps. Despite marked differences in the manner in which gastrulation proceeds in diverse animal species, the arrangement of germ layers at the end of gastrulation is comparable in all vertebrates. The process of gastrulation in higher mammals can be more readily appreciated by comparing the process of gastrulation in primitive chordates, amphibians and avian species.

Primitive chordates

The pattern of gastrulation in *Amphioxus* represents a comparatively simple model for illustrating the major cellular events in germ layer formation observed in more evolutionarily advanced species. Gastrulation in *Amphioxus* begins when the blastoderm at the vegetal pole flattens and invaginates (Fig. 5.1). The embryo then undergoes a series of morphological changes. As cells at the vegetal pole invaginate, the spherical shape of the embryo changes with the sequential formation of a cavity referred to as the archenteron or primitive gut. The opening of the archenteron to the exterior is known as the blastopore. The outer layer of cells form the ectoderm, and the inner layer the endoderm. Cells responsible for the formation of the notochord and

other mesodermal structures originally occupy a position at the edge of the blastopore. Later, these cells migrate to a position between the ectoderm and endoderm. Thus, the endodermal and mesodermal structures relocate from the surface of the embryo to its interior, forming a trilaminar embryo referred to as a gastrula.

Amphibians

Because of the presence of yolk-filled cells in the vegetal hemisphere of the amphibian blastula, invagination, as observed in *Amphioxus*, cannot occur. At the junction of the animal and vegetal hemispheres, cells from the surface move to the interior forming a cleft, the forerunner of the primitive gut. Following an influx of endodermal cells from below the cleft and mesodermal cells from above, the cleft deepens. With the constant movement of cells from the surface to the interior, a circular blastopore is formed (Fig. 5.2). The blastocoele becomes obliterated and the yolk-laden cells at the vegetal pole move to the interior. Finally, a trilaminar embryo, similar to that observed in *Amphioxus*, is formed.

Avian species

In birds, the blastoderm consists of two parts, the area pellucida and the area opaca (Fig. 5.3). The cells of the area pellucida give rise to two layers, an upper epiblast, which comprises prospective ectoderm, endoderm and mesoderm, and a lower hypoblast destined to become the extra-embryonic endoderm. The bilaminar region of the blastoderm of the chick embryo is a flat structure which corresponds to the spherical blastula observed in *Amphioxus* and in amphibians. The avian epiblast corresponds to the cells of the animal pole of the blastula; the hypoblast corresponds to the cells of the vegetal pole and the intervening space corresponds to the blastocoele. The organ-forming part of the blastoderm in birds is confined to a region of the area pellucida extending cranially from its caudal edge for about three-fifths of its length. Thickening of the blastoderm, which results from the convergence of cells in the surface layer of the blastoderm towards the midline, forms the primitive streak. At the cranial end of the primitive streak, an increased concentration of cells forms a structure referred

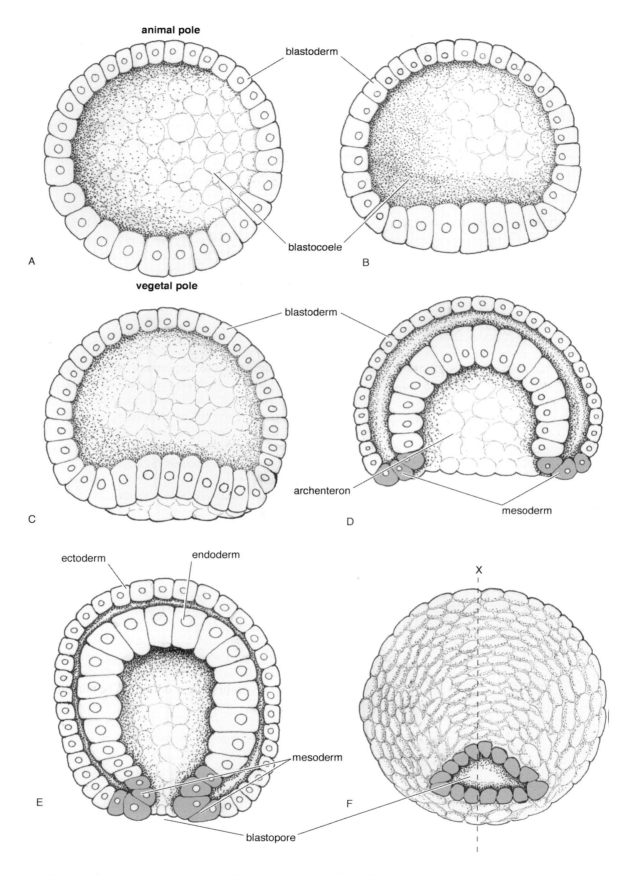

Figure 5.1 Sections showing sequential stages of gastrulation in *Amphioxus* from the blastula stage, A, to the gastrula stage, E. The section shown in E is at the level indicated in the embryo at the gastrula stage in F.

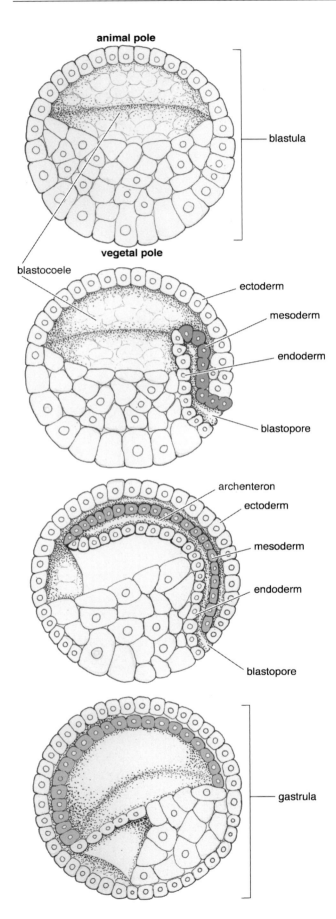

Figure 5.2 Sequential stages of gastrulation in amphibians from the blastula stage to the gastrula stage.

to as the primitive node or Hensen's node (Fig. 5.3). With the formation of the primitive streak and its associated node, the cranial-caudal axis of the embryo becomes established, dividing the embryo into right and left sides. The cells of the epiblast converging on the primitive streak do not build up but ingress into the space between the epiblast and hypoblast. The resulting depression is the primitive groove. As cells from the primitive streak move deeper into the blastocoele, they are replaced by cells from the lateral regions of the epiblast. Cells migrating from the epiblast make contact with the hypoblast and displace it forming the embryonic endoderm. As ingression of cells of the epiblast continues, areas of blastoderm which disappear from the surface are replaced by cells from the adjoining areas which divide, move towards the midline and replace the cells in the primitive streak. The newly arrived cells continue to migrate downwards and inwards. Thus, although the cells which constitute the primitive streak are constantly being replaced, the structure itself persists throughout gastrulation. Cells at the primitive node, which ingress into the interior, migrate cranially forming a column of mesodermal cells referred to as the notochord; a small cluster of mesodermal cells cranial to the notochord form the prechordal plate. The cranio-lateral movement of invaginated cells from the primitive streak gives rise to the lateral mesoderm, which is located between the epiblast and the hypoblast (Fig. 5.3).

Coincident with the development of the primitive streak, the area pellucida increases in size with growth occurring more rapidly in the cranial than in the caudal region, resulting in the formation of a pyriform structure. During this time, the primitive streak elongates to its maximum length. As the mitotic rate of the cells at the periphery of the epiblast decreases and compensation for the depletion of cells lost from the epiblast due to migration ceases, the primitive streak and primitive node cease to exist. Although the primitive streak and node recede, the node continues to form the notochord, which ultimately extends throughout the entire length of the embryo.

As cells move through the primitive streak, they undergo progressive morphological changes. Cells of the epiblast resemble typical epithelial cells resting on a basal lamina with well defined basal and apical surfaces. As these cells migrate through the primitive streak, they elongate and assume a characteristic bottle-shaped appearance and are referred to as bottle cells. On leaving the primitive streak, these cells assume the morphology and characteristics of mesenchymal cells with the ability to migrate and differentiate.

Mammals

In mammals, the blastocyst cavity is the equivalent of an empty yolk-sac cavity. The embryonic disc occupies a

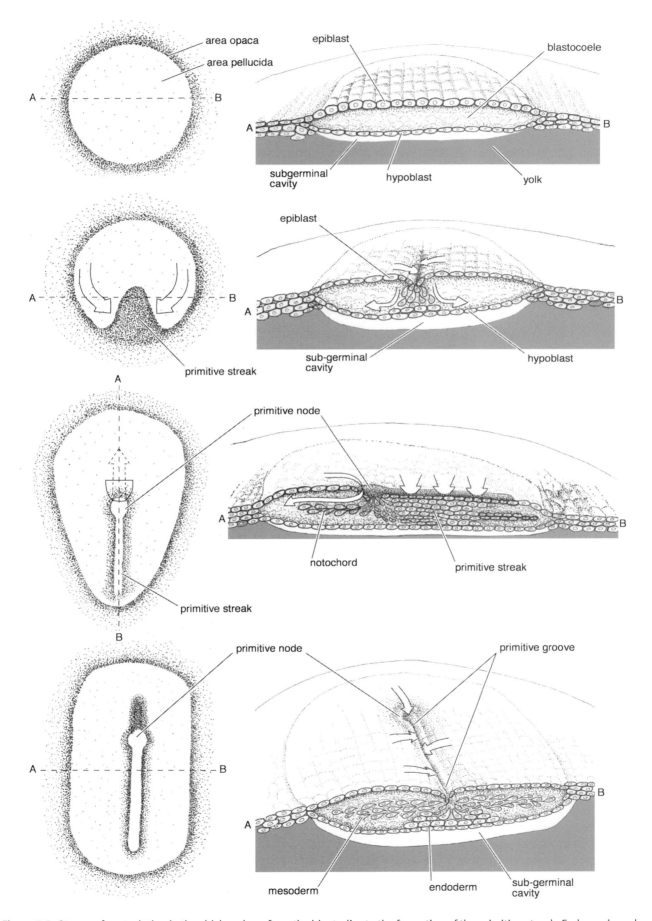

Figure 5.3 Stages of gastrulation in the chick embryo from the blastodisc to the formation of the primitive streak. Embryo viewed from a dorsal position (left) and with corresponding sections (right). Arrows indicate the direction of cellular migration.

position comparable to that of the blastoderm at the animal pole of megalecithal eggs such as those of birds, and also has a similar role in embryological development. The pattern of germ layer formation in mammals closely resembles that of birds. Although in higher mammals the yolk content is greatly diminished, gastrulation proceeds in a manner remarkably similar to that observed in megalecithal eggs. The first step in the process of gastrulation of the mammalian blastocyst is the formation of a layer of flat cells, derived from the embryonic disc, which occupy a position on its lower surface (Fig. 4.4). This layer of flat cells corresponds to the hypoblast of the chick blastoderm. The remaining cells of the inner cell mass are considered equivalent to the epiblast of the chick blastoderm. The cells of the hypoblast, which are initially found in the region of the embryonic disc, later extend along its inner surface and line the cavity of the blastocyst forming a bilaminar yolk sac. The development of the germ layers in mammals resembles that of birds with the formation of a primitive streak and primitive node. The primitive streak acts as the initiation site for gastrulation. The caudal marginal zone of the epiblast is believed to induce the formation of the primitive streak from the epiblast cells. The inductive signals are mediated by proteins such as activin, Chordin, Wnt-8c and Vg-1. However, once induction of the primitive streak takes place, adjacent epiblast cells lose their ability to respond to further inductive influences, thus ensuring that only one primitive streak is formed. Differential gene expression patterns are established along the cranial–caudal axis of the developing primitive streak. The expression domain of the gastrulation marker Fgf-8 is restricted to the dorsal layer of the primitive streak. Genes including *Not-1*, *Chordin* and *Hnf-3β* are expressed at the cranial end of the streak; *Wnt-8c*, *Nodal* and *Slug* are absent from this region. Other genes including *Brachyury* and *Vg-1* are expressed uniformly throughout the primitive streak apart from its caudal end.

Establishment of left–right symmetry in vertebrates

Organs of vertebrates are positioned asymmetrically in the thoracic and abdominal cavities. The consistency of the positioning of internal organs suggests that this arrangement is regulated by molecular processes. The left–right pattern of development is established during gastrulation. Mutations in the gene *situs inversus viscerum (Iv)* randomises the position of each organ on either side of the left–right axis. The randomised positioning of the organs is a potentially lethal anomaly. Because mutations involving the gene, termed *inversion of embryonic turning (Inv)*, cause all organs to be reversed, the resulting asymmetry has fewer deleterious consequences for the individual than mutations of the *Iv* gene.

The incidence of developmental defects relating to left–right symmetry correlates with defective or absent monocilia in the cells of the primitive node of the developing embryo. Observations of these cells have shown ciliary movement to the left around the area of the node. This evidence strongly supports the hypothesis that movement of cilia to the left increases the concentration of factors which trigger the development of left-sided structures. A process of regulated cell death which occurs along the midline of the primitive streak is also believed to play a role in the establishment of left–right symmetry. A feature of this form of cell death which distinguishes it from both necrosis and apoptosis is that cellular debris persists in the midline region. By limiting gap junction communication, this cellular debris may function as a physical barrier between the left side and the right side of the developing embryo.

In murine models, ciliary movement to the left causes activation of an unidentified factor, possibly the product of the *Inv* gene. This product, in turn, activates the *Nodal* and *Lefty 2* genes. The diffusion of Nodal and Lefty 2 proteins to the right-hand side is inhibited by the product of the *Lefty 1* gene which is secreted on the left side. *Nodal* activates *Pitx2*, a gene which induces the formation of left-sided development within the organs expressing this gene. The gene products of either *Nodal* or *Lefty 2* or both, repress the *Snail* gene, the product of which is required for right-sided development (Fig. 5.4).

Twinning

The term 'twins' identifies two individuals which develop in the same pregnancy in animals that are normally monotocous. Two distinct types of twins are recognised, dizygotic and monozygotic. Dizygotic twins arise from two ova, derived from two separate ovarian follicles, each fertilised by separate spermatozoa during a single breeding cycle. There is evidence that multiple ovulation, and therefore dizygotic twinning, has a hereditary basis. Monozygotic twins arise from a single ovum fertilised by a single spermatozoon. The two-blastomere stage is the earliest point in embryological development at which monozygotic twins can arise, each blastomere giving rise to a separate individual with its own foetal membranes (Fig. 5.5A). Genetic and obstetrical evidence indicates that approximately 30% of human monozygotic twins arise in this manner. The observation of two blastocysts within a single zona pellucida suggests that this form of twinning may occur in cattle. Moreover, it has been shown experimentally in laboratory and domestic animals that single blastomeres from the two-cell stage of cleavage are capable of developing into normal individuals following transfer to suitable recipients. The second phase of development at which monozygotic twins can arise is at the inner cell

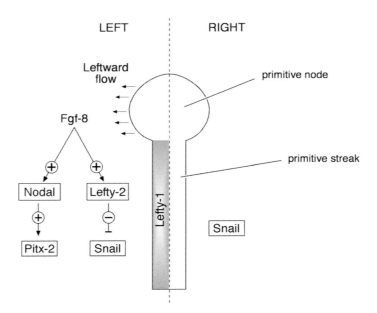

Figure 5.4 The influence of the primitive node and notochord on the distribution of signalling and transcription factors associated with left–right symmetry.

mass stage if duplication of the inner cell mass takes place (Fig. 5.5B). In this instance, twins develop with separate amnions but with a shared yolk sac and chorion. Studies of foetal membranes at birth suggest that 70% of monozygotic twins in humans arise in this way. Twin embryonic discs have been observed in human, ovine and porcine blastocysts. It has been observed *in vitro* that division of the bovine blastocyst may occur as it emerges from the zona pellucida (Fig. 5.5C). Provided that the separated portions each contain a sufficient number of both inner cell mass cells and trophoblastic cells to form two distinct blastocysts, two separate individuals can develop, each with its own foetal membranes. The third stage in development at which monozygotic twins may arise is at the embryonic disc stage with the formation of two primitive streaks each giving rise to separate individuals (Fig. 5.5D). Such twins would share a common amnion, yolk sac and chorion. Approximately 1% of human monozygotic twins are reported to arise in this manner. While a blastoderm with two or three primitive streaks has been described in the chick, no credible description of embryonic discs with more than one primitive streak has been reported in mammals. In humans, twins occur at a rate of about one in 85 births and of these, about 25% are monozygotic. In domestic animals, the incidence of twinning is influenced by species and breeds. In cattle, natural twinning occurs at a rate of 2 to 3%, while the occurrence of monozygotic twins is 0.1% or approximately 10% of same sex twins. The frequency of twin-

ning in sheep, which is from 2 to 5%, is higher in lowland breeds than in mountain breeds. In horses, the occurrence of multiple ovulations is reported to be up to 30%, yet the rate of twin births is less than 2%. This discrepancy between the high multiple ovulation rate and the low rate of twinning is attributed to the high pre-natal mortality associated with twinning in mares. There is also evidence that innate physiological mechanisms inhibit twinning in mares. Using ultrasonography, twin blastocysts are often observed in mares, yet, during the early stages of uterine migration a few days later, only one can be detected.

Twinning which occurs as a result of ova fertilised by spermatozoa from two different males in a single breeding cycle is referred to as superfecundation. In polytocous animals, offspring are referred to as litter mates.

Conjoined twins

Anomalous incomplete separation of two primitive streaks results in conjoined twins. In humans, it has been estimated that conjoined twins occur at a rate of 1 in 100,000 births. The rate in monozygotic twins is reported to be 1 in 400. The incidence of conjoined twins in cattle, which is reported to be higher than in other farm animals, occurs at a rate similar to that reported in humans. Anatomical descriptions and classification of conjoined twins are reviewed in reference sources on embryology, obstetrics and teratology.

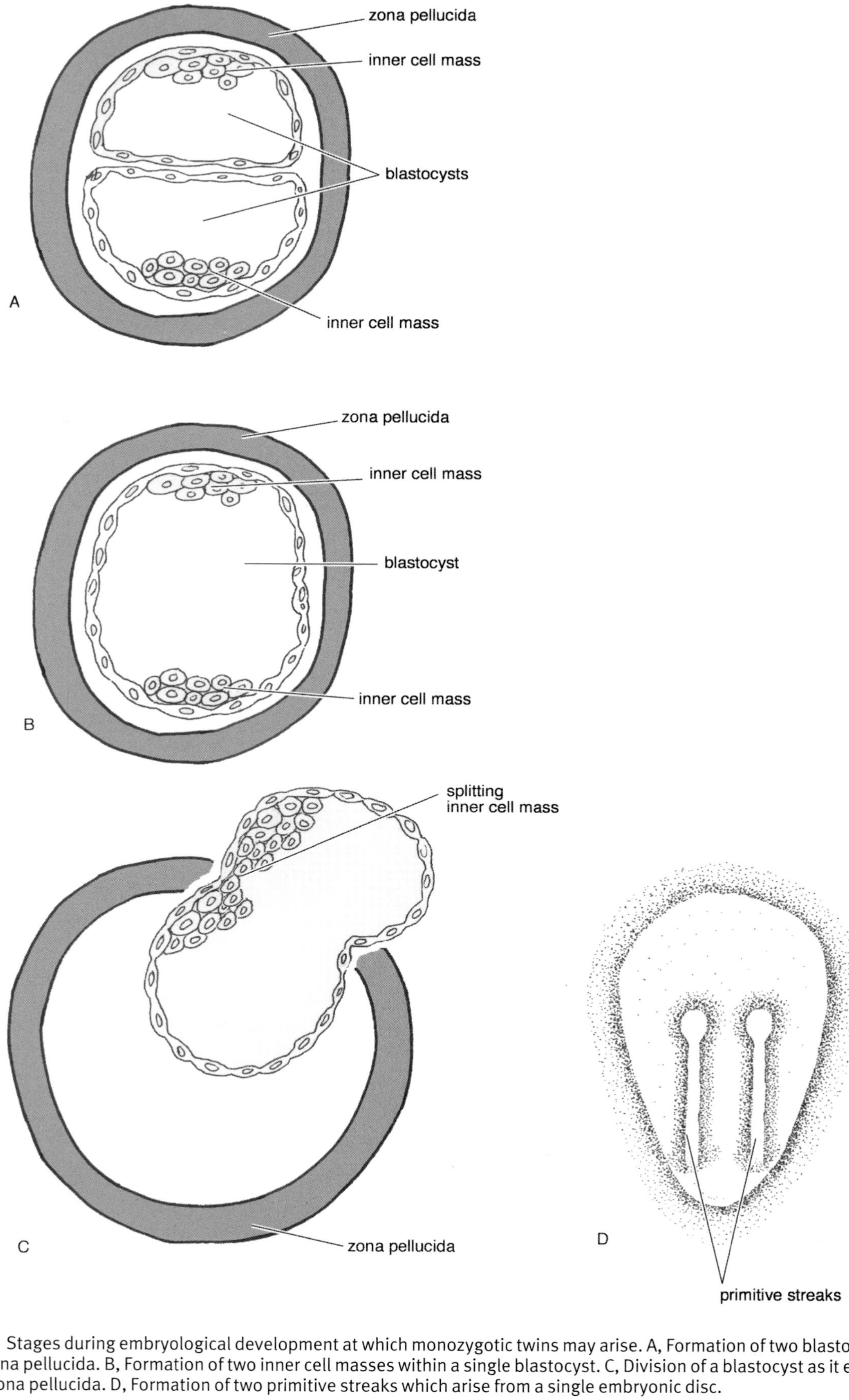

Figure 5.5 Stages during embryological development at which monozygotic twins may arise. A, Formation of two blastocysts within a single zona pellucida. B, Formation of two inner cell masses within a single blastocyst. C, Division of a blastocyst as it emerges from the zona pellucida. D, Formation of two primitive streaks which arise from a single embryonic disc.

Further reading

Levin, M. (2005) Left–right asymmetry in embryonic development: A comprehensive review. *Mechanisms of Development* **122**, 3–25.

Mercola, M. (2003) Left–right asymmetry: nodal points. *Journal of Cell Science* **116**, 3251–3257.

Mikawa, T., Poh, A.M., Kelly, K.A., Ishli, Y. and Reese, D.E. (2004) Induction and patterning of the primitive streak, an organising centre of gastrulation in the amniote. *Developmental Dynamics* **229**, 422–432.

Moore, K.L. and Persaud, T.V.N. (1998) Gastrulation: formation of germ layers. In *Before We Are Born: Essentials of Embryology and Birth Defects.* W.B. Saunders, Philadelphia, PA, pp. 62–70.

Pedersen, R.A. and Burdsal, G.A. (1994) Mammalian embryogenesis. In *The Physiology of Reproduction*, 2nd edn. Eds. E. Knobil and J.D. Neill. Raven Press, New York, pp. 319–440.

6 Aspects of Cell Signalling and Gene Functioning During Development

Cell communication is a vital part of differentiation, growth and development of the embryo. Diverse signalling mechanisms have evolved which enable complex multi-cellular organisms to develop and to function in a co-ordinated manner. These signalling mechanisms vary in their speed, duration, intensity and effect. Cell signalling is a fundamental requirement in developmental biology. The induction of cells to differentiate into tissues and organs and contribute to the formation of an independent member of a species is largely mediated by a number of cell signalling mechanisms. Although the genetic plan for an individual is determined at fertilisation, realisation of this plan requires that effective communication between cells be co-ordinated and accurate, both in timing and intensity. Disturbances of these communication processes are likely to adversely affect embryological development.

There are many different mechanisms whereby signals can be delivered to target cells within tissues or organs. Short-range signalling mechanisms, such as cell-to-cell, paracrine and autocrine signalling play a fundamental role in early embryonic development. Long-range mechanisms of cellular communication involving the endocrine and nervous systems are also a feature of embryological development; as the complexity of a developing vertebrate progresses, the necessity for long-range signalling increases.

Depending on cell type and whether a solitary signal or a combination of signals is received by the receptor of the cell, signals can be interpreted in a number of ways. The consequences of cell signalling are diverse, and, depending on the nature and interpretation of the signal, target cells may be induced to alter their function, divide, differentiate, change their morphology, or undergo apoptosis (Fig. 6.1).

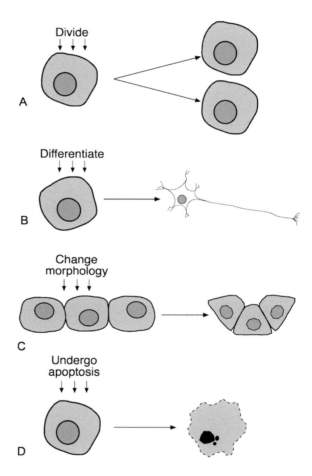

Figure 6.1 Cellular responses induced by extra-cellular signals. A, Cell division, B, differentiation, C, morphological change, D, apoptosis.

Cellular messengers and receptors

In higher organisms, chemical messages transmitted by cells are diverse. These messages are transmitted in the form of proteins, small peptides, amino acids, nucleotides, steroids, fatty acids, dissolved gases, simple molecules and ions. Broadly speaking, these chemical messengers can be divided into extra-cellular and intra-cellular signalling molecules. The molecules which mediate signalling are released by exocytosis or diffusion from the cells in which they originate.

The receptors present on the surface of the receiving cell are diverse in form. Receptors can be broadly grouped as G-protein receptors, ion channel receptors, tyrosine kinase receptors, serine–threonine receptors and members of the steroid receptor superfamily.

G-protein receptors function by activating intra-cellular G-proteins which, in turn, bind guanosine triphosphate (GTP) and influence biochemical activities by conversion of GTP to guanosine diphosphate (GDP) with the release of energy. As a family, G-protein receptors are the most diverse of all the membrane-bound receptors in terms of both structure and function. They are involved in the recognition and transduction of signals from light, proteins, calcium ions and other small molecules. Ion channel receptors influence intra-cellular activities by regulating the movement of small molecules such as potassium and sodium ions across cell membranes. Tyrosine kinase receptors, such as fibroblast growth factor receptor, activate intra-cellular proteins via tyrosine phosphorylation. Serine–threonine receptors activate intra-cellular proteins by serine or threonine phosphorylation. Members of the transforming growth factor β superfamily act through serine–threonine-type receptors.

Members of the steroid receptor superfamily, which can be present in the cytosol or on the nuclear membrane, interact with hydrophobic signalling molecules capable of diffusing across the plasma membrane. These receptors contain ligand-binding, DNA-binding and transcription-activation domains. Oestrogen and thyroid hormone receptors belong to the steroid receptor superfamily.

Types of signalling

Signalling molecules can be delivered to target cells by a number of means. These can be divided into short-range forms such as paracrine, contact-dependent, and autocrine signalling, and long-range forms, including synaptic and endocrine signalling (Fig. 6.2).

Paracrine signalling

The term 'paracrine signalling' describes short-range forms of signalling which do not require direct cell-to-cell contact (Fig. 6.2A). In this instance, the secreted messenger molecules usually reach nearby target cells by diffusion. These signalling molecules are rapidly bound by target cells in close proximity. Paracrine signalling

Paracrine signalling

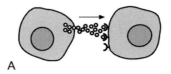

A

Contact-dependent signalling

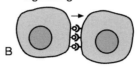

B

Autocrine signalling

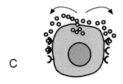

C

Synaptic signalling

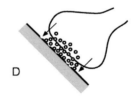

D

Endocrine signalling

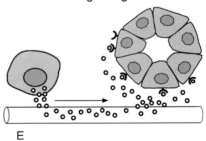

E

Figure 6.2 Short-range and long-range signalling mechanisms. Short-range mechanisms include paracrine signalling, A, contact-dependent signalling, B, and autocrine signalling, C. Long-range mechanisms include synaptic signalling, D, and endocrine signalling, E.

molecules can, however, be immobilised by the extra-cellular matrix, thereby ensuring that their effects are localised.

Contact-dependent signalling

A short-range form of communication referred to as contact-dependent signalling requires that the cell emitting the signal be in direct contact with its target cells (Fig. 6.2B). This form of signalling is of particular importance during early development. There are three variations of cell-to-cell signalling. In the first type, a signalling molecule, typically a protein in the cell membrane, binds to specific receptors on the membranes of adjacent cells. The second type of cell-to-cell signalling involves secretion of a ligand into the extra-cellular matrix which then binds to a receptor on the target cell. In the third type, a signal is transmitted directly from the cytoplasm of one cell to the cytoplasm of adjacent cells via gap junctions.

Autocrine signalling

Cells can transmit signals to cells of a similar type or sometimes to themselves (Fig. 6.2C). This type of signalling, termed autocrine signalling, has an important role during early development when groups of cells of the same type can signal clusters of similar cells to follow a common developmental pathway.

Synaptic signalling

Long-range signalling, such as that which occurs with neurons, is referred to as synaptic signalling (Fig. 6.2D). By this means, signals are transmitted rapidly and specifically to distant regions of the body.

Endocrine signalling

In common with synaptic signalling, endocrine signalling can act over long distances (Fig. 6.2E). The molecules involved in endocrine signalling can be delivered to target tissues by diffusion or haematogenously. In comparison with synaptic signalling, this type of signalling tends to be relatively slow-acting. The effects of endocrine signals are often long-lived and a relatively small number of signalling molecules can induce widespread and sustained activation of target cells.

Induction and competence

The term 'induction' describes a process whereby signals transmitted from one cell or a group of cells can change the developmental fate of other cell types. There are two forms of induction, instructive and permissive. Instructive induction refers to circumstances where a cell follows a particular developmental pathway in response to given signals, but a different pathway in the absence of these signals. Permissive induction occurs when the responding cell is already committed to a particular developmental fate but requires additional inducing signals to continue along that pathway. During induction, the signals which a cell receives depend on its microenvironment during embryonic development as well as its competence to receive, interpret and respond to appropriate signals.

Progressive complexity arises in the developing organism through a series of inductive steps termed sequential induction. Through sequential induction, the basic body plan of the early embryo becomes established. Subsequently, this plan becomes increasingly refined as it relates to enhanced function and morphology.

The term 'competence' refers to a cell's ability to respond to certain inductive signals. With paracrine or endocrine signalling, a competent cell must have the capacity to respond to the original signal in the appropriate manner. The competent cell must have a receptor capable of binding the signalling molecules. In addition to this feature it must have an intra-cellular signal-transducing apparatus capable of forming a link with the final intra-cellular target. An example of this form of interaction is the activation of individual genes or sets of genes by transcription factors. A cell which is being induced by neighbouring cells through cell-to-cell signalling mechanisms may lose its competence by breaking contact with the inducing cell as a consequence of cellular migration.

Paracrine signalling during development

Numerous fundamental developmental events are mediated by paracrine factors. These factors can be broadly grouped into four main families: the hedgehog (Hh) family, the fibroblast growth factor (Fgf) family, the Wingless (Wnt) family and the transforming growth factor (Tgf-β) superfamily.

Hedgehog family

Members of the hedgehog family of inter-cellular signalling molecules are recognised as key mediators of many fundamental processes in embryonic development. Three mammalian homologues of the *hedgehog* gene, first identified in *Drosophila*, have been characterised. These homologues are *Sonic Hedgehog* (*Shh*), *Indian Hedgehog* (*Ihh*) and *Desert Hedgehog* (*Dhh*). Hedgehog signals can function differently in different contexts. They can regulate cell fate specification, cell proliferation and cell survival. Signalling can be short or long range, direct or indirect, and also concentration dependent.

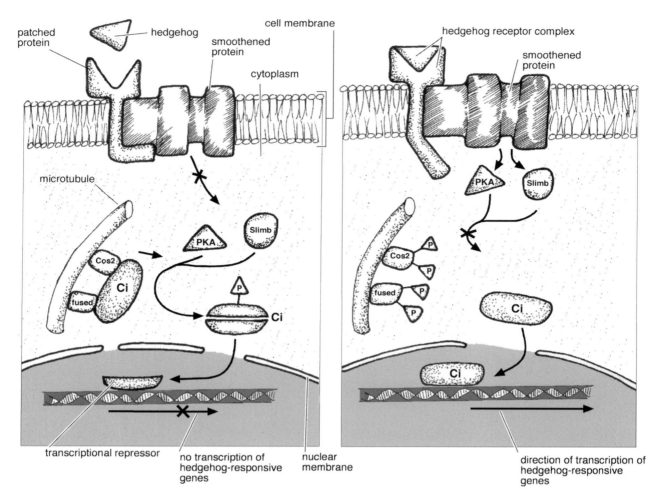

Figure 6.3 The hedgehog signalling transduction pathway illustrating the mechanisms of intra-cellular signalling in response to activation by the hedgehog protein (for explanation see text).

The gene *Shh* encodes a signalling protein which activates a number of genes instrumental in determining the body plan of the early embryo. Expression of the *Shh* gene has been detected in the primitive node and throughout the notochord, in the floorplate of the neural tube, in early gut endoderm and in the limb buds.

The cellular response to hedgehog protein is controlled by two transmembrane proteins, smoothened (Smo) and patched, the latter an inhibitor of Smo. When hedgehog protein binds to a patched receptor which acts as an inhibitor to Smo, a conformational change is induced in patched which prevents this transmembrane protein from inhibiting smoothened. Subsequently, the Smo protein releases the Cubitus interruptus (Ci) protein from microtubules, a possible consequence of the addition of phosphate groups to the Costal (Cos) and fused proteins, which form a complex with the Ci protein, binding it to the microtubules. The Smo protein also inactivates Slimb and PKA proteins, both of which cleave the Ci protein, changing it into a transcriptional repressor. In the absence of Slimb and PKA, the Ci

protein remains intact and acts as a transcriptional activator for hedgehog-responsive genes (Fig. 6.3).

Fibroblast growth factor family

A group of paracrine factors referred to as the fibroblast growth factor family consists of more than 20 structurally-related proteins. Members of the Fgf family can activate the fibroblast growth factor receptors which are of the receptor tyrosine kinase class. Receptor tyrosine kinases are proteins which protrude through the cell membrane. The ligand-binding part of the protein is positioned on the extra-cellular side, while on the intra-cellular side a dormant tyrosine kinase is present. Tyrosine kinase is an enzyme which has the ability to phosphorylate target proteins. When the Fgf binds to the extra-cellular receptor, the dormant kinase is activated and in turn phosphorylates certain intra-cellular target proteins. This leads to the activation of target proteins which can then perform new functions within the cell (Fig. 6.4).

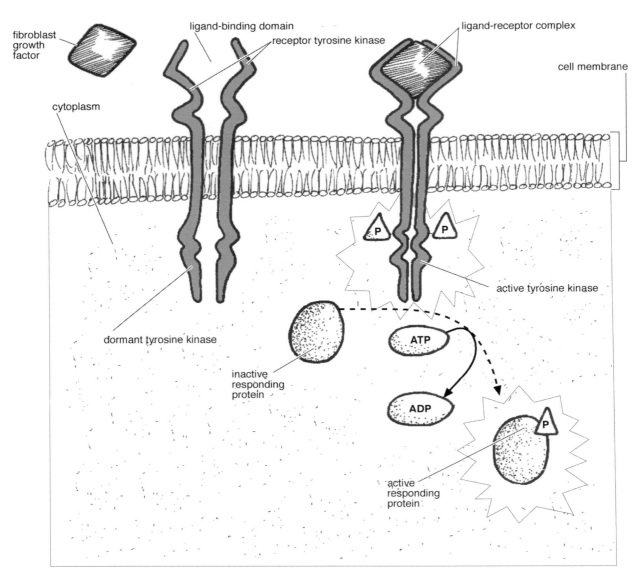

Figure 6.4　The fibroblast growth factor signal transduction pathway which operates through the phosphorylation of intra-cellular proteins, leading to their activation (for explanation see text).

Wingless family

The Wingless (Wnt) gene family consists of structurally related genes encoding cysteine-rich secreted glycoproteins which act as extra-cellular signalling factors. *Wnt* genes are implicated in a wide variety of biological processes including cell fate determination. These genes can influence the body plan early in embryological development and also cell growth and differentiation post-natally. Members of the Wnt family of paracrine factors interact with transmembrane receptors which are members of the frizzled family of proteins. In most instances, binding of Wnt signalling factor to a frizzled protein causes the latter to activate dishevelled protein. Activated dishevelled protein inhibits the activity of the enzyme glycogen-synthase-kinase-3 (GSK-3). Active GSK-3 inhibits the dissociation of β-catenin from the

adenomatous polyposis coli (APC) protein. However, when GSK-3 is inhibited, β-catenin can dissociate from the APC protein and enter the nucleus. Once in the nucleus, the β-catenin can form a complex with the DNA-binding proteins LEF or TCF. Following binding to β-catenin, these complexes become active transcription factors, capable of activating Wnt-responsive genes (Fig. 6.5).

Transforming growth factor superfamily

The transforming growth factor-β superfamily contains over 30 distinct proteins which function as inducers during embryological development. The carboxy-terminal region of these proteins contains the mature peptide. These peptides, which can form homodimers or heterodimers with other Tgf-β peptides, are secreted from

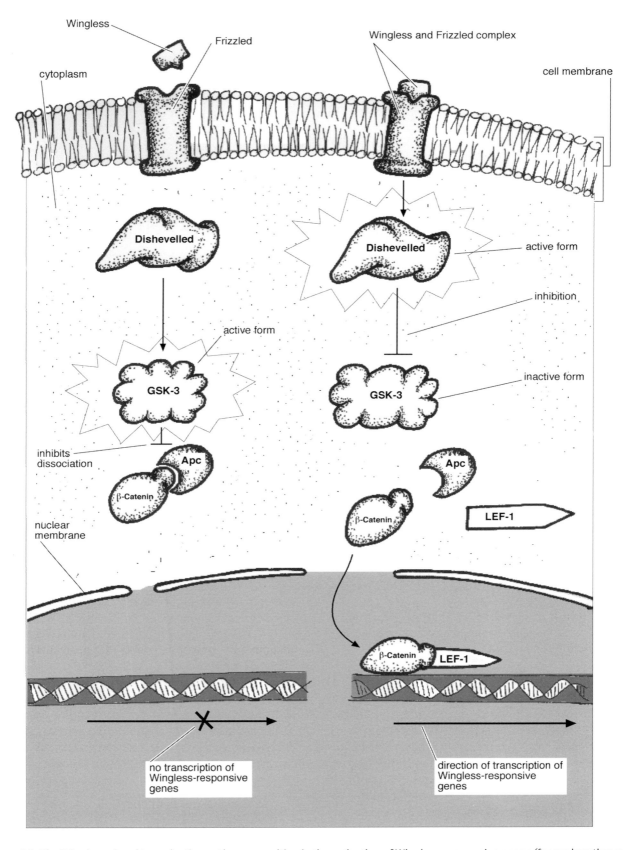

Figure 6.5 The Wingless signal transduction pathway, resulting in the activation of Wingless-responsive genes (for explanation see text).

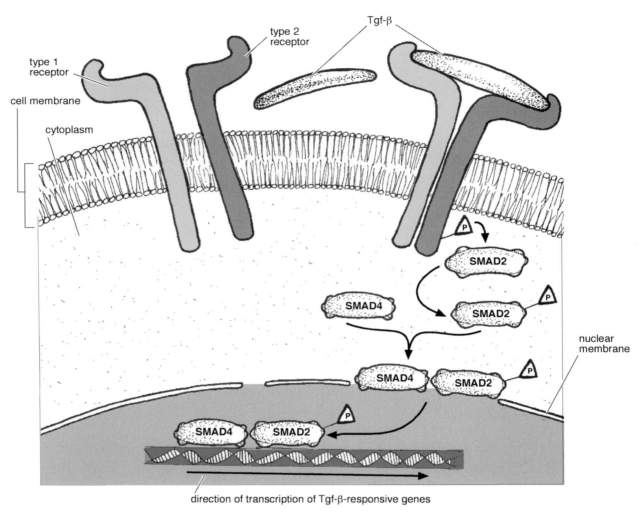

Figure 6.6 The transforming growth factor signal transduction pathway leading to activation of Tgf-β-responsive genes via SMAD proteins (for explanation see text).

the cell. The Tgf-β superfamily of proteins, which has a diverse range of functions, includes proteins such as the bone morphogenic proteins and paramesonephric inhibitory hormone.

Members of the Tgf-β superfamily activate SMAD transcription factors. The Tgf-β ligand binds to a type II Tgf-β receptor which allows that receptor to bind to a type I Tgf-β receptor. When the two receptors are in close proximity, the type II receptor activates the type I receptor by phosphorylation of serine or threonine on the receptor. The activated type I receptor can then phosphorylate the SMAD proteins which subsequently function as transcription factors (Fig. 6.6).

Apoptosis

Programmed cell death, referred to as apoptosis, occurs in many cell types during normal development. Cell death due to apoptosis is distinct from necrosis, which

can occur as a result of acute non-specific injury to the cell. Many different apoptotic pathways exist in mammals. Extra-cellular or intra-cellular stimuli can trigger apoptosis. Caspases are the principal intra-cellular mediators of apoptosis. This family of proteases cleaves target proteins at specific aspartic acid sites. When synthesised, caspases exist as inactive precursors. Once activated, their innate proteolytic activity is amplified through the activation of additional caspases, a process referred to as the caspase cascade. Activated caspases can cleave proteins essential for the survival of the cell such as nuclear lamin. They can also trigger the release of the DNA-degrading enzyme, DNase. Apoptosis plays a central role in the remodelling of interdigital tissue. Survival factors can act by binding to receptors which repress the apoptotic pathway; absence of survival factors can result in the activation of apoptosis. These factors act on members of the Bcl-2 family of intra-cellular proteins, some of which are inhibitors of apoptosis.

Morphogens

A morphogen is a substance which can specify a cell's differentiation pathway as a function of its concentration in the microenvironment of the target cell. This form of signalling, a fundamental mechanism during early development, is best characterised in *Drosophila* where morphogens controlling development diffuse along the anterior–posterior axis of the blastoderm. Gradation in the concentration of transcription factors enables spatial domains in the *Drosophila* larva to be sequentially defined. In response to the morphogen gradient, regionally activated genes in turn act on other genes further defining cranial–caudal orientation of the developing *Drosophila* embryo and, subsequently, segment specialisation.

In vertebrates, a number of developmental processes are under the influence of morphogens. The signalling molecule Shh acts as a morphogen during limb development where it is produced at high levels in a discrete region of the developing limb, called the zone of polarising activity (ZPA). During neural tube development, Shh secreted from the notochord acts as a morphogen in this region.

There are many mechanisms by which morphogens can form gradients. These mechanisms include diffusion, signal relay, transport via cytonemes, surface transport by proteoglycans and cyclical endocytosis and exocytosis.

Differentiation

The term 'differentiation' describes a progressive process whereby cells and tissues develop specific structural and functional roles characterised by their specialised physiological or biochemical activities. Differentiation of cells occurs through the interaction of many cell types mediated by a variety of cell signals. The co-ordination which takes place can result in both transient and permanent cellular changes. The process of differentiation takes place gradually in vertebrates and may continue over a long period during development. The capability of an individual somatic cell to develop into different cell types is determined by its degree of differentiation. Although all somatic cells within an individual animal have the same complement of genes, the gene expression pattern is reflected in the function and morphology of each cell type.

Gene structure and organisation

In the nucleus of eukaryotic cells, DNA is present in the chromosomes. Genomic DNA does not exist in a pure form within the nucleus, as it is bound to histones.

Chromatin represents a complex of DNA and protein. Genes in eukaryotic cells are contained within the chromatin. Two types of chromatin are recognised, a highly condensed form, termed heterochromatin and a less condensed form termed euchromatin. Genes, if present in heterochromatin, are in an inactive form.

Genes consist of regions of DNA which eventually become transcribed by RNA polymerase II into mRNA. These DNA regions are termed exons. Non-coding regions, termed introns, may interrupt the genomic sequence of exons. When exons are spliced together they form the template for mRNA transcription from which the final protein product is translated.

X-chromosome inactivation

In addition to their species-specific autosomal complement of chromosomes, female mammals normally carry two X-chromosomes in their genomes. Potentially this could result in the genes carried on the two X-chromosomes being expressed simultaneously in the female as compared to the male, with undesirable consequences. To maintain the normal level of X-chromosome gene expression in females, one of the X-chromosomes is inactivated in each somatic cell at an early stage of development. The inactive X-chromosome, termed a Barr body, can be observed near the nuclear membrane in somatic cells. Either the paternally derived or maternally derived X-chromosome may be inactivated. Transcriptional inactivation of the X-chromosome starts at what is termed the inactivation centre and spreads throughout the X-chromosome, thereby inactivating the majority of genes present on that particular chromosome. The inactivation of X-chromosomes occurs at the blastocyst stage of development. At this stage, X-chromosomes are inactivated in a random fashion. The effects of this random X-chromosome inactivation can be observed in female tortoiseshell cats. In these cats, allelic variants of pigment genes, which encode either black or orange pigment, are present on the X-chromosomes. The tortoiseshell pattern can be attributed to random inactivation of maternally-derived and paternally-derived allelic variants of the pigment genes.

DNA methylation and parental imprinting in mammals

The cytosine residues in DNA can be methylated by methyltransferase enzymes, forming 5-methylcytosine. In mammals, about 5% of the cytosine residues are methylated. Methylation of cytosine is generally confined to regions containing cytosine/guanosine (CpG) dinucleotide repeats. DNA methylation, which correlates with transcriptional repression, is a prominent feature in X-chromosome inactivation and has a role in parental imprinting. Methylated DNA can remain unaltered following successive rounds of nuclear division.

The term 'imprinting' describes differential allelic expression or repression depending on whether the allele is of paternal or maternal origin. Imprinted genes are generally organised in large domains within the chromosome. Imprinting control regions (ICRs) can span several kilobases and are rich in CpG dinucleotides. Another feature of ICRs is that there is methylation of these regions in one of the two parental alleles. The pattern of methylation is different for male and female gametes. In spermatocytes the pattern of methylation is similar to that observed in mature spermatozoa. However, this pattern changes after fertilisation. In female gametes, the methylation pattern is established during the meiotic stage of oogenesis.

In diploid somatic cells, copies of each allele are expressed in an equivalent manner. In contrast, imprinted genes may behave differently, depending on whether they are carried on the paternal or maternal chromosome. Many genes which are subject to imprinting are associated with embryonic growth.

Promoters, enhancers and silencers

In addition to the protein-coding regions of a gene, a number of regulatory sequences also exist within the genome. Promoters are sites on DNA where RNA polymerase II and other transcription factors bind, initiating transcription. Promoters are generally located directly upstream from the start of the coding area of the DNA. Most promoter regions contain a thymine–adenine–thymine–adenine (TATA) box, a region of DNA which contains the sequence TATA. Eukaryotic RNA polymerases require the presence of transcription factors for binding effectively to the promoter region. At least

six nuclear proteins which are required for the initiation of transcription by RNA polymerase II have been identified. These proteins are termed basal transcription factors and, together with RNA polymerase II, form the transcription initiation complex. By stabilising the transcription initiation complex, cell-specific transcription factors function in gene activation.

An enhancer is a DNA sequence which activates promoter utilisation by RNA polymerase. Enhancers can only activate promoters which are present on the same chromosome, a process referred to as cis activation. However, enhancers may be present up to 50 kilobases away from the promoter. Regulatory proteins bound to the enhancer can interact with transcription factors bound either to the promoter or to RNA polymerase. Enhancers can regulate the tissue-specific expression of differentially regulated genes. Silencers act as inhibitors of transcription in a manner comparable to enhancers.

Transcription factors

Proteins which bind to the enhancer or promoter regions of DNA are termed transcription factors (Table 6.1). These factors function by increasing (up-regulating) or decreasing (down-regulating) the final quantity of the mRNA transcript. Transcription factors have three major domains, a DNA binding domain, a trans-activating domain, and in addition, they may have a protein–protein interacting domain.

Gene systems essential for development

Hox genes and segmental identity in Drosophila

In Drosophila, the process of segmentation is controlled by Gap, Pair-Rule and Segment Polarity genes. These genes, however, do not establish regional differences

Family	Representative transcription factors	Areas of development in which these factors participate
High mobility group	Sry, Sox	Sex determination
Homeodomain	Hox	Establishment of regional identity
MADs box	Mef-2	Muscle development
Paired domain	Pax-6	Neural specification, eye development
PolI	Oct-4	Maintenance of pluripotency
T box family	Tbx-5	Limb specification
Winged helix	Foxa-1	Pancreatic development
Zinc finger	Steroid receptors	Early embryonic implantation

Table 6.1 Major families of transcription factors and examples of their roles in vertebrate development.

Table 6.2 Genes within the homeotic complex of *Drosophila* species, their domains of expression and roles in development, based on data derived from mutant phenotypes.

Gene complex/gene	Domain of expression	Role in development
Antennapedia complex		
Labial	Intercalary segment of the head	Inhibition of labial development in prosencephalon
Proboscipedia	Maxillary and labial segments of the head	Specification of proboscis and maxillary palps
Deformed	Mandibular and maxillary segments of the head	Specification of mouth region
Sex combs reduced	Labial segment of head and first thoracic segment	Specification of labial and first thoracic segments
Antennapedia	Anterior boundary parasegment 6	Specification of second thoracic segment
Bithorax complex		
Ultrabithorax	Anterior boundary parasegment 6	Specification of parasegments 5 and 6
Abdominal A	Anterior boundary parasegment 7	Specification of parasegments 7 to 9
Abdominal B	Anterior boundary parasegment 10	Specification of parasegments 10 to 13 and parasegment 14

between segments. A family of genes referred to as Homeobox (Hox) genes encode transcription factors which provide the basis for this cranial–caudal axis development throughout the animal kingdom (Table 6.2). These genes exist in clusters termed the homeotic complex (Fig. 6.7). Since the discovery of Homeobox genes in *Drosophila*, paralogous genes have been identified in vertebrates. In both mice and humans, Hox genes have been identified as four unlinked homeotic complexes which are designated Hoxa, Hoxb, Hoxc and Hoxd (Fig. 6.7). It is postulated that the additional Hox gene clusters arose as a result of duplications of a single Hox cluster. These genes contain a highly conserved coding region termed a homeodomain, a region encoding a 60 amino acid DNA-binding motif, which folds into three alpha helices.

The structure and function of Hox genes are highly conserved throughout the animal kingdom. The fundamental role which these genes play in development may explain some of the dramatic morphological evolutionary changes observed across species. The four Hox clusters identified in mammals contain a total of 39 genes.

Hox clusters, which are located on separate chromosomes, show considerable homology with each other and retain the same order within their respective complexes. The position along the length of the embryo where Hox genes are expressed, as identified by *in situ* hybridisation experiments, matches the chromosomal order of the genes within each complex. Hox genes located at the 3′ end of the complex are expressed in the more cranial regions of the developing embryo, and genes at the 5′ end of the cluster are expressed at the more caudal regions. The expression level of Hox genes in each region of the developing embryo is negatively regulated by the homeotic gene products expressed in more posterior regions, a phenomenon termed posterior dominance. There is evidence that the nested overlapping expression of the Hox genes provides a combinatorial key which triggers specific downstream expression of genes associated with embryonic regional development, thus conferring positional identity on those regions.

In mammals, the products of Hox genes impart directional instructions relating to early development, particularly evident in segmented regions such as the developing central nervous system. Because of the complexity of a mammal and the fact that the mammalian Hox gene complex contains multiple copies of genes with overlapping functional activity, Hox mutants provide equivocal information on the role of genes within the Hox gene complex. Accordingly, the developmental anomalies seen in Hox gene mutants are often subtle or morphologically inapparent.

Due to the relative simplicity of *Drosophila*, the Hox genes are well characterised in this insect. Because *Drosophila* has a short generation time and owing to the fact that only one homeotic complex exists within its genome, a more comprehensive analysis of its Hox genes can be carried out than is possible in mammals. Loss-of-function studies of Hox mutants have elucidated the roles of individual Hox genes in *Drosophila*.

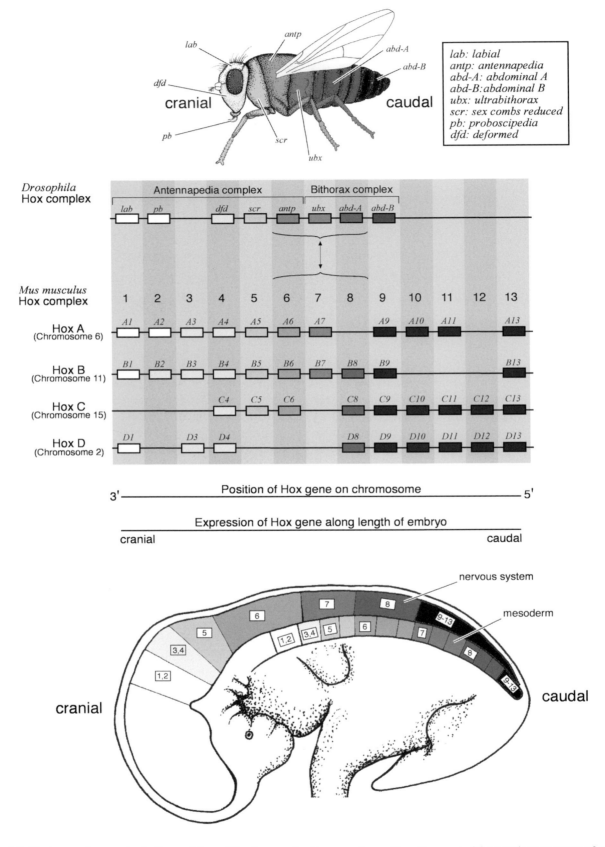

Figure 6.7 The homeotic complex in *Drosophila* and the four murine Hox complexes. The alignment of the paralogous groups from each complex illustrates the evolutionary conservation of these gene sequences across species and the homology of genes in different complexes within the same animal.

Experimental measurement of gene expression

Many techniques for measuring gene expression are available. Molecular biology techniques such as real-time polymerase chain reaction (RT–PCR) and micro-array technology allow RNA expression levels to be measured empirically. The technique of RT–PCR is generally used for measuring relative gene expression levels of individual genes, while micro-arrays can be used for measuring expression of vast subsets of genes simultaneously. Other techniques such as Western blotting and two-dimensional gel electrophoresis can be used for exploring the profile of expressed proteins in a particular cell type.

The function of regulatory components such as promoter regions can be explored by incorporating a reporter gene, such as a gene encoding green fluorescent protein, luciferase or β-galactosidase, downstream from the promoter region. The level of activation of the reporter gene reflects the efficiency of the regulatory component being studied.

Experimental evaluation of gene function

Gene function can be evaluated by the development of chimeric mice. First, the zona pellucida is removed from a fertilised ovum at an early cleavage stage and then two cleavage-stage embryos, each possessing a different genotype, are combined forming a composite embryo called a chimera. Specific genes together with genes encoding antibiotic resistance markers can be integrated into the genome of embryonic stem (ES) cells. These ES cells can then be cultured, selected and injected directly into a blastocyst forming a chimera. If such ES cells provide progenitors for spermatozoa and ova in the chimeric mice, the progeny will be heterozygous for the gene of interest. Sibling matings can then produce homozygous mice for the gene in question. As the genes incorporated can be non-functional versions of a wild-type gene, these 'knockout' studies can provide an understanding of the function of normal genes in the developmental process.

Recently, a new technique, termed RNA interference, has been employed to target and destroy specific RNA transcripts. An enzyme called a dicer cleaves double stranded RNA (ds RNA) into small ds RNA fragments (approximately 21 bp) referred to as small interfering RNA (si RNA). The si RNA assembles into RNA polymerase-containing structures called RNA-induced silencing complexes, which bind to complementary RNA and identify it for destruction. Silencing of specific RNA transcripts is a useful tool for exploring gene function.

Concluding comments

Cell signalling and gene functioning are fundamental processes involved in the differentiation, organisation and ultimately formation of tissues, organs and systems. The signalling mechanisms which exist in mammals are diverse in form and function. Many signalling processes, though highly regulated, must also be adaptable so that the ability to respond in a context-dependent way is retained. Efficient signalling mechanisms relating to stage of development and embryonic site are requirements for normal embryogenesis.

Further reading

Alberts, B., Johnson, A., Lewis, J., Raff, M., Roberts, K. and Walter, P. (2002) *Molecular Biology of the Cell*, 4th edn. Garland Science, New York.

Bockaert, J. and Pin, J.P. (1999) Molecular tinkering of G protein-coupled receptors: an evolutionary success. *European Molecular Biology Organisation Journal* **18**, 1723–1729.

Freeman, M. and Gurdon, J.B. (2002) Regulatory principles of developmental signalling. *Annual Review of Cell and Developmental Biology* **18**, 515–539.

Gilbert, S.F. (2003) *Developmental Biology*, 7th edn. Sinauer Associates, Sunderland, Mass.

Ingham, P.W. and McMahon, A.P. (2001) Hedgehog signalling and animal development: paradigms and principles. *Genes and Development* **15**, 3059–3087.

Lodish, H., Berk, A., Zipursky, S.L., Matsudaira, P., Baltimore, D. and Darnell, J.E. (2000) *Molecular Cell Biology*. W.H. Freeman and Company, New York.

Ogden, S.K., Manuel, A.J., Stegman, M.A. and Robbins, D.J. (2004) Regulation of hedgehog signalling: a complex story. *Biochemical Pharmacology* **67**, 805–814.

Rousseaux, S., Caron, C., Govin, J., Lestrat, C., Faure, A. and Khochbin, S. (2005) Establishment of male-specific epigenetic information. *Gene* **345**, 139–153.

Sontheimer, E.J. (2005) Assembly and function of RNA silencing complexes. *Molecular Cell Biology* **6**, 127–138.

Tabata, T. and Tekei, Y. (2004) Morphogens, their identification and regulation. *Development* **131**, 703–712.

Twyman, R.M. (2001) *Instant Notes: Developmental Biology*. BIOS Scientific Publishers, Abingdon.

7 Establishment of the Basic Body Plan

At the end of gastrulation, the developing embryo has a pear-shaped outline and is composed of an outer ectodermal layer, a middle mesodermal layer and an inner endodermal layer. A longitudinal column of mesoderm, the notochord, which arose from the primitive node, establishes the cranial–caudal axis of the developing embryo (Fig. 7.1).

Using the notochord as a reference axis, the embryo can be considered to have a right and a left side. Ectoderm directly above the notochord proliferates in response to factors emanating from the notochord, giving rise to the neural plate, a layer of ectoderm known as neuro-ectoderm. Subsequently, the neural plate forms the neural groove, which in turn becomes detached from the overlying ectoderm and gives rise to the neural tube. Following formation of the neural tube and associated structures, the superficial layer of cells is referred to as surface ectoderm. Some neuroectodermal cells migrate from the lateral margins of the developing neural tube and occupy a position dorso-lateral to the neural tube. In this location, these neuroectodermal cells are referred to as neural crest cells. The central nervous system (brain and spinal cord) arise from the neural tube; the peripheral nervous system develops from both the neural tube and the neural crest (Fig. 7.1D).

Under the inductive influence of the neural tube and neural crest, some surface ectodermal cells in the cephalic region form discrete thickenings known as placodes. These placodes include the nasal, lens and otic placodes, which give rise to the nasal chambers, lens and inner ear respectively. In addition, a small number of neurogenic placodes develop which contribute to the formation of the sensory components of some cranial nerves.

The endoderm gives rise to the epithelial lining of the primitive gut and respiratory tract and their associated mural glands, and also to the epithelial lining of the bladder, middle ear and auditory tube. The parenchymal cells of the liver, pancreas, thyroid and parathyroid glands also arise from endoderm.

The mesoderm, which arises from the primitive streak, forms a sheet of cells which spreads laterally and cranially between the epiblast and the hypoblast. During formation of the neural tube, however, mesoderm adjacent to the developing tube forms a thickened column of cells, the paraxial mesoderm. With the exception of the cephalic region, a chord of cells which extends along the length of the embryo lateral to the paraxial mesoderm forms the intermediate mesoderm. On either side of the neural plate, cells of the paraxial mesoderm form whorl-like aggregations called somitomeres. Development of somitomeres, which begins in the cephalic region, proceeds caudally in association with the regression of the primitive node. The first seven somitomeres contribute mesodermal components to some structures in the head region. Caudal to the seventh, somitomeres become organised into discrete blocks of paraxial mesodermal tissue, referred to as somites (Fig. 7.2). These blocks of paraxial mesoderm are first observed in the cephalic region, caudal to the otic vesicle, and continue to develop sequentially in a cranio-caudal direction. The majority of components of the axial skeleton, associated musculature and overlying dermis derive from somites. From the second to the fourth week of gestation in domestic animals, somites may be observed beneath the surface ectoderm as paired structures on either side of the developing neural tube. During this stage of development, the approximate age of an embryo can be estimated from the number of somites observed. The total number of somite pairs which develop is usually constant for a given species; the canine embryo has four occipital, eight cervical, 13 thoracic, seven lumbar, three sacral and ten to 20 caudal pairs of somites.

Mesoderm lateral to the somites forms a column of cells referred to as intermediate mesoderm, which contributes to components of the urinary and reproductive systems. The mesodermal tissue occupying a position lateral to the intermediate mesoderm, which remains largely unsegmented in mammals, is referred to as lateral mesoderm. Spaces which develop in the lateral mesoderm coalesce and divide it into an outer somatic

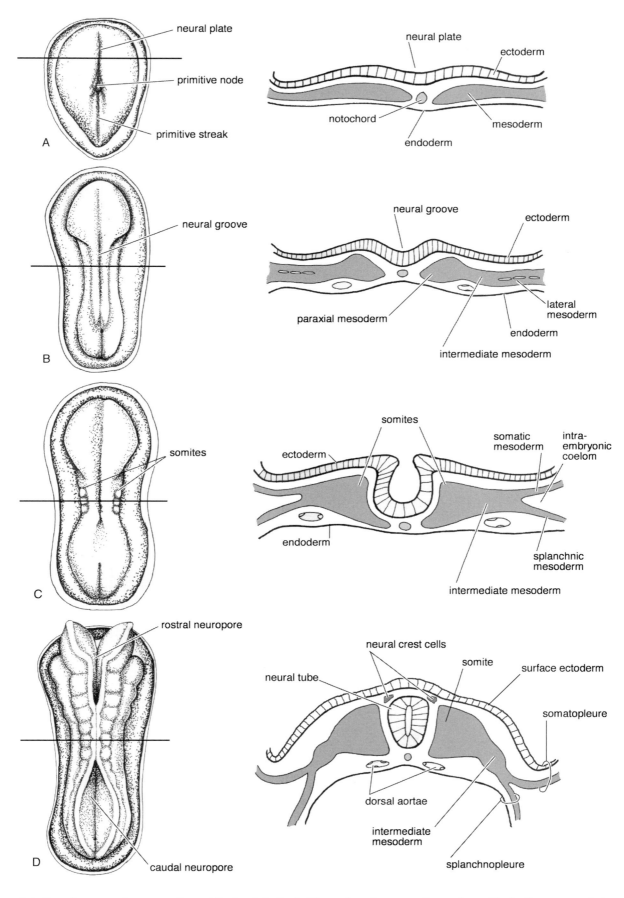

Figure 7.1 Dorsal views and cross-sections at the levels indicated through early mammalian embryos illustrating progressive developmental changes leading to the establishment of the basic body plan.

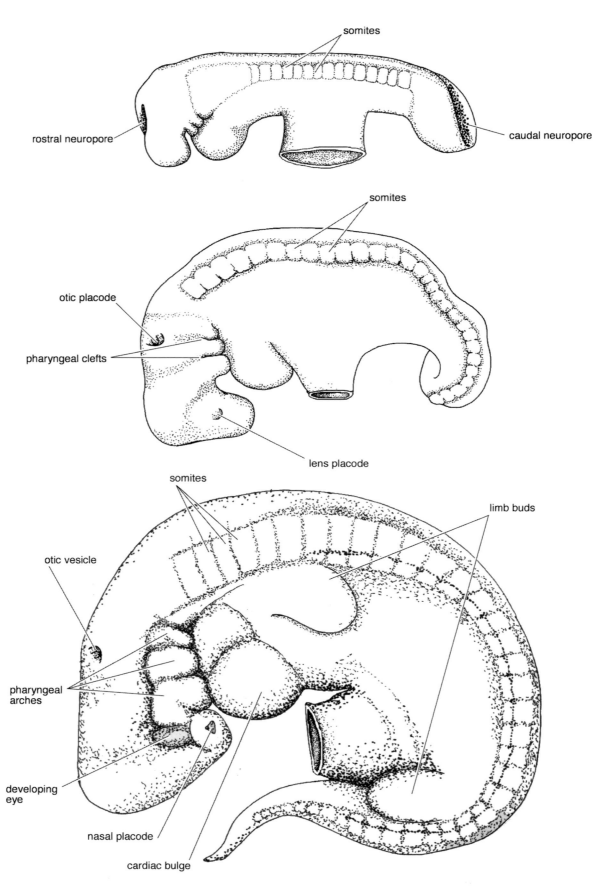

Figure 7.2 Lateral views of a mammalian embryo at different stages of development showing recognisable structures.

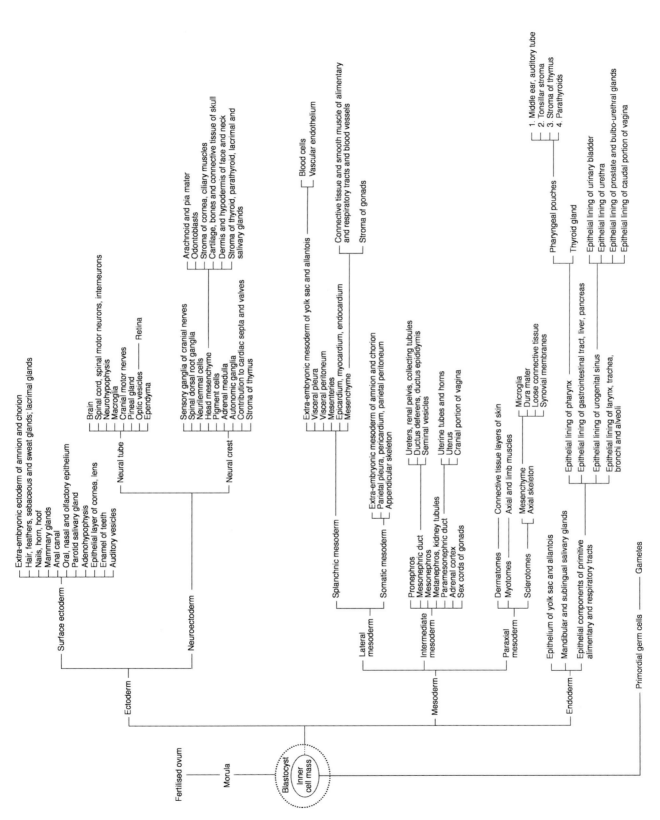

Figure 7.3 The progressive differentiation of cells which arise from the blastocyst and form the three germ layers. From these germ layers the cells, tissues and organs of the body are formed.

layer and an inner splanchnic layer. The somatic layer fuses with the ectoderm forming the somatopleure. Fusion of the splanchnic layer with the endoderm forms the splanchnopleure. The space between the somatopleure and splanchnopleure is referred to as the embryonic coelom and from it the body cavities, namely the pleural, pericardial and peritoneal cavities arise (Fig. 7.1). From the mesoderm which lines the coelomic cavity a simple squamous epithelium, the mesothelium, arises. Mesothelium forms the serous membranes which line body cavities.

After gastrulation, the trilaminar embryonic disc is transformed by the formation of head, tail and lateral folds into a three-layered tube. The inner endodermal layer forms the lining of the embryonic gut, the ectoderm gives rise to the nervous system and the epidermis of the skin and its derivatives, and from the mesodermal layer structural and connective tissue components of the body are formed. As a result of body wall folding, a portion of the blastocyst does not become incorporated into the embryo proper and remains attached to the embryo at the umbilicus as the extra-embryonic or foetal membranes.

Changes associated with the internal organisation of the embryo are reflected in its external appearance. The embryo becomes C-shaped with a prominent row of somites located on either side of the midline (Fig. 7.2). The optic vesicles and otic placodes are prominent structures at this time. Six paired segmental mesenchymal blocks of neural crest origin, the pharyngeal arches, develop in the cephalic region in a cranio-caudal sequence, between the foregut and surface ectoderm. Between each arch, the surface ectoderm invaginates forming five pharyngeal clefts. Internally, the endoderm of the foregut evaginates between the arches, forming five pharyngeal pouches.

Differentiation of the somitomeres, pharyngeal arches, clefts and pouches is described in association with the development of structures in the head region.

At this time, the developing heart causes a well defined cardiac bulge in the thoracic region. From the third week onwards, the fore and hind limb buds are recognisable. In the developing embryo, the cephalic region exhibits precocious growth and differentiation associated with brain development. Subsequently, equilibrium is established between the growth rate in the cephalic region and other regions of the developing embryo.

From the fertilised ovum totipotential stem cells in the blastocyst give rise to the three germ layers, ectoderm, mesoderm and endoderm. The cells, tissues and organs of the body are derived from these three germ layers (Fig. 7.3).

Further reading

Bryden, M.M., Evans, H.E. and Binns, W. (1972) Embryology of sheep: extraembryonic membranes and development of body form. *Journal of Morphology* **138**, 169–206.

Carlson, B.M. (2004) Establishment of the basic embryonic body plan. In *Human Embryology and Developmental Biology*, 3rd edn. Mosby, Inc., Philadelphia, PA, pp. 103–128.

Johnson, K.E. (1988) Establishment of the basic body plan and primitive circulation. In *Human Developmental Anatomy*. Harwal Publishing Company, Malvern, PA, pp. 79–82.

Latshaw, W.K. (1987) Development of the general body form. In *Veterinary Developmental Anatomy*. D.C. Dukes, Toronto, pp. 75–86.

Patten, B.M. (1952) The early development of the body form and the establishment of the organ systems. In *Embryology of the Pig*, 3rd edn. Blakiston, New York, pp. 60–93.

Wolpert, L. (1978) Vertebrate body plan. 1. Axes and layers. In *Principles of Development*. Oxford University Press, Oxford, pp. 61–96.

8 Coelomic Cavities

At the end of gastrulation, the embryonic mesoderm consists of three regions, paraxial, intermediate and lateral mesoderm. As development proceeds, clefts develop in the right and left lateral mesoderm. Later, these clefts coalesce forming a cavity which splits the lateral mesoderm into an outer layer of somatic mesoderm and an inner layer of splanchnic mesoderm (Fig. 8.1). The cavities between the two layers of mesoderm on the left and right sides are referred to as coelomic cavities. The left and right developing coelomic cavities located on either side of the midline, extend cranially, meet and fuse in front of the developing neural and cardiogenic plates, forming a horseshoe-shaped coelomic cavity (Fig. 8.2). The lateral walls of the coelomic cavity are composed of somatic mesoderm which fuses with ectoderm forming somatopleure. The medial walls are composed of splanchnic mesoderm which fuses with endoderm, forming splanchnopleure. The mesodermal cells lining the coelomic cavity differentiate into a simple squamous epithelium, referred to as mesothelium. Following cranial, caudal and lateral folding of the embryo, the convex region of the horseshoe-shaped coelom occupies a position ventral to the foregut and

the developing heart, and gives rise to the primordium of the pericardial cavity. The right and left limbs of the coelomic cavity are connected to the pericardial cavity by the pericardial–peritoneal canals (Fig. 8.3). Lateral body folding results in division of the developing embryonic coelom into an intra-embryonic and an extra-embryonic region. Subsequently, the intra-embryonic coelom gives rise to the pericardial, pleural and peritoneal cavities. The extra-embryonic coelom is associated with the developing foetal membranes. The intra-embryonic and extra-embryonic coelomic cavities, which are initially continuous at the umbilicus, subsequently become separated from each other.

Pleural and pericardial cavities

The primordia of the developing lungs and heart are surrounded by the left and right segments of the pleuro-pericardial cavity (Fig. 8.4). Gradually, folds of mesoderm, the pleuro-pericardial folds, containing the left and right common cardinal veins and left and right phrenic nerves, grow medially into the left and right segments of the pleuro-pericardial cavity. When these

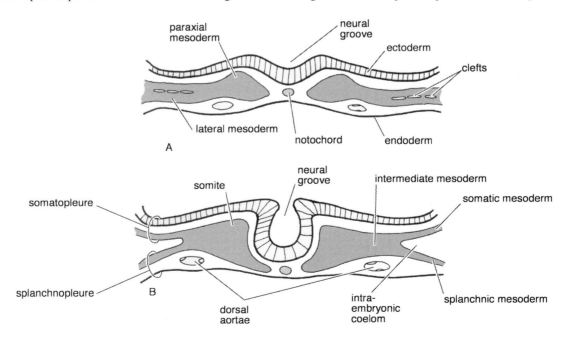

Figure 8.1 Cross-sections through embryos at early stages of development showing formation of the intra-embryonic coelom.

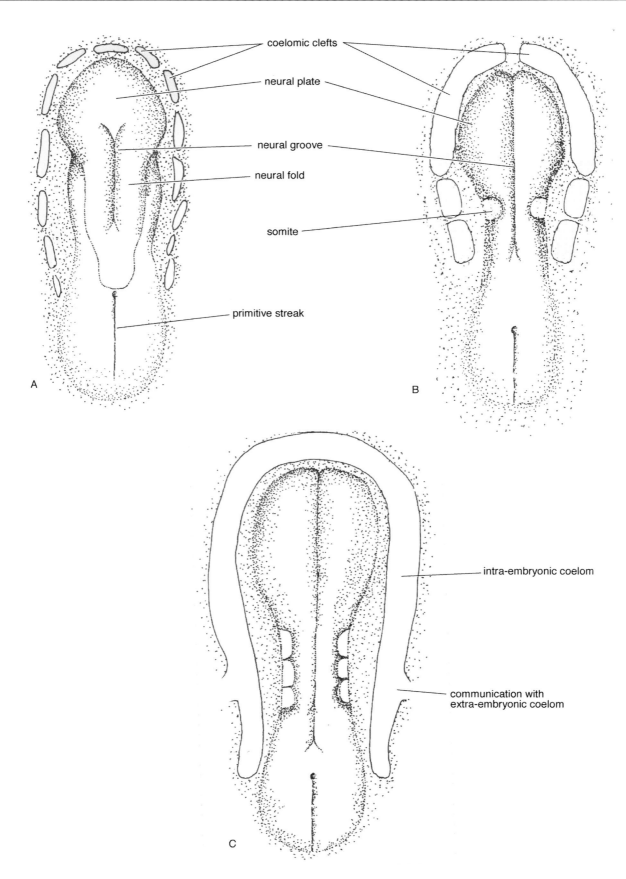

Figure 8.2 Dorsal views of embryos at early stages of development, A, B and C, showing the formation of the horseshoe-shaped coelomic cavity.

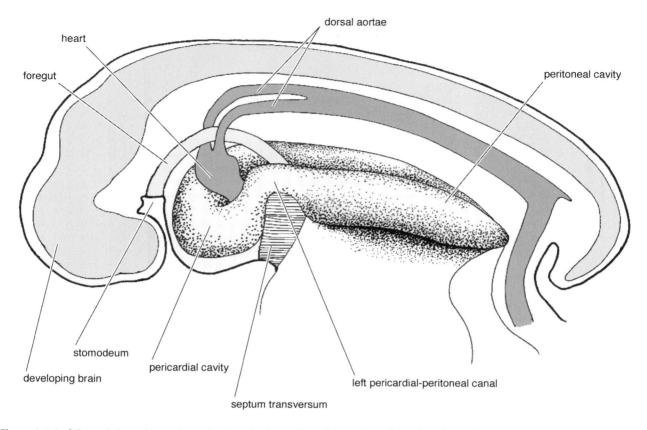

Figure 8.3 Left lateral view of an embryo showing the formation of the pericardial and peritoneal cavities and the pericardial–peritoneal canal.

folds meet, they divide the left and right segments of the pleuro-pericardial cavity into pleural cavities dorsally, and pericardial cavities ventrally. The heart is initially suspended by a double dorsal fold of mesothelium, the dorsal mesocardium, and anchored by a double ventral fold, the ventral mesocardium. The ventral mesocardium atrophies soon after its formation and this change is followed later by atrophy of the dorsal mesocardium, resulting in the formation of a single pericardial cavity. At this stage, the heart is suspended within the pericardial cavity solely by the blood vessels entering and leaving the heart. The pericardial sac thus formed consists of an inner visceral layer surrounding the heart and an outer parietal layer lining the thoracic wall. The left and right pleural cavities remain separate and communicate with the left and right limbs of the intra-embryonic coelom, located on either side of the developing foregut, by means of the left and right pleuro-peritoneal canals. The developing lungs, which grow into the pleural cavities, subsequently expand into the pleuro-peritoneal canals. The mesothelium in direct contact with the developing lungs is referred to as visceral pleura while the mesothelium in contact with the wall of the pleural cavity is called the parietal pleura. As the lungs continue to enlarge, the pleural cavities extend into the lateral body walls dividing them into thin inner layers and thicker outer layers, the latter destined to become the

definitive thoracic walls (Fig. 8.4C). The inner layers, which are continuous with the pleuro-pericardial folds, extend ventrally around the parietal layer lining the pericardial cavity and fuse, forming the fibrous layer of the pericardium. This fibrous layer, which anchors the pericardium either to the developing diaphragm or to the ventral thoracic wall, depending on species, encloses the left and right phrenic nerves. In dogs and cats, this structure is referred to as the phrenico-pericardial ligament and in horses and cattle as the sterno-pericardial ligament. Because the pleural surface of the pleuro-pericardial fold is covered by parietal pleura, in its final form the outer wall of the pericardium is composed of parietal pericardium, a middle fibrous layer and an outer layer of parietal pleura. The mesenchymal tissue which forms a septum separating the pleural cavities is referred to as the mediastinum. All the structures within the thoracic cavity, with the exception of the lungs, caudal vena cava and right phrenic nerve, are contained within the mediastinum, which extends from the developing vertebral column to the developing sternum.

Diaphragm

Initially, the pleuro-pericardial cavity communicates with the two limbs of the embryonic coelom. As a consequence of cranio-caudal folding, an aggregation of mesoderm,

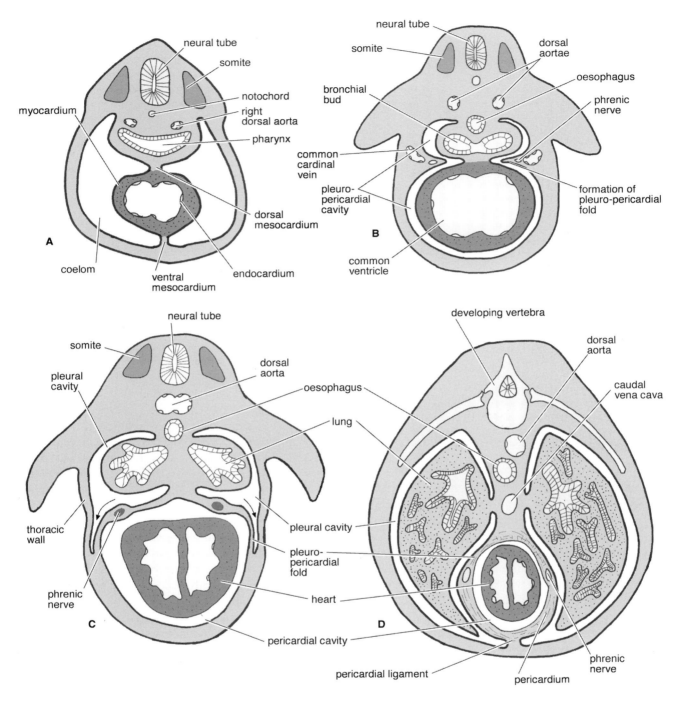

Figure 8.4 Sections through the thoracic regions of embryos at different stages of development, A to D, showing the formation of the pleural and pericardial cavities. In C, arrows indicate extension of pleural cavities into the body wall.

referred to as the septum transversum, moves from a position in front of the developing heart to a location caudal to it, forming a ventral partition, the diaphragm, which partially separates the pleuro-pericardial cavity from the developing peritoneal cavity. Subsequently, closure of the communication between the pleural cavity and the peritoneal cavity results from the formation of pleuro-peritoneal folds which develop from the lateral body wall and grow medially, fusing dorsally with the mesothelial fold suspending the oesophagus, the

mesoesophagus, and ventrally with the septum transversum. The partition formed by fusion of the pleuro-peritoneal folds, the dorsal mesothelial fold suspending the oesophagus and the septum transversum, constitutes the primordial diaphragm (Fig. 8.5). During subsequent enlargement of the thoracic cavity, mesoderm derived from the body wall forms the muscular rim of the diaphragm. By this means, matching growth of both diaphragm and thoracic wall occurs. The musculature of the diaphragm derives from myoblasts which originate

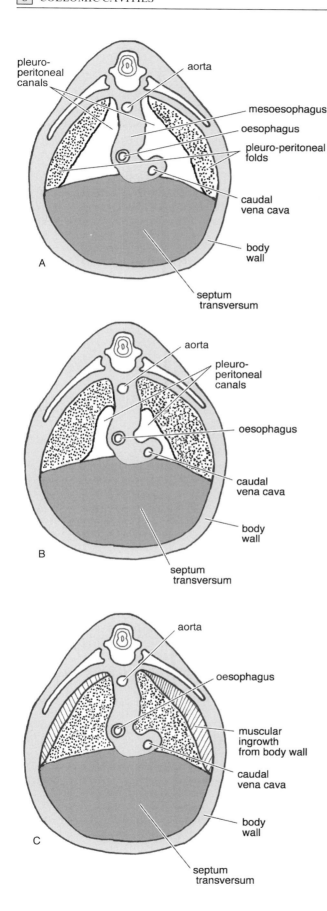

in cervical and thoraco-abdominal somites. Associated with the change in position of the septum transversum, myoblasts from the caudal cervical somites migrate into the septum. Ventral branches of the cervical spinal nerves innervate these myoblasts. Thus, the musculature of the central region of the diaphragm is innervated by ventral branches of caudal cervical nerves which form the left and right phrenic nerves. Ventral branches of thoracic and lumbar spinal nerves innervate the muscular rim of the diaphragm. Structures pass between the thoracic and abdominal cavities at three sites in the diaphragm. These sites, in dorso-ventral order, are: the aortic hiatus, through which the aorta, azygos vein and cysterna chyli pass; the oesophageal hiatus, through which the oesophagus and dorsal and ventral branches of the vagus nerves pass; and the foramen venae cavae, through which the caudal vena cava passes.

Anomalies of the diaphragm

Congenital anomalies of the diaphragm occur due to failure of the embryonic components of the developing diaphragm to unite and form a complete partition between the abdominal and thoracic cavities. This failure results in a persistent opening between the abdominal and thoracic cavities. When abdominal viscera pass through this opening into the thoracic cavity, the condition is referred to as congenital diaphragmatic herniation. Two forms of congenital diaphragmatic herniation occur in domestic animals, pleuro-peritoneal herniation and peritoneal-pericardial herniation.

Pleuro-peritoneal herniation is due to failure of one or both pleuro-peritoneal folds to develop or to fuse with the mesoesophagus and septum transversum resulting in failure of the pleuro-peritoneal canal to close. This defect usually occurs on the left side with the communication between the abdominal cavity and the thoracic cavity in a dorso-lateral position. Pleuro-peritoneal herniation is the most common form of congenital diaphragmatic defect in humans and results in the presence of abdominal viscera, usually the stomach and intestines, in the pleural cavity.

Peritoneal-pericardial herniation is more common in domestic animals, especially in dogs and cats, than pleuro-peritoneal herniation. This condition is considered to be due to a defect in the development of the septum transversum which results in an abnormal communication between the peritoneal and pericardial cavities. Incomplete fusion of the thoracic wall during lateral body folding is considered to be a contributing factor in the development of this anomaly. As a consequence of this defect, herniation of abdominal viscera, usually the liver, the pyloric region of the stomach and the intestines, into the pericardial cavity occurs.

Figure 8.5 Sequential stages in the development of the diaphragm.

The most common form of diaphragmatic herniation observed in small animal veterinary practice usually results from traumatic injury, often a consequence of road traffic accidents.

Peritoneal cavity

As already described, the lateral folding of the body wall results in the formation of left and right intra-embryonic coeloms, which surround the developing gut (Fig. 8.6). In the developing abdominal cavity, the gut is suspended by folds of splanchnic mesoderm between the left and right coelomic cavities. The mesothelium lining the abdominal cavity is referred to as peritoneum. Initially, the primordial digestive tract and its derivatives in the abdominal cavity are suspended from the dorsal body wall and anchored to the ventral body wall by a double layer of peritoneum. Folds of peritoneum which surround the intestine and connect it to the body wall are referred to as mesenteries. The folds of peritoneum which attach organs to each other, or attach organs to the body wall, are referred to as ligaments.

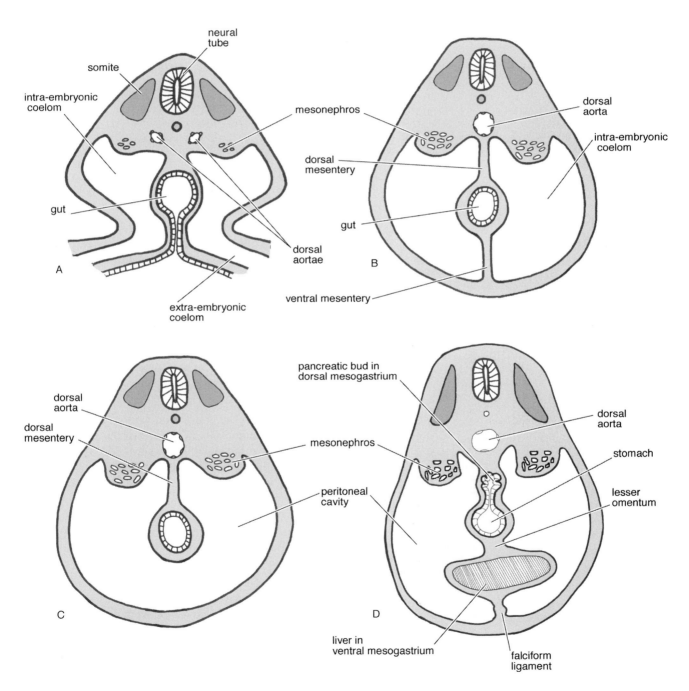

Figure 8.6 Sections through the abdominal regions of embryos at different stages of development, at the level of the gut, A, B and C, and at the level of the stomach, D.

Early in its development, the gut is a relatively straight tube and is attached to the wall of the abdominal cavity by both dorsal and ventral mesenteries. Later, the ventral mesentery caudal to the commencement of the duodenum and cranial to the rectum atrophies. In these regions, the gut remains suspended by a dorsal mesentery. Atrophy of the ventral mesentery allows the gut to increase in length and to undergo partial rotation, and also results in coalescence of the left and right coelomic cavities forming a single peritoneal cavity. Later in development, evaginations of peritoneum which extend into the developing inguinal canals form a left and a right tunica vaginalis.

Organs may be classified as intra-peritoneal if they are enclosed by a fold of peritoneum; those organs which are located against the abdominal wall and are covered by peritoneum on their surfaces not in contact with the abdominal wall are referred to as retro-peritoneal. In reality no organ is located within the peritoneal cavity which, in normal circumstances, contains only a thin film of peritoneal fluid of mesothelial origin.

Omenta

The term 'omentum' refers to a fold of peritoneum which attaches an organ to the stomach. The dorsal and ventral folds of peritoneum which suspend and anchor the stomach are referred to as the dorsal mesogastrium and ventral mesogastrium respectively. As a consequence of the partial rotations of the developing stomach, the original arrangement of these attachments becomes altered. During rotation of the stomach to the left, the dorsal mesogastrium elongates and is also drawn to the left, forming a pouch-like double fold enclosing a cavity referred to as the omental bursa. The enlarged dorsal mesogastrium continues to elongate and occupies a position between the abdominal viscera and the abdominal wall. At this stage of development, the structure, which is referred to as the greater omentum, consists of a superficial and a deep fold of peritoneum. The omental bursa communicates with the peritoneal cavity

through an opening, the epiploic foramen. The spleen primordium develops from aggregations of mesoderm which form within the superficial layer of the greater omentum. The fold of omentum which attaches the spleen to the stomach is referred to as the gastro-splenic ligament; the fold which attaches the spleen to the kidney is known as the lieno-renal ligament.

The dorsal bud of the pancreas extends into the superficial fold of the greater omentum. The lesser omentum becomes modified by the developing liver, which grows into the ventral mesogastrium and subdivides it into two regions. The resulting fold which extends from the lesser curvature of the stomach to the liver forms the lesser omentum, while the fold extending between the liver and ventral body wall forms the falciform ligament (Fig. 8.6D).

Further reading

Carlson, B.M. (2004) Digestive and respiratory systems and body cavities. In *Human Embryology and Developmental Biology*. Mosby, Philadelphia, PA, pp. 353–391.
Evans, M.S. and Biery, D.N. (1980) Congenital peritoneopericardial diaphragmatic hernia in the dog and cat: a literature review and 17 additional case histories. *Veterinary Radiology* 21, 108–116.
Latshaw, W.K. (1987) Mesenteries and compartmentalization. In *Veterinary Developmental Anatomy*. B.C. Decker, Toronto, pp. 169–180.
Liem, K.F., Bemis, W.E., Walker, W.F. and Grande, L. (2001) Development of the coelomic cavity and mesenteries. In *Functional Anatomy of the Vertebrates*, 3rd edn. Harcourt College Publishers, Fort Worth, TX, pp. 146–158.
Romer, A.S. (1962) The body cavities. In *The Vertebrate Body*. W.B. Saunders, Philadelphia, PA, pp. 288–296.
Wensing, C.J.G. (1975) Celomic cavities and serous membranes. In *The Anatomy of Domestic Animals*, Vol. 1, 5th edn. Ed. R. Getty. Saunders, Philadelphia, PA, pp. 87–103.

9 | Foetal Membranes

Primitive reproduction in lower vertebrates is characterised by females of the species laying large numbers of small, yolk-laden eggs in an aquatic environment with subsequent discharge of sperm by males in the same location. Fertilisation in these circumstances is described as external. The yolk provides the nutritional requirements for the developing zygote while oxygen is obtained from the aquatic environment and metabolic waste is discharged into the same watery habitat. In species in which the embryo is provided with a limited supply of nutrients, an intermediate free-feeding larval stage develops which subsequently undergoes metamorphosis and grows to the adult form. The large number of eggs produced in these circumstances compensates for the high mortality associated with this type of reproduction.

Species which produce a small number of large eggs, with high yolk content and in which the young are at a more advanced stage of development when emerging from the egg, have an enhanced probability of survival. In this type of development, which is commonly encountered in cartilaginous fish, some bony fish, reptiles, birds and mammals, a larval stage does not occur.

Species at a more advanced stage of evolutionary development produce eggs which are retained within the body of the female. The male deposits sperm into the female tract and fertilisation is internal. In these species, the yolk content of the egg is relatively low and the embryo receives its nutritional and oxygen requirements from the maternal vascular system. This pattern of reproduction is found in most vertebrate species with the exception of birds. Species in which the developing embryo is retained within the body of the female and the young are born alive are termed viviparous. The term oviparous is used to describe those species in which embryos hatch from eggs incubated outside the body. A number of species exhibit an intermediate developmental pattern between oviparity and viviparity. In these species, termed ovo-viviparous, yolk-laden eggs are retained within the mother's body and the embryo receives its nutritional requirements from the egg itself, its respiratory needs supplied by the maternal vascular system.

Embryos which develop in an aquatic environment rely on their own egg-derived food supply as they acquire oxygen from the water and their metabolic waste diffuses into their aquatic surroundings. The yolk is stored either within the endodermal cells of the ventral gut wall as in amphibians with medialecithal eggs, or as an extra-cellular mass ventral to the developing embryo as in fish, reptiles and birds with megalecithal eggs (Fig. 9.1). In embryos which develop from megalecithal eggs, the body wall of the embryo grows around the yolk mass forming a trilaminar sac, the yolk sac. The mesoderm of the trilaminar yolk sac becomes vascularised and the enclosed nutrients are absorbed via the endodermal layer and then transported to the embryo by the vitelline vessels. The development of the head, tail and lateral body folds raises the embryo above the yolk, so that a demarcation becomes evident between the embryo itself and the yolk sac. The initial broad connection between the embryo and the yolk sac becomes constricted until they are connected only by a stalk. As the yolk is consumed, the sac diminishes in size until it is eventually withdrawn into the abdominal cavity through the umbilicus.

The evolution of terrestrial vertebrates necessitated changes in the developing embryos to enable them to survive in non-aquatic environments. Although some species, such as amphibians, have evolved to a terrestrial existence, they return to an aquatic environment for egg laying. Other species, such as turtles, lay in damp surroundings from which the eggs can derive water. Birds and reptiles have adapted to their non-aquatic environment by laying eggs with protective membranes or shells secreted by their reproductive tracts. In addition, albumen, also secreted by the female reproductive tract as an additional source of nutrients, is enclosed in the shell. Terrestrial species also evolved additional extra-embryonic membranes, the amnion, the chorion and the allantois, to provide further protection, conserve water and store waste products.

In mammals, there is a tendency towards a reduction in protective egg membranes and in yolk content. The eggs of most eutherian mammals are 80–140 μm in diameter and miolecithal.

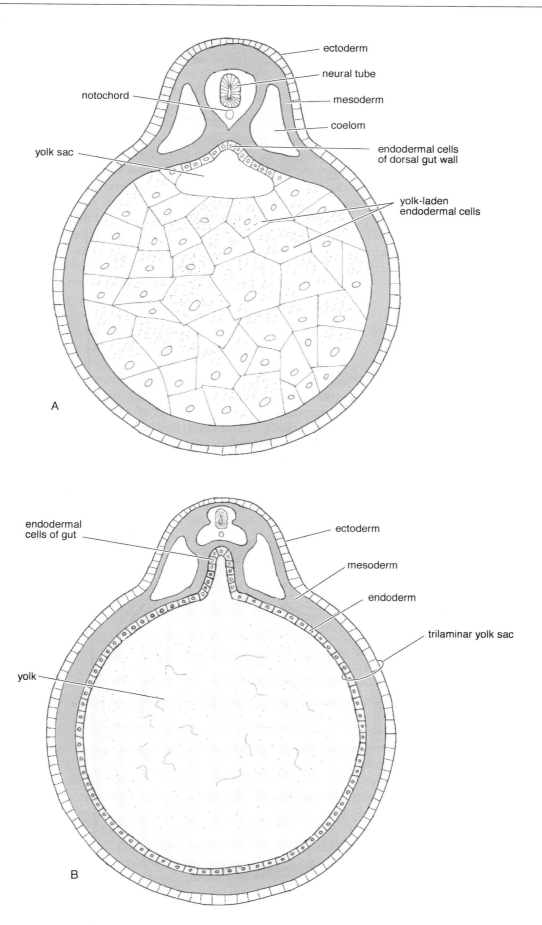

Figure 9.1 A, Amphibian embryo with yolk stored within endodermal cells of ventral gut wall. B, Avian embryo with yolk stored as extra-cellular ventral mass.

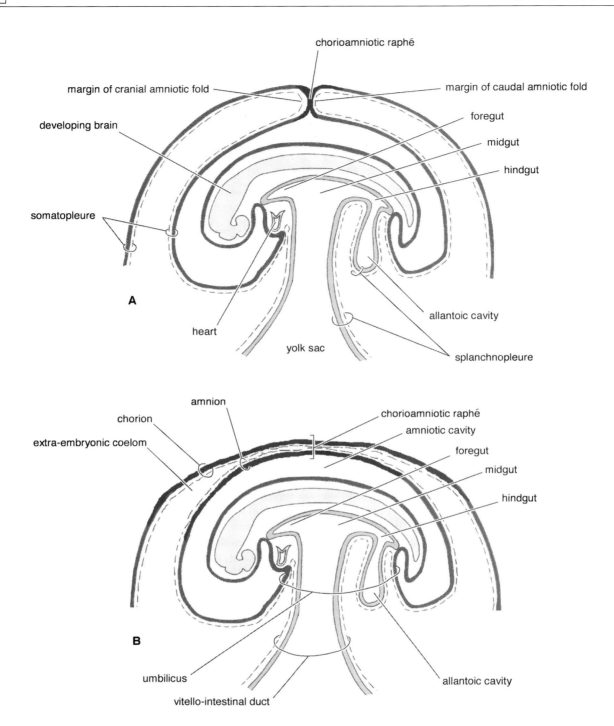

Figure 9.4 Chick embryos showing dorsal folding of the extra-embryonic somatopleure, A. Fusion of the amniotic folds leading to the formation of outer chorionic membranes and inner amniotic membranes, B.

During incubation, the albumen loses water, becomes more viscous and rapidly decreases in volume. The expanding extra-embryonic membranes force the albumen distally where it becomes surrounded by the splanchnopleure of the yolk sac and allantois. The portion of the chorio-allantoic membrane enclosing the albumen is known as the albumen sac (Fig. 9.5). Around the 12th day, a narrow communication, the amniotic duct, which develops between the albumen sac and the amniotic sac, allows albumen to enter the amniotic cavity where it mixes with the amniotic fluid and can be swallowed by the embryo and utilised as a source of nourishment (Fig. 9.5). Incubation periods for domesticated birds are shown in Table 9.1.

Mammals

The extra-embryonic or foetal membranes of domestic mammals consisting of yolk sac, amnion, chorion and allantois develop in a manner similar to those of birds.

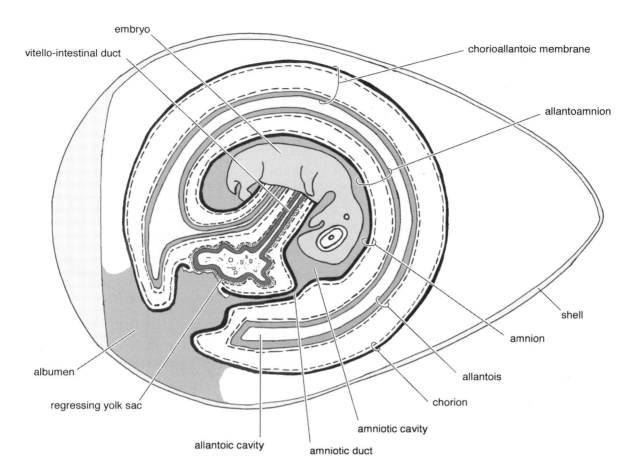

Figure 9.5 Chick embryo showing enlargement of the allantois between the chorion and amnion and formation of amniotic duct.

Table 9.1 Incubation periods for domesticated birds.

Species	Incubation period (days)
Budgerigar	18–20
Chicken	21
Duck	28
Goose	28
Pheasant	28
Turkey	28

The yolk sac in higher mammals, however, is devoid of yolk. In viviparous animals, the foetal membranes become apposed to uterine maternal tissue forming the placenta, an anatomical structure which functions as an organ of physiological exchange between mother and foetus.

Yolk sac

At the end of cleavage, the blastocyst which is enclosed within the zona pellucida consists of an inner cell mass and a layer of trophoblastic cells. As gastrulation proceeds, endodermal cells separate from the embryonic disc and line the blastocyst cavity leading to the formation of a bilaminar yolk sac (Fig. 9.6A). Mesodermal cells then migrate from the primitive streak and occupy a position between the inner endodermal layer and the outer trophoblastic layer. This trilaminar structure is termed the trilaminar yolk sac (Fig. 9.6B). The mesodermal layer becomes vascularised, and the union of the vascular trilaminar layer with the uterine epithelium forms a choriovitelline placenta. The mesoderm of the trilaminar yolk sac gradually splits into an outer somatic and an inner splanchnic layer (Fig. 9.6C). With the formation of the embryonic body wall folds, a portion of the splanchnopleure becomes enclosed within the embryo and forms the embryonic gut, while that portion which remains outside the embryo is the definitive yolk sac (Fig. 9.6D). The embryonic gut and yolk sac communicate with each other at the umbilicus by means of the vitello-intestinal duct. In horses, the vascular yolk sac possesses a well-defined terminal sinus similar to that in birds.

Amnion and chorion

In domestic mammals, the amnion and chorion form by folding in a manner similar to that described for birds

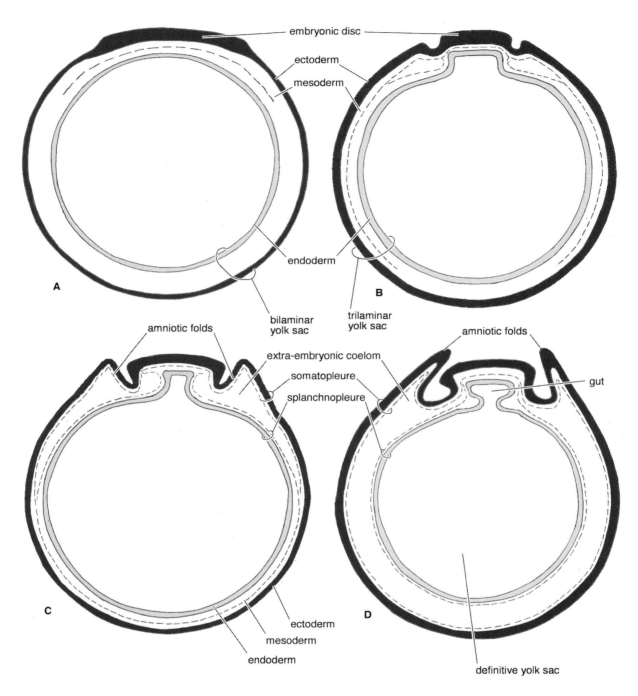

Figure 9.6 Stages in the formation of a bilaminar yolk sac, A, and trilaminar yolk sac, B, in domestic mammals. C, Formation of somatopleure and splanchnopleure. D, Convergence of amniotic folds and formation of definitive yolk sac.

(Fig. 9.4). The zona pellucida ruptures during the second week of development and allows the blastocyst to leave its confined space and elongate. The elongating blastocyst may reach a length of 60–100 cm in cattle, sheep and pigs. The embryonic disc itself is minimally affected in this process of elongation, which involves the trophoblast, and to a lesser extent, the inner endodermal lining. Soon after the appearance of the primitive streak, the trophoblast folds around the embryonic disc. As the embryo grows, its head and tail push deeper into the trophoblast, which becomes lined by a layer of somatic

mesoderm forming the extra-embryonic somatopleure. The folds are known as the amniotic or chorioamniotic folds. The amniotic folds extend centripetally above the embryo where they meet and fuse. Later, the outer layer of the somatopleure separates from the inner layer leaving the embryo surrounded by two membranes. The inner somatopleure membrane, which remains attached to the embryo at the umbilicus, forms the amnion, and the outer somatopleure membrane, which completely surrounds the embryo, the amnion and the yolk sac, forms the chorion (Fig. 9.7). Where the amniotic folds

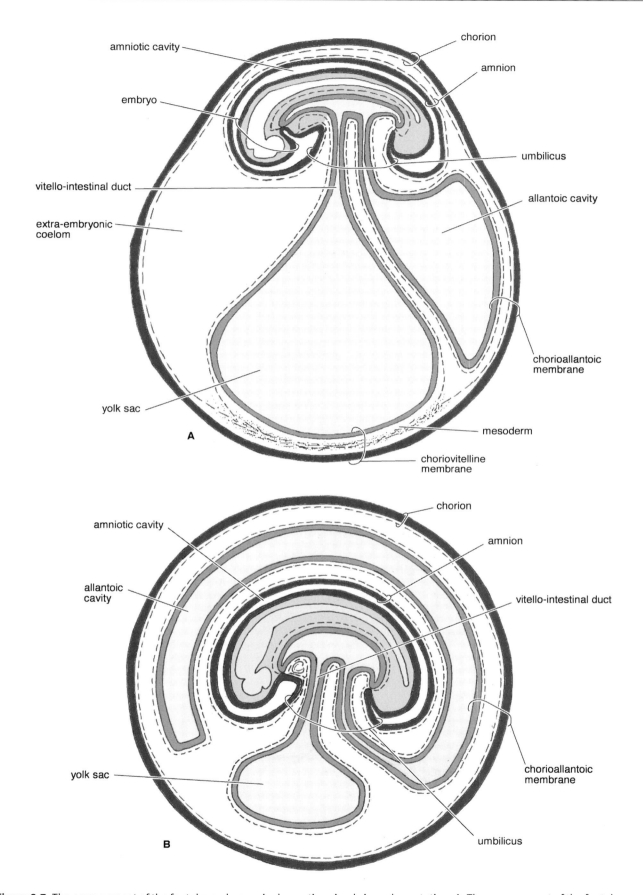

Figure 9.7 The arrangement of the foetal membranes in domestic animals in early gestation, A. The arrangement of the foetal membranes in horses and carnivores at mid-gestation, B.

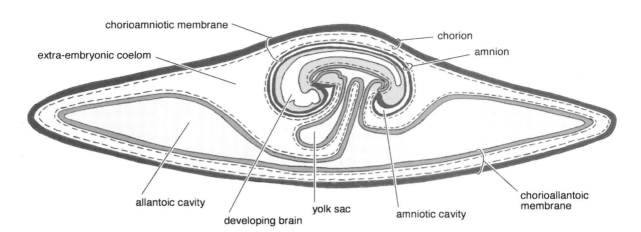

Figure 9.8 The arrangement of the foetal membranes in ruminants and pigs at mid-gestation.

fuse, a cord-like chorioamniotic raphé is present for a short time and then breaks down resulting in complete separation between the amnion and the chorion. The space between the amnion and the chorion is the extra-embryonic coelom.

The amnion is a thin, tough membrane which forms the wall of a fluid-filled sac in which the embryo develops. The volume of amniotic fluid increases rapidly until mid-pregnancy and then decreases gradually. The amnion has a primarily protective role.

Formation of the amnion by folding, which occurs in birds, reptiles and domestic mammals, is considered to be the most primitive form of amniogenesis. In higher primates and humans, the amnion forms by a process of cavitation of the inner cell mass, which is considered to be the most specialised form of amniogenesis. The method of amnion formation influences the type of implantation: early implantation is associated with cavitation amniogenesis and late implantation with formation of the amnion by folding.

Allantois

In domestic animals, the allantois develops as a diverticulum of the hindgut (splanchnopleure), which grows into the extra-embryonic coelom. In cattle, sheep and pigs, this vesicular diverticulum is anchor-shaped (Fig. 9.8), while in dogs, cats and horses, it is a tube-shaped structure which, as it grows, becomes completely interposed between the amnion and chorion (Fig. 9.7B). The vascular allantoic mesoderm, when fused to the chorion, forms the vascular chorioallantoic membrane. The area of contact between this vascular chorioallantoic membrane and the endometrium forms the chorioallantoic placenta. The volume of fluid in the allantoic sac increases gradually during the first third of pregnancy and thereafter rises rapidly.

The primary function of the allantois is to vascularise the chorion so that the chorioallantoic placenta provides nutrients and a respiratory pathway for the developing embryo. It also functions as an extension of the bladder facilitating the storage of renal waste.

In humans and higher primates, the allantois is a narrow, tube-like outgrowth of the hindgut which grows into the connecting body stalk but does not contain fluid.

Foetal fluids

In domestic mammals the total volume of foetal fluid in both the amniotic and allantoic sacs increases and, by the end of gestation in cattle, may be up to 20 litres (Fig. 9.9). However, the volumes of amniotic and allantoic fluids do not increase at an equal rate. In cattle, the volume of allantoic fluid increases gradually during the first third of pregnancy and then rises rapidly until the end of gestation. The amniotic fluid volume increases relatively rapidly up to mid-pregnancy and then gradually declines (Fig. 9.9). Similar variations in the volumes of these fluids are observed in other domestic mammals.

In early pregnancy, the composition of foetal fluids is similar to foetal and maternal plasma and may be considered a dialysate of the maternal or foetal extracellular fluids. In addition, secretions of the respiratory tract and fluid from the skin, prior to keratinisation, are present in the amniotic fluid. Similarly, secretions of the allantoic membrane are added to the allantoic fluid. As the developing kidneys become functional during the early foetal period, urine is passed from the bladder via the urachus to the allantoic cavity. Later in gestation, when the foetal urethra becomes patent, the foetus can pass urine into the amniotic cavity. At this stage, the foetus can swallow amniotic fluid which is absorbed from the foetal gut and transferred across the placenta for excretion by the mother. This accounts in part for

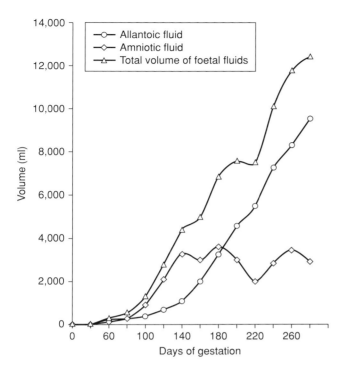

Figure 9.9 Changes in the volumes of bovine foetal fluids at different stages of gestation.

the perceived stabilisation of amniotic fluid volume in the last third of pregnancy.

In cattle, both allantoic and amniotic fluids have a pale, urine-like appearance at mid-pregnancy. As gestation proceeds, the allantoic fluid acquires a brownish tinge while the amniotic fluid changes to a colourless, slightly viscous, lubricating fluid.

Amniotic fluid provides an aqueous medium in which the fragile embryo can develop symmetrically, free from distortion that could arise from pressure of its own weight against surrounding structures. This fluid also prevents adhesion of the embryo to the amniotic membrane. During implantation, the increasing volume of foetal fluids assists the elongating chorionic sac to appose the uterine epithelium. At parturition, the pressure from the fluid-filled sacs aids dilation of the cervix. With rupture of the sacs, the foetal fluids lubricate the birth canal for the passage of the foetus.

At parturition in horses, dogs and cats, the chorioallantoic membrane ruptures intravaginally releasing the allantoic fluid. The chorionic sac, however, remains attached to the endometrium and is not immediately expelled. The amniotic sac then ruptures, but having no attachment to the chorion due to the disposition of the allantois in these species, the foetus is born surrounded by the amnion. In ruminants and pigs, the allantois does not completely surround the amnion, and as a result a

wide area of the amnion fuses to the chorion. Thus, the amniotic sac is usually retained and the foetus is born without its amniotic membrane.

The term 'conceptus' is used to describe the embryo or foetus and associated fluid-filled membranes. The growing conceptus can be detected in the uterus of the mare and cow from approximately 15 days of gestation using ultrasonic scanning and by palpation per rectum in both species after 30 days.

Structures associated with foetal membranes

Calculi are found in the allantoic fluid in a number of species. In the mare, these calculi, which occur as small brown masses up to 4 cm in diameter, are referred to as hippomanes. Morphological and histological studies have revealed that hippomanes, which first appear around 90 days, are allantoic calculi consisting of central nuclei of desquamated cellular debris surrounded by allantoic precipitates. The so-called pedunculated hippomanes which are found in the chorioallantoic membrane of the mare, and which are derived from the endometrial cups, are more appropriately referred to as chorioallantoic pouches.

Epithelial thickenings known as amniotic plaques form on the inner ectodermal surface of the amnion in ruminants and horses from the tenth week of gestation. They are especially prominent in the region of the umbilical cord. These epithelial cells have high glycogen content but their functional significance is uncertain.

Umbilical cord

The umbilical cord is the connecting stalk between the foetus and the placenta. The body of the cord consists of foetal mucoid connective tissue, surrounding two umbilical arteries, two umbilical veins, the urachus, and the vestige of the yolk sac (Fig. 9.10). In horses, dogs and cats, the umbilical cord is divided into an amniotic and allantoic portion due to the arrangement of the foetal membranes in these species. In cattle, sheep and pigs, the amnion is reflected on to the surface of the umbilical cord. In these animals, the cord is short and breaks at birth. As the umbilical vessels emerge from the body of the cord, their branches diverge and continue to opposite poles of the chorionic sac. In the early stages of development, a pouch of peritoneum containing the mid-gut loop of intestines occupies the proximal portion of the cord, resulting in a physiological congenital umbilical hernia.

The umbilical arteries, present in the umbilical cord, descend in a spiral fashion in the cord around the urachus (Fig. 9.10). They give off branches to the amniotic sac

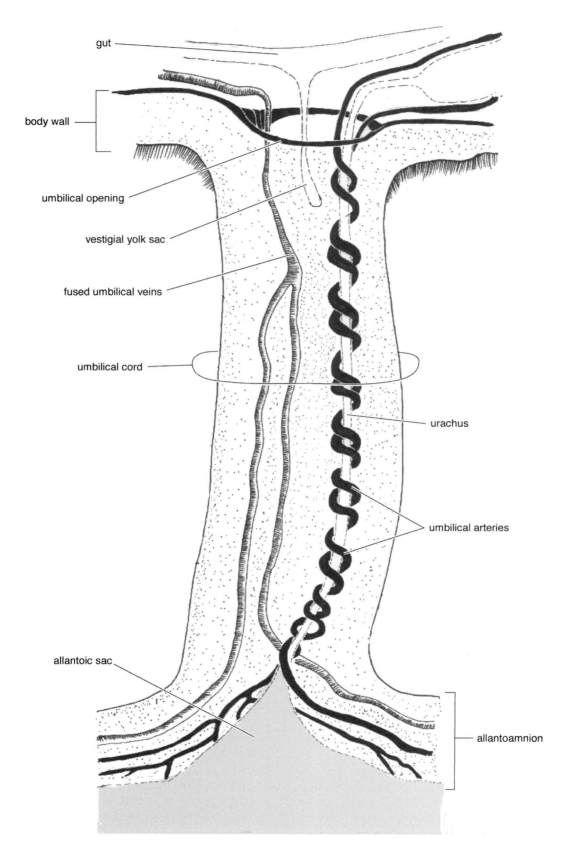

gut

body wall

umbilical opening

vestigial yolk sac

fused umbilical veins

umbilical cord

urachus

umbilical arteries

allantoic sac

allantoamnion

Figure 9.10 The arrangement of the blood vessels and urachus in the umbilical cord in the mare and in the sow.

Table 9.2 Umbilical cord lengths at birth in different species.

Species	Umbilical cord length
Cat	Approximately one-third of length of foetus
Cow	30–40 cm
Dog	Approximately half of length of foetus
Horse	50–100 cm
Pig	20–25 cm
Sheep	20–30 cm

and terminate in the chorioallantoic membrane. In horses and pigs, the umbilical veins fuse within the amniotic part of the cord, while in other species they fuse on entering the abdominal cavity. Umbilical cord lengths in different species of domesticated animals are presented in Table 9.2.

In cattle, sheep and pigs, the cord ruptures as the foetus passes through the birth canal. In horses, dogs and cats, the cord normally breaks as a result of the action of the dam after the foetus has been born. The point of rupture is 3–5 cm from the umbilicus. The ruptured umbilical arteries retract within the abdomen and the recoil of the elastic fibres in their walls seals their lumina thus preventing haemorrhage. The umbilical veins lack elastic tissue and remain open for a time and may allow entry of bacteria leading to joint ill. The urachus usually closes at this time; failure to close can lead to leakage of urine at the umbilicus and may predispose to infection. This condition, known as persistent urachus, can be corrected surgically.

Anomalies associated with foetal membranes

In cattle, excessive accumulation of foetal fluids can occasionally occur in either the amniotic or allantoic sacs. This condition is referred to as hydrops of the foetal sacs. In hydrops of the allantois, hydrallantois, the condition becomes clinically evident between the sixth and ninth months of gestation; up to ten to 40 times the normal volume of allantoic fluid may be produced. Clinically, it presents as a progressive distension of the right abdominal wall. Pathological changes in the placenta are considered to be responsible for this condition. Hydramnion, an abnormal condition in the cow resulting in levels of eight to ten times the normal amniotic fluid volume, is usually associated with malformations of the foetal digestive system such as oesophageal atresia. The condition is rare in sheep, pigs, dogs and cats, and has not been reported in horses.

Further reading

Amoroso, E.C. (1952) Placentation. In *Marshall's Physiology of Reproduction*, Vol. 2, 3rd edn. Ed. A.S. Parkes. Longmans, Green and Co., London, pp. 127–311.

Arthur, G.H. (1969) The fetal fluids of domestic animals. *Journal of Reproduction and Fertility* **9**, 45–52.

Bongso, T.A. and Basrur, P.K. (1976) Fetal fluids in cattle. *Canadian Veterinary Journal* **17**, 38–41.

Boyd, J.D. and Hamilton, W.J. (1952) Cleavage, early development, and implantation of the egg. In *Marshall's Physiology of Reproduction*, Vol. 2, 3rd edn. Ed. A.S. Parkes. Longmans, Green and Co., London, pp. 1–126.

Brace, R.A. (1999) Amniotic fluid. In *Encyclopedia of Reproduction*, Vol. 1. Eds. E. Knobil and J.D. Neill. Academic Press, San Diego, pp. 149–153.

Brazer, F.W. (1999) Allantochorion (chorioallantois). In *Encyclopedia of Reproduction*, Vol. 1. Eds. E. Knobil and J.D. Neill. Academic Press, San Diego, pp. 256–264.

Brazer, F.W. (1999) Allantoic fluid. In *Encyclopedia of Reproduction*, Vol. 1. Eds. E. Knobil and J.D. Neill. Academic Press, San Diego, pp. 93–95.

Bryden, M.M., Evans, H.E. and Binns, W. (1972) Embryology of the sheep 1. Extraembryonic membranes and the development of the body form. *Journal of Morphology* **138**, 168–186.

Ewart, J.C. (1898) *A Critical Period in the Development of the Horse*. Adam and Charles Black, London.

Ginther, O.J. (1992) Placentation and Embryology. In *Reproductive Biology of the Mare*, 2nd edn. Equiservices, Cross Plains, Wisconsin, pp. 345–418.

Latshaw, W.K. (1987) Extraembryonic membranes and placentation. In *Veterinary Developmental Anatomy*. B.C. Decker, Toronto, pp. 49–74.

Mossman, H.W. (1987) *Vertebrate Fetal Membranes*. Rutgers University Press, New Brunswick, NJ.

Noakes, D. (2001) Development of the conceptus. In *Arthur's Veterinary Reproduction and Obstetrics*, 8th edn. Eds. D.E. Noakes, T.J. Parkinson and G.C. England. W.B. Saunders, London, pp. 57–68.

Perry, J.S. (1981) The mammalian fetal membranes. *Journal of Reproduction and Fertility* **62**, 321–335.

Rothchild, I. (2003) The yolkless egg and the evolution of eutherian viviparity. *Biology of Reproduction* **68**, 337–357.

Struss, J.F. and Budak, E. (1999) Fetal membranes. In *Encyclopedia of Reproduction*, Vol. 2. Eds. E. Knobil and J.D. Neill. Academic Press, San Diego, pp. 326–337.

Van Nierkerk, C.H. (1965) The early diagnosis of pregnancy, the development of the foetal membranes and nidation in the mare. *Journal of the South African Veterinary Medical Association* **36**, 483–488.

Whitwell, K.E. and Jeffcott, L.B. (1975) Morphological studies on the foetal membranes of the normal singleton foal at term. *Research in Veterinary Science* **19**, 44–55.

10 Forms of Implantation and Placentation

Following fertilisation, the zygote, as it undergoes cleavage, moves along the uterine tube and enters the uterus. The developing embryo, suspended in tubal fluid, is transported by a combination of ciliary and muscular action and takes up to three days to reach the uterus in most mammals. The nutritional requirements of the embryo are supplied initially by its own yolk and by the secretions of the maternal reproductive tract. The developing embryo is protected from maternal cellular defences by the zona pellucida within which it appears to carry no electrical charge. In addition, the zona pellucida is immunologically inert as it does not express major histocompatibility complex antigens. Because the blastocyst is enclosed within an intact zona pellucida, implantation cannot occur as it moves through the uterine tube. On reaching the uterus, the blastocyst hatches from the zona pellucida and remains free for a short period in the uterine lumen. During this time, it receives nourishment from secretions of the uterine glands. Subsequently, the blastocyst attaches to the uterine mucosa, a process referred to as implantation.

Implantation

The term implantation is used to describe the attachment of the developing embryo to the endometrium. This process, which occurs in three stages in domestic animals, is gradual, with apposition of the blastocyst or foetal membranes to the uterine epithelium followed by adhesion. Depending on the species, the final stage involves firm attachment or actual invasion of the endometrium. As a fertilized ovum remains relatively independent of maternal influences prior to implantation, it can be grown to the blastocyst stage *in vitro*. However, from the time of implantation onwards, the viability of the embryo is greatly influenced by maternal factors, and embryonic survival is dependent on hormonal and immunological adaptation of the dam to pregnancy.

The intervals between fertilisation and implantation in humans and different species of animals are presented in Table 10.1. The form of implantation differs from one species to another. In primates and guinea-pigs, the blastocyst burrows through the uterine epithelium to the uterine stroma where the embryo develops. This form of implantation is referred to as interstitial implantation (Fig. 10.1A and B). In rodents, implantation involves the blastocyst becoming lodged in a uterine cleft with proliferation of the surrounding uterine mucosa. This form of implantation is known as eccentric implantation (Fig. 10.1C). In horses, cattle, sheep, pigs, dogs, cats and rabbits, the fluid-filled sacs surrounding the embryo expand so that the extra-embryonic membranes become apposed to the uterine epithelium and attach to it. This form of implantation, the most common example of attachment in mammals, is referred to as centric or superficial implantation (Fig. 10.1D). In animals with either interstitial or eccentric implantation, the three stages of attachment occur within a short time interval and it is possible to accurately estimate the time of implantation. With centric or superficial implantation, the stages of attachment extend over a longer time period than in interstitial implantation and wide variation has

Table 10.1 The times, from ovulation, during which implantation occurs in humans and in different species of animals.

Species	Time (days)
Rodents	5 to 6
Humans	6 to 7
Rabbits	7 to 8
Cats	12 to 14
Pigs	12 to 16
Dogs	14 to 18
Sheep	14 to 18
Cattle	17 to 35
Horses	17 to 56

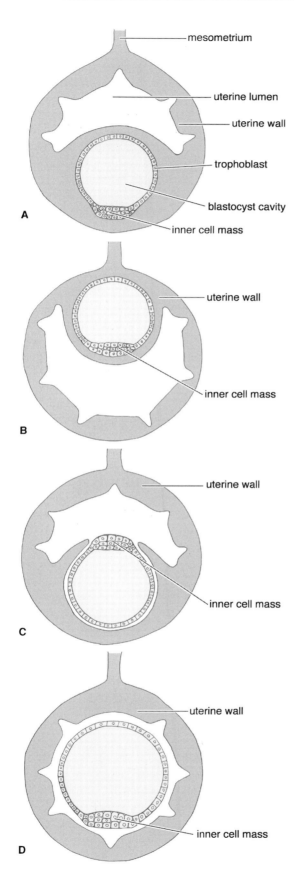

Figure 10.1 Cross-sections through pregnant uteri showing three different forms of implantation. A, Interstitial, anti-mesometrial implantation. B, Interstitial, mesometrial implantation. C, Eccentric, anti-mesometrial implantation. D, Centric or superficial implantation.

been reported for the time of implantation in ruminants and horses.

In eccentric or interstitial implantation, the site of blastocyst attachment is described by relating its position in the uterus to the mesometrium. When the blastocyst implants in the endometrium on the same side as the attachment of the mesometrium, this is referred to as mesometrial implantation (Fig. 10.1B). When implantation occurs at a site opposite to the attachment of the mesometrium, this is referred to as anti-mesometrial implantation (Fig. 10.1A). The orientation of the blastocyst is similarly described by relating the position of the inner cell mass to the mesometrium (Fig. 10.2).

In utero *spacing and embryo orientation*

After reaching the uterus, blastocysts are moved to their implantation sites. In cattle and sheep, when a single ovum is fertilised, the blastocyst attaches to the middle or upper third of the uterine horn adjacent to the ovulating ovary. In sheep, when two blastocysts derive from one ovary, one blastocyst usually migrates to the contralateral

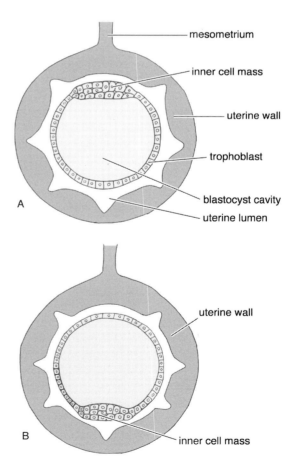

Figure 10.2 Cross-sections through pregnant uteri showing orientation of blastocyst at time of implantation. A, Mesometrial orientation of inner cell mass. B, Anti-mesometrial orientation of inner cell mass.

horn, where it becomes implanted. As intra-uterine migration is rare in cattle, when twins arise from ovulation involving one ovary, both embryos usually develop in the same horn. In mares, ultrasonography has demonstrated that, irrespective of which ovary ovulates, the blastocyst migrates between the left and right uterine horns between the 11th and the 17th days. After this time mobility ceases and the blastocyst implants in either the left or right horn close to the body of the uterus.

In polytocous animals, the blastocysts are evenly spaced within the uterine horns. Although the underlying mechanism responsible for the spacing of implanting blastocysts is unclear, oestrogen produced by the developing blastocyst is considered to have an important role in embryo spacing.

Endocrine control of implantation

Implantation requires co-operative interaction between the dam and the blastocyst. The high levels of oestrogen produced during the follicular stage of the oestrous cycle cause proliferation of the endometrium and, in addition, progesterone produced during the luteal stage renders the endometrium receptive to the blastocyst. In all mammals, progesterone is essential for both the establishment and the maintenance of pregnancy. For maintenance of pregnancy in domestic mammals, continued functioning of the cyclical corpus luteum is a requirement and this is achieved through the production of anti-luteolysin by the conceptus which inhibits the production of luteolytic uterine secretions. This response to the presence of the conceptus is referred to as maternal recognition of pregnancy. While the basic strategy is to maintain and prolong the cyclical corpus luteum by inhibiting or reducing the secretion of prostaglandin $F_{2\alpha}$ ($PGF_{2\alpha}$), the factors which control the process show species variation. In species in which the life span of the corpus luteum is similar in pregnant and non-pregnant animals, recognition of pregnancy may occur by different means.

Delayed implantation

In a number of species, there is an unusually long delay between the entry of the blastocyst into the uterus and the time at which implantation occurs. In these species, the blastocyst enters a period of decreased cell division and metabolic quiescence, referred to as diapause, a state characterised by decreased protein and nucleic acid synthesis and a decline in carbon dioxide output. In mink and ferrets, the interval is comparatively short, usually a matter of weeks, whereas in roe deer, bears, badgers and seals, the interval may be substantially longer, up to four months in some instances. Delayed implantation increases the probability that offspring are born at a time of year favourable for survival. Although there is limited information on the underlying mechanisms which operate in delayed implantation, both uterine and hypothalamic factors are implicated. When blastocyst development is slowed as a consequence of seasonal influences, this type of diapause is referred to as seasonal or obligative delayed implantation. In addition to those animals in which delayed implantation is a normal occurrence, a similar but shorter delay may occur in certain species of rodents and insectivores. The delay in implantation in these species is attributed to the influence of stress factors, such as lactation, which inhibit implantation. If rodents become pregnant during a post-partum oestrus, blastocyst implantation is delayed until weaning occurs. The delay is influenced by litter size. With a litter size of one or two, implantation is not delayed, whereas with six or more offspring, there may be a delay of up to six days. This mechanism, which ensures that the dam does not have to support two litters contemporaneously, is referred to as facultative or lactational delayed implantation.

Ectopic pregnancy

Implantation and subsequent embryonic development in an extra-uterine location is referred to as ectopic pregnancy. Sites of abnormal implantation include the ovary, the uterine tube and the peritoneal cavity. Ectopic pregnancy, which occurs more frequently in humans than in domestic animals, usually leads to death of the embryo or foetus and may be accompanied by severe maternal haemorrhage and sometimes death.

Embryonic mortality

In the absence of infectious diseases and despite optimal nutrition, early embryonic mortality is a frequent occurrence in all domestic species. Most of these early embryonic deaths, which occur around the time of maternal recognition of pregnancy or the time of implantation, are attributed to defective interaction between the conceptus and the dam.

There is a 10–15% fertilisation failure rate in heifers bred under optimal conditions. By 28 days post-fertilisation, the rate of embryonic death is reported to be approximately 25%, with the highest mortality occurring between days eight and 18. By day 17, embryonic death in sheep is reported to be 33%. Exceptionally high embryonic mortality rates, up to 50%, are reported in mares by the 28th day of gestation. Embryonic mortality in pigs is reported to be in excess of 41%, with up to 21% of losses occurring before day ten. Embryonic loss is reported to be higher in the human population than in the animal population, with 62% of pregnancies confirmed at day 12 ending in embryonic or foetal death.

Survival of the developing embryo depends on the establishment of a placenta, the formation of which, in turn, depends on cooperative interactions between the blastocyst and the uterus. These interactions are affected by complex factors, which involve adequate hormonal stimulation of the endometrium, environmental stimuli and the nutritional status of the mother. Factors which may contribute to early embryonic mortality are hormonal imbalance, maternal rejection and chromosomal abnormalities in the developing embryo.

Placentation in mammals

When the blastocyst reaches the uterus, it is initially sustained by uterine secretions and after a short delay it attaches to uterine tissue with the subsequent formation of a placenta. This complex structure allows selective exchange of nutrients, gases and waste products. It also functions as a site of hormone production. Based on the relationship between foetal membranes and maternal tissue, two basic types of placentae are recognised, choriovitelline and chorioallantoic. When the fused vascular choriovitelline membranes become attached to the endometrium, the resulting placenta is known as a choriovitelline or yolk sac placenta. This type of placentation is commonly encountered in marsupials. When the chorioallantoic membrane becomes attached to the endometrium, the resulting placenta is referred to as a chorioallantoic placenta. While this is the definitive form of placentation in higher mammals, it may be preceded by and co-exist with a temporary choriovitelline placenta (Fig. 10.3).

Choriovitelline placenta

The yolk sac is formed early in development in higher mammals, usually while the blastocyst is still unattached in the uterine cavity. In most mammals, with the exception of humans, the endoderm of the early yolk sac combines with the trophoblastic layer of the blastocyst, forming the bilaminar yolk sac. When the vascular mesoderm becomes interposed between the chorion and the endoderm, the bilaminar structure becomes a trilaminar yolk sac which functions as the embryonic component of the choriovitelline placenta (Fig. 10.3). While the choriovitelline placenta persists as the definitive placenta in most marsupials, among domestic mammals the choriovitelline placenta exists only as an early temporary structure, losing its exchange function when the extra-embryonic coelom extends into the mesoderm of the trilaminar yolk sac, separating the mesoderm into splanchnic and somatic layers. As these changes take place rapidly in cattle, sheep and pigs, this functional yolk sac placenta is of short duration. In dogs and cats, the choriovitelline placenta functions up to the 21st day of pregnancy, whereas in horses it functions up to the eighth week of pregnancy. The choriovitelline placenta does not establish an extensive and intimate contact with the endometrium.

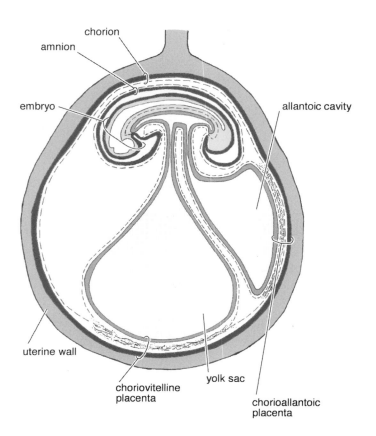

Figure 10.3 Components of a choriovitelline placenta and of a chorioallantoic placenta.

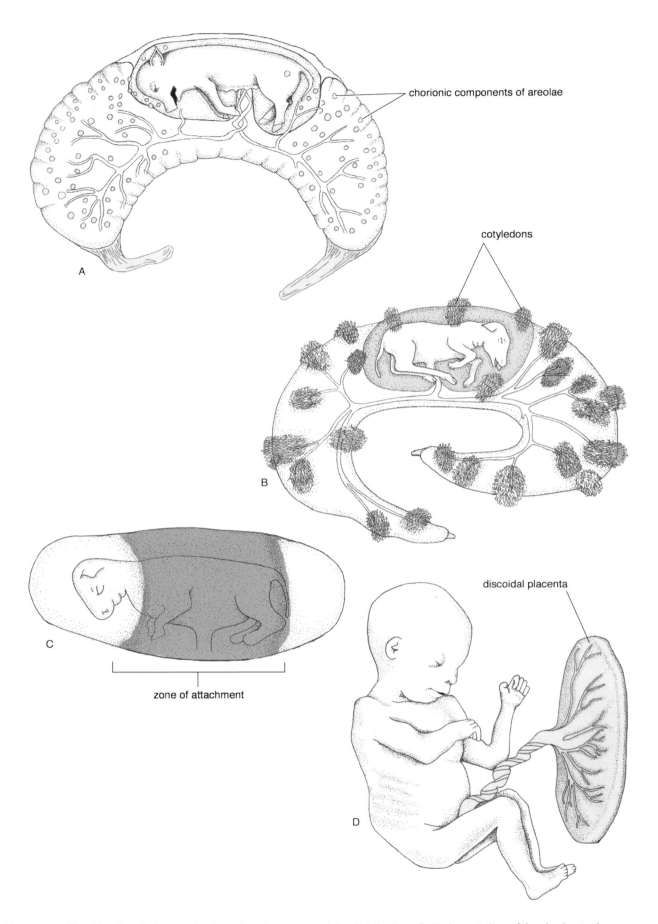

Figure 10.4 Classification of placentation based on the shape and the distribution of attachment sites of the chorion to the endometrium. A, Diffuse form of placentation which occurs in horses and pigs. B, Cotyledonary form of placentation which occurs in ruminants. C, Zonary form of placentation which occurs in carnivores. D, Discoidal form of placentation which occurs in humans, monkeys and rodents.

Chorioallantoic placenta

The embryonic component of a chorioallantoic placenta is formed by the attachment and fusion of the outer wall of the expanding allantoic sac with the adjacent chorion (Fig. 10.3). This is the definitive form of placentation which occurs in higher mammals and is characterised by an extensive area of contact between the embryonic placental component and the endometrium. Increased surface contact is achieved through folding of the chorioallantois and the endometrial surface, formation of chorionic villi and the establishment of chorionic labyrinths.

Classification of chorioallantoic placentation

Chorioallantoic placentae can be classified according to their shapes and the relationship of the extra-embryonic membranes to the endometrium. Formation of chorionic villi, their distribution on the surface of the chorionic sac and their relationship with the endometrium are used to define some placental characteristics. Placental morphology and areas of chorionic villous attachment can be described as diffuse, cotyledonary, zonary or discoidal. Diffuse placentation, which occurs in horses and pigs, is characterised by uniform distribution of villi on the outer surface of the chorion (Fig. 10.4A). In cotyledonary placentation, which occurs in ruminants, chorionic villi are restricted to defined areas referred to as cotyledons, which are distributed over the surface of the chorionic sac (Fig. 10.4B). Zonary placentation, which occurs in domestic carnivores, is characterised by chorionic villi which are confined to a girdle-like structure around the middle of the chorionic sac (Fig. 10.4C). In discoidal placentation, which occurs in humans, monkeys and rodents, villi are restricted to disc-shaped areas on the chorionic sac (Fig. 10.4D).

The degree of contact between foetal tissue and uterine mucosa varies and may involve merely the loose apposition of these two tissues, termed apposed placentation, or their intimate fusion, termed conjoined placentation. With an apposed placenta, there is no fusion of the maternal and foetal tissue, and separation is easily achieved at parturition without damage to maternal tissue. This form of placentation is termed non-deciduate. In conjoined placentation, an intimate connection is formed between maternal and embryonic tissue, and at birth, some maternal tissue is lost with the foetal tissue. This type of placentation is termed deciduate. The placentae of horses, ruminants and pigs are described as apposed and non-deciduate; in humans, dogs, cats and rodents, they are conjoined and deciduate.

Histological classification of placentation

Based on the number of tissue layers interposed between the foetal and maternal bloodstream, four basic types of placentation can be described. In the simplest form, maternal endothelium, maternal connective tissue, maternal uterine epithelium, foetal (chorionic) epithelium, foetal connective tissue and foetal endothelium separate the maternal blood and foetal blood. In the most complex form, the maternal layers are successively broken down until the chorionic epithelium (trophoblast) comes in direct contact with the maternal blood supply. By using the name of the maternal tissue which is contiguous with the chorion, the following types of placentation, based on histological features, can be described: epitheliochorial, synepitheliochorial, endotheliochorial and haemochorial (Fig. 10.5).

In epitheliochorial placentation, the endometrial epithelium remains intact and is apposed to the chorionic epithelium (Fig. 10.5A). This type of placentation occurs in horses, donkeys, pigs and whales.

The term 'syndesmochorial', which describes removal of uterine epithelium leaving the chorion in contact with maternal connective tissue, was formerly used to describe the histological form of placentation in ruminants. Electron microscope studies, however, have demonstrated that an attenuated layer of combined maternal and foetal epithelium persists in ruminant placentae. Consequently, the term 'syndesmochorial' has been replaced by the term 'synepitheliochorial' (Fig. 10.5B). The prefix 'syn' implies a union of foetal and maternal cells in the cryptal epithelium. The term 'syndesmochorial' is an inappropriate description of ruminant placentation.

In endotheliochorial placentation, the uterine epithelium and connective tissue are removed and the chorionic epithelium comes in direct contact with the endometrial capillaries (Fig. 10.5C). Placentae of this type are found in dogs, cats and elephants.

With haemochorial placentation, the maternal endothelium is removed and chorionic epithelium comes in direct contact with maternal blood (Fig. 10.5D). This type of placentation is found in some rodents and in higher primates.

A current classification of placentation, based on histological criteria, is presented in Table 10.2. Placental classification, based on the number of tissue layers interposed between the foetal and maternal circulations, does not relate directly to the functional efficiency of placentae.

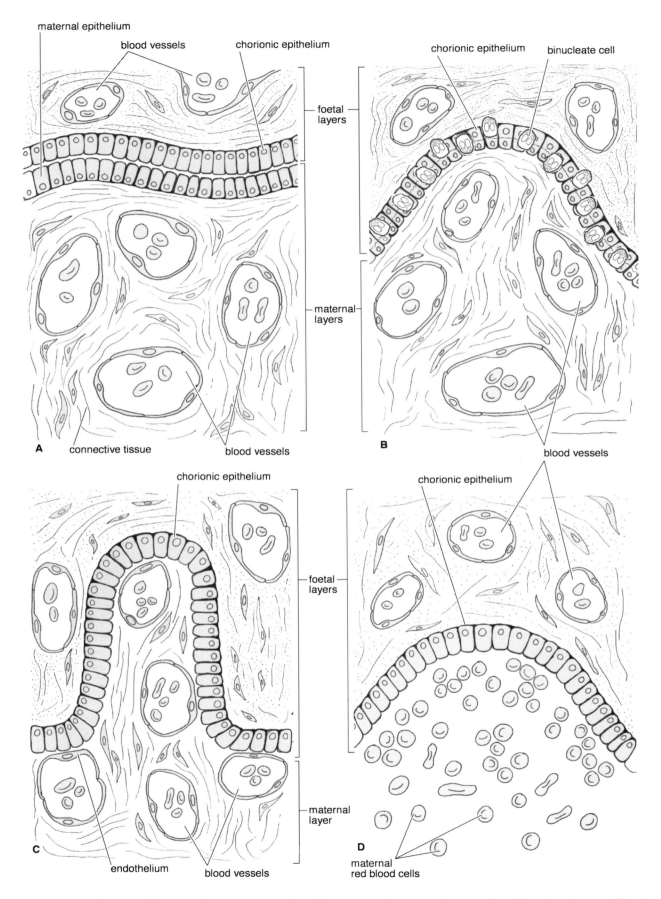

Figure 10.5 Classification of placentae based on the number of tissue layers interposed between foetal blood and maternal blood. A, Epitheliochorial. B, Synepitheliochorial. C, Endotheliochorial. D, Haemochorial.

Table 10.2 Description and histological classification of placentae of domestic animals and humans. The foetal layers are listed in accordance with their position relative to the maternal circulation.

| Species | Type of placentation | Placental layers | | | | | |
| | | Maternal layers | | | Foetal layers | | |
		Endothelium	Connective tissue	Epithelium	Epithelium	Connective tissue	Endothelium
Pigs	Epitheliochorial	Present	Present	Present	Present	Present	Present
Horses	Epitheliochorial	Present	Present	Present	Present	Present	Present
Cattle	Synepitheliochorial	Present	Present	Present[a]	Present	Present	Present
Sheep	Synepitheliochorial	Present	Present	Present[a]	Present	Present	Present
Goats	Synepitheliochorial	Present	Present	Present[a]	Present	Present	Present
Dogs	Endotheliochorial	Present	Absent	Absent	Present	Present	Present
Cats	Endotheliochorial	Present	Absent	Absent	Present	Present	Present
Humans	Haemochorial	Absent	Absent	Absent	Present	Present	Present

[a] combined maternal and foetal epithelium.

Placental haemophagous organs

Localised accumulations of maternal blood occur between the chorion and endometrium in the placentae of carnivores and ungulates. These areas are referred to by various names including haematomata, haemophagous organs, green border and brown border. These blood-filled spaces are considered to be a source of iron for the foetus. Despite the extensive use of the term 'haematoma' in the literature relating to these structures, it is an inappropriate description as it more correctly describes a pathological accumulation of extravasated blood. The folded columnar epithelium of the trophoblast, which is in direct contact with the accumulated blood, possesses microvilli which enhance uptake of red blood cells and other nutrients. It is reported that these columnar cells engulf maternal red blood cells which are utilised as a source of iron by the developing embryo. The breakdown products of haemoglobin account for the green and brown coloration of canine and feline haemophagous organs, respectively. The relative prominence and gross appearance of placental haemophagous organs show species variation.

Haemotrophe and histotrophe

The nutritional material supplied to the embryo from the circulating maternal blood is referred to as haemotrophe. Products absorbed by the embryo from the endometrium are known as histotrophe.

Implantation and placentation in pigs

Porcine embryos enter the uterus at the 4-cell to 8-cell stage 48 hours after ovulation. They remain near the tip of the uterine horn until about day six, after which they are moved to their sites of implantation. Intra-uterine migration may continue until the 11th day. During the pre-implantation period, the blastocyst changes from a spherical structure 0.5–2 mm in diameter on the ninth day, to an ovoid sac 5 cm long with a distinct embryonic disc evident by the 11th day. By day 13, the blastocyst is an elongated filamentous structure up to 100 cm in length (Fig. 10.6). Because elongation of blastocysts is not synchronous, both spherical and elongated blastocysts may be found at the same stage of pregnancy. Irrespective of their length, blastocysts become regularly spaced in the uterine horns (Fig. 10.7). Elongation of blastocysts is due to cellular reorganisation and remodelling of trophoblastic cells rather than hyperplasia, with minimal change in the size of the embryonic disc during this period. Changes in the blastocyst are attributed to growth factors released by the conceptus and uterine tissue. Endoderm from the primitive streak lines the trophoblastic cavity forming a bilaminar yolk sac. Mesoderm derived from the primitive streak occupies a position between the two layers and forms a trilaminar yolk sac, the embryonic component of a short-lived choriovitelline placenta. The extra-embryonic coelom expands rapidly into the trilaminar yolk sac and separates the endoderm from the trophoblast, thereby terminating the function of the choriovitelline

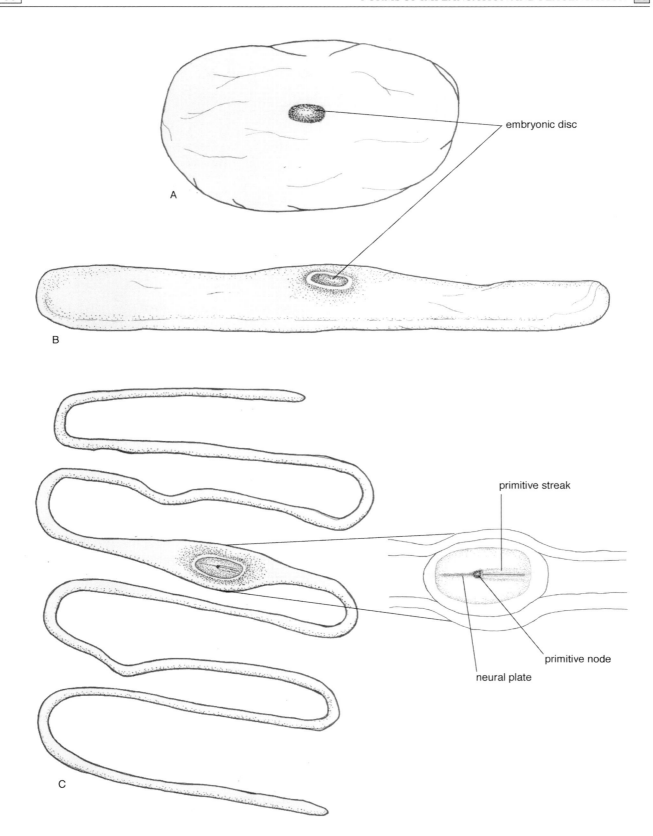

Figure 10.6 Morphological changes in the porcine blastocyst showing the marked elongation which occurs between the ninth and thirteenth days of gestation. Enlarged view of the disc shows the primitive streak, primitive node and neural plate.

Figure 10.7 Spacing of porcine blastocysts, A, and spacing of developing embryos enclosed in extra-embryonic membranes, B, within the uterus.

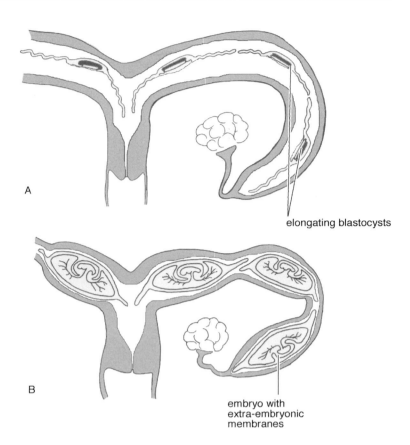

elongating blastocysts

A

B

embryo with extra-embryonic membranes

placenta. Amniotic folds develop at about the 12th day and fuse by the 16th day, forming the inner amniotic and outer chorionic sacs. On the 15th day, the allantoic sac forms as an outgrowth of the hindgut and expands into the extra-embryonic coelom. By the 30th day, the allantois becomes anchor-shaped and expands towards both extremities of the chorionic sac (Fig. 10.8). The allantois, which vascularises the chorion, does not expand to the tips of the chorionic sac and consequently the tips remain avascular. Shortly afterwards, the avascular ends of the chorionic sac become necrotic, a feature characteristic of porcine extra-embryonic membranes (Fig. 10.9). The necrotic tips of chorionic sacs of adjacent embryos form an avascular zone which prevents inter-embryonic vascular anastomosis.

Implantation, which is centric, is a gradual process beginning around the 12th day. The elongated blastocyst exhibits a slight dilatation in the region of the embryonic disc which ensures close apposition and adhesion of the trophoblast to the endometrium. As the extra-embryonic sacs expand and fill with fluid, the area of contact between maternal and embryonic tissue increases. Firm attachment is observed by the 18th day, with interdigitation of microvilli between embryonic and maternal epithelium. As most of the chorionic sac is apposed to the endometrium, this form of placentation is termed diffuse.

Maternal recognition of pregnancy in pigs

During the oestrous cycle, endocrine secretion of $PGF_{2\alpha}$ by the uterus exerts a luteolytic effect. By the 12th day of pregnancy, oestrogens, produced by the blastocyst, prevent the release of luteolytic quantities of $PGF_{2\alpha}$. In these circumstances, $PGF_{2\alpha}$ is secreted into the uterine lumen but is unable to exert its luteolytic effect. In the absence of the luteolytic effect of $PGF_{2\alpha}$, the corpus luteum persists. It is possible that the oestrogens also have a direct luteotrophic effect on the corpus luteum. Thus, oestrogen produced by the blastocyst is a key factor for the continuation of pregnancy. At least four embryos, two in each horn, are required to produce a sufficient level of oestrogen for the avoidance of luteolysis.

Porcine choriovitelline placenta

In the sow the choriovitelline placenta is a transient structure. The yolk sac reaches its maximum development by day 18 and regresses rapidly.

Porcine chorioallantoic placenta

In the sow, the chorioallantoic placenta is diffuse, non-deciduate and epitheliochorial. By the 13th day of development, the chorionic epithelium becomes apposed

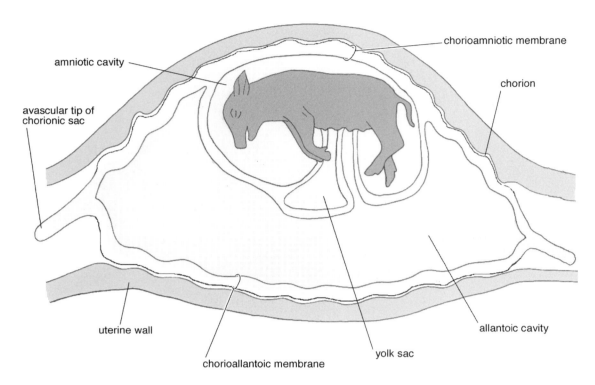

amniotic cavity

chorioamniotic membrane

avascular tip of
chorionic sac

chorion

uterine wall

chorioallantoic membrane

yolk sac

allantoic cavity

Figure 10.8 Arrangement of porcine foetal membranes *in utero* at day 30 of gestation showing anchor-shaped allantois and avascular tips of the chorionic sac.

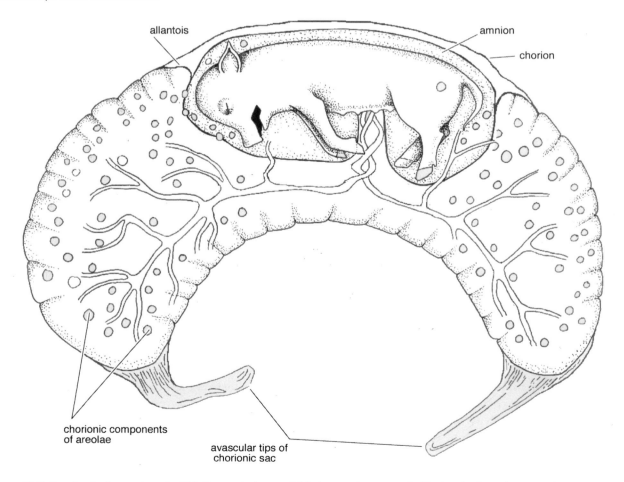

allantois

amnion

chorion

chorionic components
of areolae

avascular tips of
chorionic sac

Figure 10.9 Porcine foetus enclosed within its amniotic sac which, in turn, is surrounded by its chorion. The avascular tips of the chorion and the chorionic portions of areolae are shown.

to the uterine mucosa, and follows the folding of the maternal epithelium. Adhesion gradually occurs between the maternal and foetal epithelium with the formation of microvilli resulting in an interdigitation of both tissues. This process, which is well advanced by the 18th day, is completed by the 24th day. Around the 17th day, areas of the trophoblast overlying the openings of the uterine glands, which do not become attached to the uterine mucosa, form elevations usually less than 3 mm in diameter, known as areolae (Figs. 10.9 and 10.10). The chorion of the domes of the areolae is folded and lined with tall columnar epithelium, and projects into the areolar cavity containing the secretions of the uterine glands. The chorionic epithelium of the areolae absorbs secretions and has a special role in iron transportation. As pregnancy proceeds, the apposing surfaces of the placenta form primary and secondary interdigitating folds, which together with the microvilli hold the two surfaces in close contact.

Throughout gestation, the endometrium is lined by dark-staining, simple cuboidal epithelium, with spherical nuclei containing small nucleoli. During the first half of pregnancy, the epithelium of the chorioallantois is of a simple columnar type. About mid-gestation, the epithelium of the chorioallantois over the summits of the maternal folds becomes converted into tall columnar cells. Foetal capillaries often push deeply into the cuboidal epithelium of the trophoblast and are referred to as intra-epithelial capillaries. The capillaries, however, do not come into direct contact with the maternal epithelium but remain separated from it by a thin layer of the flattened foetal epithelium.

Implantation and placentation in cattle and sheep

In cattle and sheep, the zygote at the 8-cell stage enters the uterus on the third or fourth day post-ovulation. By the sixth day in sheep and the eighth day in cattle, the blastocyst has formed and emerges from its zona pellucida. In sheep the blastocyst, which has a spherical shape, is 1 mm in diameter. It elongates to 100 mm by the 14th day of gestation. The bovine blastocyst elongates from approximately 2 mm on the 12th day to 100 mm by the 16th day. During this period of elongation, the embryonic disc, which is approximately 0.3 mm × 0.2 mm on the 14th day, undergoes little development. The elongating blastocyst extends into the non-pregnant horn on the 14th day in sheep and on the 18th day in cattle. By the 22nd day, the bovine blastocyst extends to the tip of the contralateral horn (Fig. 10.11). In sheep, the allantois commences to grow into the extra-embryonic coelom on the 16th day and the amniotic folds fuse on the 17th day. In cattle, the amniotic folds fuse on the 18th day and the allantois is evident by the 19th day. At this stage in cattle and sheep, the allantois becomes anchor-shaped and extends to the tips of the chorionic sac (Fig. 10.12). As the tips of adjacent chorionic sacs overlap, vascular anastomosis between adjoining extra-embryonic membranes occurs in 90% of bovine twins. In sheep, the incidence of comparable vascular anastomoses is low.

Maternal recognition of pregnancy in ruminants

In ruminants, the factors responsible for the maternal recognition of pregnancy, which extend the functional life of the corpus luteum, exert their effect prior to the commencement of implantation. Removal of the ovine blastocyst from the uterus up to the 12th day of pregnancy does not alter the length of the oestrous cycle. After this time, the life of the corpus luteum is extended whether or not the blastocyst is removed. As the bovine blastocyst does not appear to influence survival of the corpus luteum up to the 15th day of pregnancy, removal of the conceptus before this time does not extend the functional life of the corpus luteum. The bovine conceptus produces a trophoblastic protein, bovine interferon-tau (bIFN-τ), between the 16th and 24th days of pregnancy, which acts on endometrial cells, inhibiting the production of oxytocin receptors. As oxytocin receptors are not expressed on endometrial cells, oxytocin secreted by the corpus luteum and/or neurohypophysis cannot stimulate $PGF_{2\alpha}$ synthesis by the endometrium. In the absence of $PGF_{2\alpha}$ the corpus luteum persists. The ovine conceptus also secretes a protein, ovine interferon-tau (oIFN-τ) between the 12th and 16th days of pregnancy, which inhibits the secretion of $PGF_{2\alpha}$ by the endometrium, thereby preventing luteolysis. An interferon with similar biological activity is secreted by the caprine blastocyst between the 16th and 21st days of pregnancy.

Choriovitelline placenta in ruminants

In cattle and sheep, the yolk sac forms a choriovitelline placenta for a few days until it is replaced by the chorioallantoic placenta.

Chorioallantoic placenta in ruminants

The chorioallantoic placenta of cattle and sheep is cotyledonary, non-deciduate and synepitheliochorial. The endometrium of cattle and sheep is composed of caruncles and inter-caruncular areas. The caruncles of non-pregnant cattle are small, raised, non-glandular areas approximately 0.5–1 cm in diameter. During the oestrous cycle, they become more prominent and in pregnancy they reach a diameter of up to 10 cm. The number of caruncles ranges from 80 to 140 in cows and 80 to 100 in ewes. Bovine caruncles have a convex surface with a distinct stalk, whereas ovine caruncles are

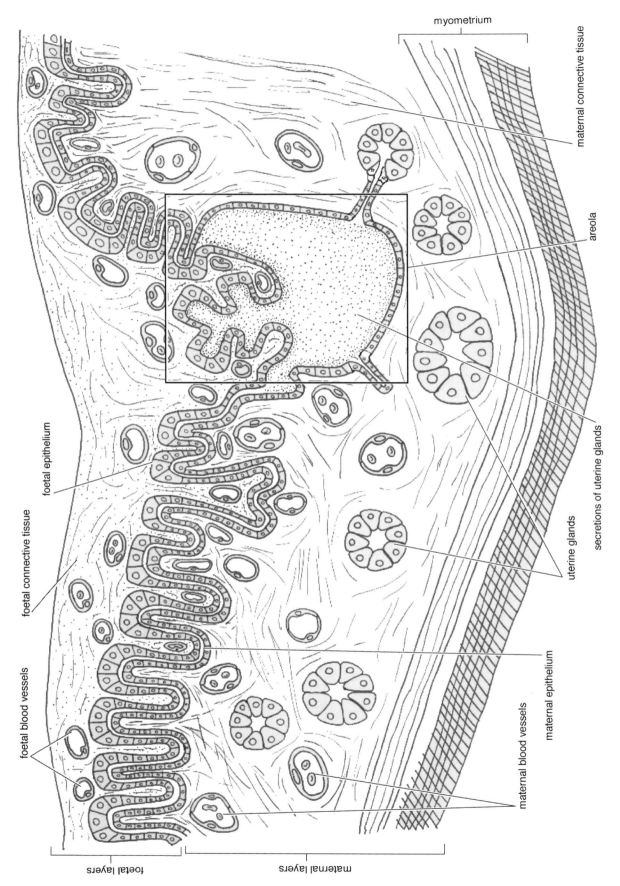

Figure 10.10 Microscopic appearance of porcine chorioallantoic placenta close to mid-gestation illustrating the apposition of folded foetal and maternal epithelium and an areola.

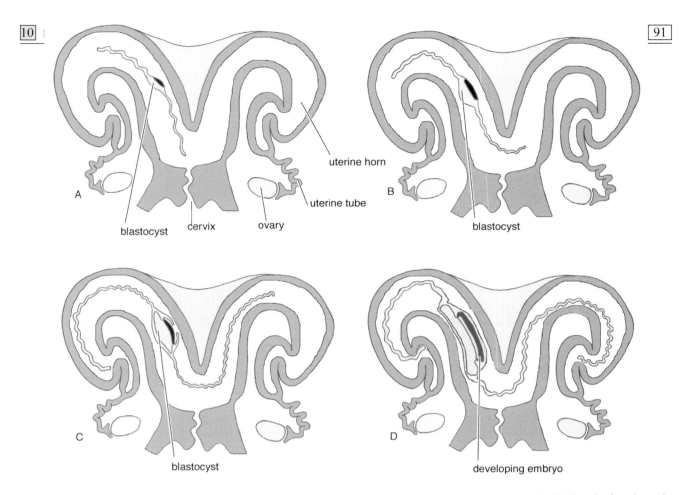

A

uterine horn

uterine tube

blastocyst   cervix   ovary

B

blastocyst

C

blastocyst

D

developing embryo

Figure 10.11 Sequential changes in the developing bovine blastocyst and its location in the uterus from the third to the fourth week of gestation, showing the marked elongation of the blastocyst and its extension into the non-pregnant horn.

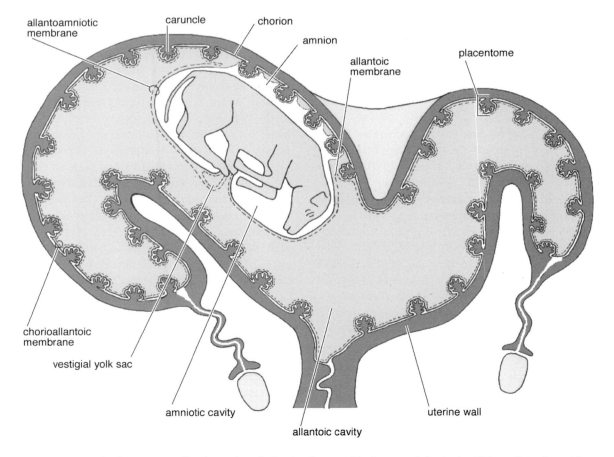

allantoamniotic membrane

caruncle

chorion

amnion

allantoic membrane

placentome

chorioallantoic membrane

vestigial yolk sac

amniotic cavity

allantoic cavity

uterine wall

Figure 10.12 Late stage in the process of implantation of a bovine foetus with clusters of chorionic villi interdigitating with maternal caruncles, forming placentomes.

concave with broad attachments. The bovine chorion becomes apposed to the endometrium around the 17th day of gestation. Adhesive contact occurs by the 18th day with the proliferation of trophoblastic papillae which penetrate the openings of uterine glands. These papillae appear first in the area close to the embryonic disc. However, around the 30th day in sheep, and 36th day in cattle, villous processes develop on the chorioallantoic membrane apposed to the caruncles (Fig. 10.12). Aggregations of these villi, referred to as cotyledons, fit into crypts in the caruncles analogous to fingers fitting into a glove. The combined cotyledon and caruncle form a specialised physiological unit known as a placentome (Fig. 10.13). As gestation proceeds, the primary villous processes form secondary and tertiary villi, which fit into corresponding crypts in caruncles. Chorioallantoic villi consist of vascular allantoic mesenchyme covered by a simple layer of epithelium composed of two cell types, columnar cells with rounded or irregularly shaped nuclei with large nucleoli, and binucleate cells. Binucleate giant cells, a characteristic of ruminant placentae, are formed from trophoblastic cells when their nuclei undergo mitotic division without accompanying cytoplasmic division. Epithelial cells of the maternal crypts are cuboidal with spherical nuclei and distinct nucleoli. Among the cuboidal cryptal cells, binucleate cells of trophoblastic origin are present. Interdigitation of microvilli occurs between the trophoblastic and cryptal cells, increasing the extent of foetal–maternal contact. Ovine cryptal cells lose their distinct cellular appearance forming a syncytium of maternal cells and binucleate trophoblastic cells.

Binucleate cells first appear in the trophoblast during the third week of pregnancy in cattle, sheep and goats. These cells constitute up to one-fifth of the total trophoblastic cell population beyond mid-pregnancy; subsequently their numbers decrease. Binucleate cells migrate through microvillar junctions and fuse with the maternal cryptal cells forming a syncytium (Fig. 10.14). In cattle, migration of binucleate cells to the cryptal maternal epithelium ceases around the 40th day of gestation, whereas, in sheep, migration continues throughout pregnancy. The binucleate cells release granules by exocytosis into the maternal connective tissue. Their function may include the transfer of complex molecules from foetal to maternal tissue. Binucleate cells in cattle and sheep have been shown to contain placental lactogens. In early pregnancy, binucleate cells synthesise substantial amounts of protein including pregnancy-associated glycoproteins and pregnancy-specific protein B. The presence of these proteins, which first appear in maternal serum by the 28th day of pregnancy, may be used as a confirmatory test for pregnancy.

In the inter-caruncular areas of bovine and ovine uterine tissue, the intact chorion and maternal epithelium are in intimate contact except for areas associated with the openings of uterine glands. The foetal–maternal attachment in the inter-caruncular areas resembles that found in the diffuse porcine placenta.

Following parturition, the chorionic villi are withdrawn from the crypts. Separation occurs at the interdigitation of the microvilli, and the foetal and maternal epithelia remain intact. When the foetal villi separate from the maternal crypts, expulsion of the foetal membranes occurs. Failure of this separation results in the retention of the foetal membranes, a common complication of parturition in cattle. Factors contributing to retention of bovine foetal membranes include dystocia, uterine inertia and metritis.

Implantation and placentation in horses

The equine zygote enters the uterus at the morula stage between the fifth and sixth day after ovulation. A unique feature of reproduction in the mare is that only fertilised ova enter the uterus; unfertilised ova are retained in the uterine tubes. A possible mechanism whereby the developing embryo enters the uterus relates to secretion of appreciable quantities of prostaglandin E_2 by the morula, which acts locally, relaxing the circular muscle of the uterine tube thereby facilitating its entry into the uterus. By the sixth day, the blastocyst becomes enclosed by a thin acellular membrane or capsule of trophoblastic origin composed of glycoprotein molecules. At the eighth day, the blastocyst is approximately 0.5 mm in diameter and the zona pellucida is lost. The capsule, which expands with the blastocyst, persists up to the 20th day of gestation and may prevent attachment of the blastocyst to the endometrium during the period of intra-uterine migration. The equine blastocyst, unlike that of ruminants and pigs, remains almost spherical until the time of implantation. Studies utilising ultrasonography demonstrate that the equine conceptus moves from one uterine horn to the other at least once per day, between the 11th and 15th days. At approximately the 17th day of gestation, the conceptus becomes apposed to the endometrium in one of the uterine horns, close to the body of the uterus. The shape of the conceptus changes from a spherical structure at day 11 to an oblong structure at day 17, as observed by ultrasonography. Between days 18 and 21, the conceptus assumes a triangular shape and between days 24 and 48 it has an irregular appearance. From the 56th day, the extra-embryonic membranes have expanded into the uterine body, and into the non-pregnant horn by the 77th day. The embryo itself can be detected by ultrasonography by the 21st day of gestation. The amniotic folds, which form

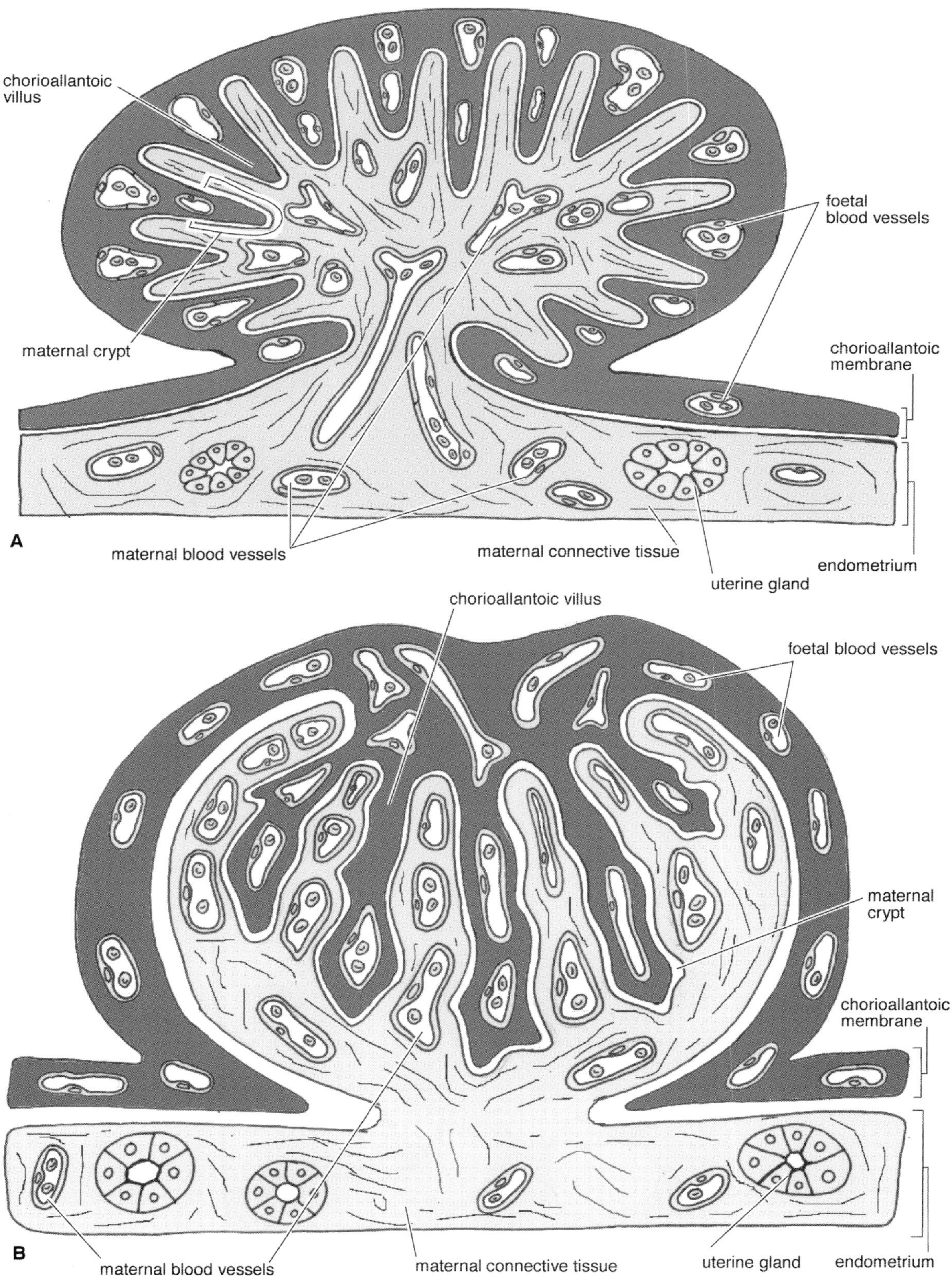

Figure 10.13 Section through a bovine placentome, A, and ovine placentome, B, illustrating distinguishing features of these two specialised structures involved in maternal–foetal exchange. The bovine placentome is convex, whereas the ovine placentome is concave.

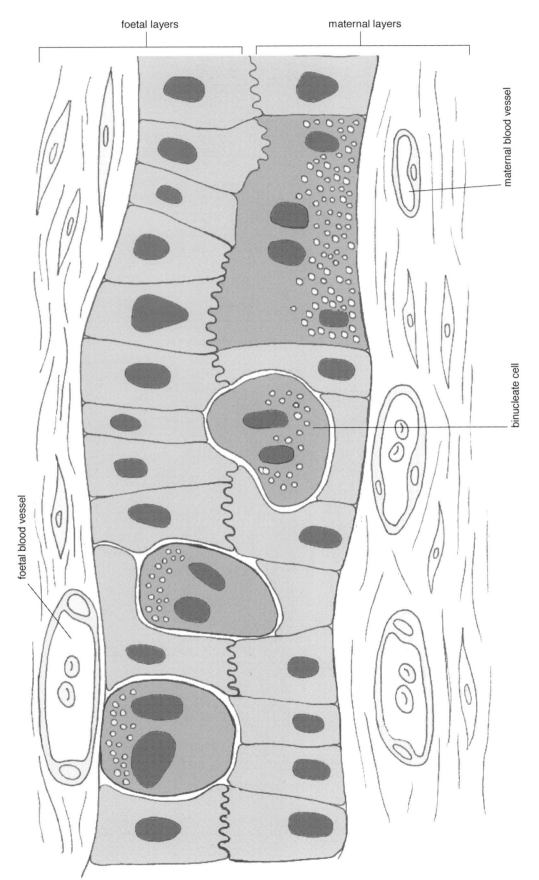

Figure 10.14 Microscopic appearance of bovine foetal–maternal placental interface illustrating the migration of binucleate foetal cells into uterine epithelium.

around the 16th day, fuse by the 20th day. The allantois extends into the extra-embryonic coelom by the 21st day, and by the 28th day it becomes interposed between the chorion and the amnion. By the 42nd day the allantois begins to partially surround the yolk sac. Formation of foetal fluids, close to the time of foetal membrane development, causes the membranes to expand and establish contact with the uterine wall. Hippomanes up to 3–4 cm in diameter may be observed in the allantoic fluid after the 60th day of gestation.

Maternal recognition of pregnancy in horses

The critical period for maternal recognition of pregnancy is from the 14th to 16th days post-ovulation. Although the exact mechanism for the maintenance of pregnancy is not clearly defined, it is suggested that the conceptus secretes factors which exert their effect locally, thereby inhibiting endometrial release of prostaglandin. Intra-uterine migration of the equine conceptus may enhance the local distribution of these inhibiting factors.

Equine choriovitelline placenta

A functional choriovitelline placenta which develops during the second week of pregnancy persists up to the eighth week. The vascular yolk sac has a well defined terminal sinus. During the fourth week, the allantois is in contact with the chorion and the chorioallantoic placenta begins to develop. The chorioallantoic placenta and the choriovitelline placenta co-exist for approximately four weeks and, subsequently, the functional role of the choriovitelline placenta ceases (Fig. 10.15).

Equine chorioallantoic placenta

The chorioallantoic membrane is apposed to the endometrium by the 17th day of gestation. The area of attachment is at first confined to a girdle of chorionic villi adjacent to the yolk sac. This discrete white annular band, referred to as the chorionic girdle, occupies a position at the boundary of the chorioallantois and the trilaminar yolk sac, a position it continues to occupy until the 40th day of gestation (Fig. 10.15). Around the 25th day, the width of the girdle is approximately 1 mm, at 27 days it is approximately 3 mm, and at 34 days it is approximately 7 mm. By 40 days, it is diffuse and fragmented. At first the chorionic epithelium is in contact with the uterine epithelium only in the region of the chorionic girdle. Later, when the allantois fuses with the chorion forming the chorioallantoic membrane, the area of attachment remote from the girdle increases until the entire chorioallantoic membrane becomes attached to the endometrium. The attachment at first is in the form of a simple diffuse apposition of foetal and

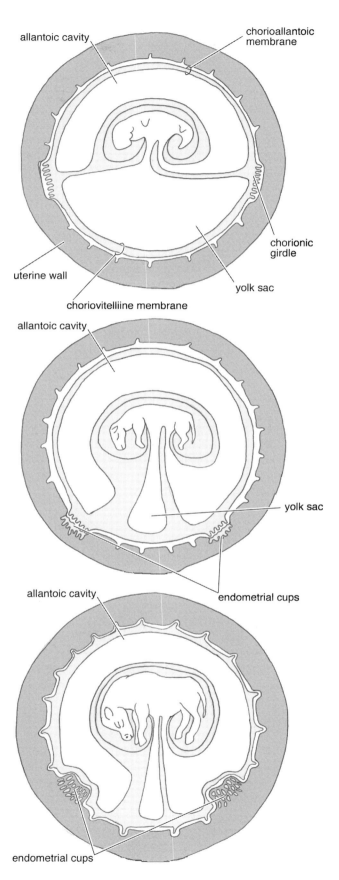

Figure 10.15 Changes in the arrangement of equine foetal membranes from the 30th to the 70th days of gestation and the development of endometrial cups.

maternal tissue similar to that in pigs. Between the seventh and eighth weeks of gestation, villi develop on the chorioallantoic membrane which fit into crypts in the endometrium. The changes which occur in equine foetal membranes from the 30th to the 70th days of gestation are illustrated in Fig. 10.15. Initially, the villi have a simple structure. Later, secondary and tertiary villi are formed from the primary villi up to the fourth month of pregnancy. The villi and their corresponding crypts form microscopic inverted dome-like structures referred to as microcotyledons (Fig. 10.16). The villi consist of an outer layer of simple columnar epithelium with a core of vascular mesoderm. The maternal crypts are lined by simple cuboidal epithelium. Microvillous interdigitations occur between the foetal and maternal epithelial layers. The ducts of uterine glands present in the stroma between adjacent microcotyledons open on to the surface of inter-microcotyledonary areas. The trophoblast located over openings of uterine glands is comparable in function and structure to areolae in pigs.

Endometrial cups

A distinguishing feature of equine placentation is the formation of ulcer-like structures termed endometrial cups, which develop in the endometrium in the region of the chorionic girdle. These cups, which develop at approximately the 35th day of gestation and reach diameters from 2 mm to 5 cm, atrophy around the 120th day (Figs. 10.15 and 10.17A).

Close to the 35th day of gestation, columnar epithelial cells of the chorionic girdle penetrate and destroy the endometrial epithelium. After they migrate through the basement membrane into the endometrial stroma, these cells lose their migratory ability and develop into large epithelioid cells referred to as endometrial cup cells (Fig. 10.17B). These cells, which are polyhedral in shape with pale-staining foamy cytoplasm, are up to 100 μm in their cross-sectional dimensions. Their nuclei are ovoid with prominent nucleoli. Many of these cells are binucleate. Endometrial cups, which are first macroscopically evident at about the 40th day, appear as discrete, pale, slightly raised plaques in the endometrium. The cups continue to enlarge and become crater-like due to continuing growth at their periphery with accompanying central necrosis. After the 80th day, the endometrial cup cells become increasingly pale and necrotic. Hypertrophied endometrial glands discharge their copious secretion into the crater-like depressions of endometrial cups, which are covered by the chorioallantoic membrane. Endometrial cup cells have been shown by *in vitro* and *in vivo* experiments to be the principal source of equine chorionic gonadotrophin (eCG), formerly known as pregnant mare serum gonadotrophin (PMSG).

The concentration of eCG in maternal serum rises rapidly from the 40th day of gestation reaching a level of 40–200 i.u./ml between the 50th and 70th days. Thereafter, levels decline steadily and become undetectable by the 120th day of gestation. The presence of eCG in the serum of mares during this period forms the basis of a pregnancy test.

As endometrial cup cells are of foetal origin, they are foreign to the mare and, accordingly, induce a maternal immunological response which results in lymphocytic infiltration of the uterine stroma (Fig. 10.17B). Invasion by cytotoxic T lymphocytes which destroy endometrial cup cells, together with the production of antibodies directed against paternal antigens on the cup cells, correlates with the cessation of eCG secretion around the 120th day of gestation. Once endometrial cups are formed, subsequent termination of pregnancy, either surgically or as a consequence of abortion, does not alter the continued development and subsequent regression of endometrial cups. Mares in which pregnancy has been terminated during the time when endometrial cups are present do not revert to oestrus until the cups have regressed and eCG levels have disappeared. Even after termination of pregnancy, the continued secretion of eCG by endometrial cup cells can give a positive reaction in a pregnancy diagnostic test based on detection of eCG in the serum.

Foetal genotype is reported to exert a profound effect on endometrial cup development and on the duration and level of eCG secretion. Among the *Equidae*, the offspring of inter-species breeding show considerable variation in the serum output of eCG. In donkeys, the endometrial cups are smaller and the eCG levels lower than those found in horses. In a mare carrying a mule foal, the cups are small and degenerate by the 80th day, and the eCG levels are approximately one-tenth of that normally found in a mare carrying an intra-species offspring. In donkeys carrying hinny foals, the cups are similar in size and duration to those in mares, as are the eCG levels.

Implantation and placentation in dogs and cats

During the luteal stage of the oestrous cycle, the uterine mucosa of dogs and cats becomes extensively folded with hypertrophy of the superficial and deep uterine glands. At this stage, canine and feline uterine mucosa can be histologically divided into two zones, a superficial compact zone and a deep spongy zone. The superficial zone is composed of many glands and ducts, whereas, in the deeper zone, glands are more sparsely distributed.

In dogs and cats, the developing embryo reaches the uterus at the 16-cell to 32-cell stage, between the sixth

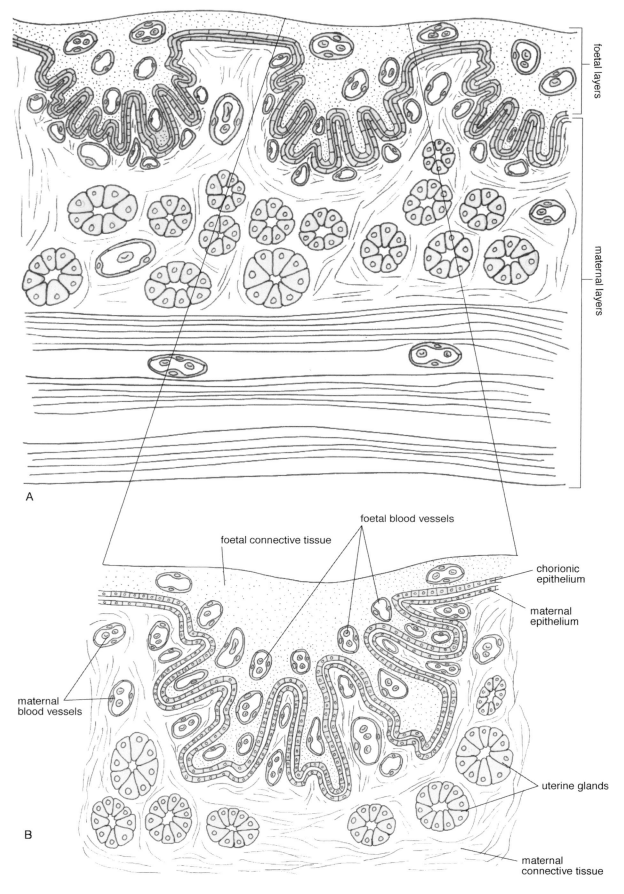

Figure 10.16 Microscopic appearance of equine foetal–maternal placental interface at mid-pregnancy showing microcotyledons, A. Details of an individual microcotyledon are also shown, B.

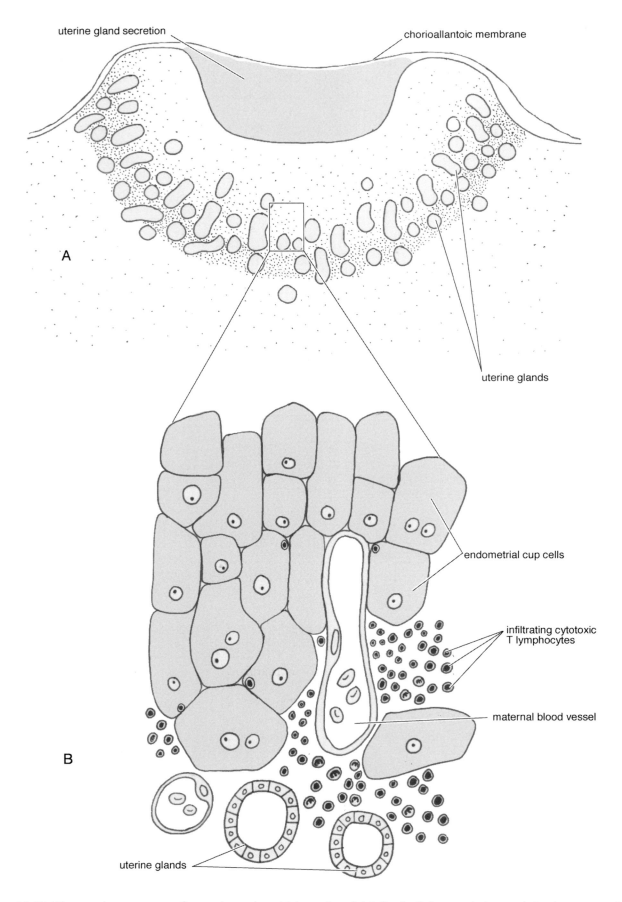

Figure 10.17 Microscopic appearance of an equine endometrial cup, A, and details of cellular morphology and structures present, B.

and seventh days after ovulation. Blastocysts remain free in the uterine horns for up to 13 days and may reach a diameter of 2.6 mm prior to implantation. Before implantation, intra-uterine migration, which allows for appropriate spacing of embryos within the uterine horns, may occur. Endoderm lines the trophoblast in the early blastocyst stage forming a bilaminar yolk sac, which subsequently becomes a trilaminar yolk sac with the migration of mesoderm between the endoderm and the trophoblast. The amniotic folds fuse around the 15th day and the allantois gradually expands into the extra-embryonic coelom.

Maternal recognition of pregnancy in dogs and cats

Unlike other domestic animals, the duration of the functional corpus luteum in dogs and cats is of similar length in pregnant and non-pregnant animals. Accordingly, in bitches and queens, signalling from the blastocyst does not appear to be a requirement for the maintenance of pregnancy.

Choriovitelline placentae in dogs and cats

A trilaminar yolk sac forms in both dogs and cats before the blastocyst becomes anchored to the uterine mucosa. The choriovitelline placenta formed by the apposition of uterine and foetal tissue is established by the 13th day of gestation in cats and by the 14th day in dogs. Breakdown of the trilaminar yolk sac by the expanding extra-embryonic coelom allows the expanding allantois to fuse with the chorion and form a chorioallantoic placenta, which co-exists with the choriovitelline placenta. During the fourth week of gestation, the role of the choriovitelline placenta as an organ of respiratory and nutritional exchange ceases. However, the yolk sac continues to be an important site of erythropoiesis until late in gestation. Remnants of the yolk sac are present until birth. Although the presence of implanted blastocysts is detectable by a number of diagnostic procedures by the 13th day in cats and the 15th day in dogs, developing blastocysts are not palpable until after 20 days. Initially, the choriovitelline placenta consists of trophoblastic villi which erode the uterine epithelium and invade the stroma. At this stage, foetal villi are poorly vascularised.

Chorioallantoic placentae in dogs and cats

The chorioallantoic placenta of the bitch and queen is zonary, deciduate and endotheliochorial. The allantois, which expands into the extra-embryonic coelom by the 15th day of gestation, surrounds the amnion and fuses with the chorion on the 18th day in cats and the 20th day in dogs (Fig. 10.18A). Chorioallantoic villi invade the endometrium with many of the villi projecting into openings of uterine glands. Uterine tissue response to

the presence of the trophoblastic villi is characterised by proliferation and enlargement of cells and by vasodilation. As the cells of the invaded uterine epithelium lose their outlines, they form a homogeneous mass of protoplasm with fragmented nuclei. This amorphous material is referred to as symplasma. During its advance into the maternal tissue, the trophoblast destroys not only the surface epithelium and glandular epithelium but also the sub-epithelial stroma. Apart from some blood vessels at the periphery of the zone of attachment, the maternal blood vessels remain intact and become completely surrounded by trophoblastic cells. However, vascular damage at the periphery of the zone of attachment leads to accumulation of maternal blood between the chorion and the endometrium. Although the chorionic sac expands beyond the zonary area of villous attachment and penetration, it does not invade the uterine mucosa. Accordingly, the invasive placental area remains as a girdle-like band around the middle of the chorionic sac. Four distinct zones are present in a cross-section through the uterus of domestic carnivores at the zonary area of attachment: placental labyrinth, junctional zone, glandular or spongy zone and myometrium (Fig. 10.18B). By mid-pregnancy, the labyrinth is comparatively thick and comprises two-thirds of the depth of the zonary area. The trophoblast covering the surface of the villi consists of two layers. The lightly staining cellular layer, the cytotrophoblast, is located closest to the foetal stroma while the basophilic syncytiotrophoblast is located closest to the maternal tissue. The villous cores consist of allantochorial connective tissue with thin-walled foetal blood vessels. Between neighbouring syncytial layers, thick-walled maternal blood vessels and randomly distributed maternal deciduate cells with pale cytoplasm, large nuclei and prominent nucleoli are present. Deciduate cells of maternal origin are less obvious in dogs than in cats. The feline placental labyrinth consists of vertical villi enclosing maternal capillaries. In dogs, the villi of the placental labyrinth are extensively branched and have a lobular appearance.

The junctional zone consists of invading villous tips, maternal vessels, uterine gland secretions and maternal cell debris. Trophoblastic cells in this zone absorb histotrophe. In dogs, there is a prominent layer of connective tissue interposed between the superficial and deep uterine glands which forms a well-defined boundary between the junctional zone and the deep spongy zone.

In the deep spongy zone, the uterine glands become greatly hypertrophied and have a sponge-like appearance. The lumina of the glands become dilated and filled with secretion and necrotic material sloughed from surface glandular cells. Although the connective tissue in this region is scanty, it is highly vascular. Towards the

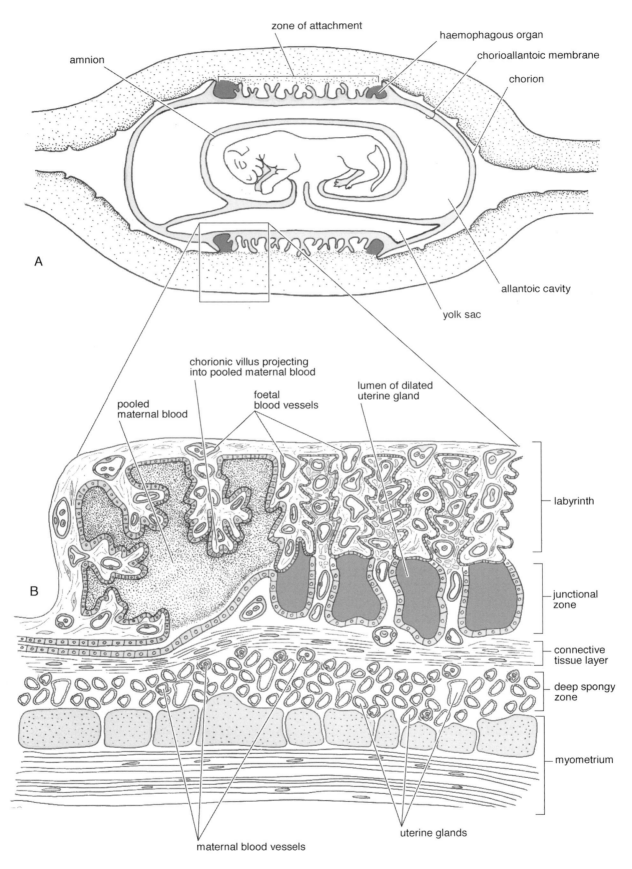

Figure 10.18 A, Arrangement of canine foetal membranes within the uterus illustrating the zonary nature of chorioallantoic attachment to the endometrium and the position of haemophagous organs at the borders of the zonary region. B, Microscopic appearance of a section through the border of the zonary region of attachment.

end of gestation, only the deep secretory portions of glands remain intact.

In dogs, haemophagous organs, which have a characteristic green appearance, are present along the margins of the zone of attachment. Smaller central haemophagous organs may also be present. In cats, haemophagous organs, which have a brown appearance, occur irregularly in the zonary area.

Functional aspects of the placenta

The placenta is an organ for physiological exchange between foetus and dam which acts as a selective barrier and as an endocrine organ. Its structure enables foetal nutrition, excretion and respiration to take place without permitting transfer of molecules of high molecular weight, particulate matter and blood cells. Transfer of molecules of low molecular weight across the placental barrier may be by simple diffusion, by facilitated diffusion or by active transport. Oxygen, carbon dioxide, water and electrolytes, which are essential for foetal life, readily cross the placental barrier by simple diffusion. More complex substances of nutritional importance such as glucose, amino acids, lipids and vitamins are actively transported. The placenta is permeable to many low molecular weight drugs. Some drugs which cross the placenta can cause serious developmental defects during the late embryonic or early foetal period. One such example, thalidomide, formerly administered as a mild sedative to pregnant women, can cause severe developmental limb defects in humans.

In some species such as humans, rabbits and guinea-pigs, and to a lesser extent, dogs and cats, antibodies are actively transported across the placenta. A number of viruses, pathogenic bacteria and protozoa may reach the embryo by various routes, sometimes causing breakdown of the placental barrier, and leading to congenital infection.

Red cell incompatibility between mother and foetus can result in haemolytic diseases in newborn animals. In humans, the disease occurs when Rhesus-positive foetal red blood cells inherited from the father sensitise a Rhesus-negative mother during birth. In subsequent pregnancies, when there is a Rhesus-positive foetus, antibodies produced by the mother can cross the placenta and bind to Rhesus-positive red cells in the foetal circulation resulting in red cell damage and haemolytic disease, evident at birth.

In horses, isoimmunisation can occur at the birth of the first foal when the foal's red blood cells, which are antigenically distinct from those of the mare, enter the maternal circulation. Foals born following second or subsequent pregnancies, with foetal red blood cell antigens inherited from the stallion which are absent from the mare's red blood cells, are at risk of acquiring isoimmune haemolytic anaemia. In horses, unlike humans, antibodies are not transferred *in utero* and foals are born without evidence of haemolytic disease. The antibodies, with specificity for red blood cells, are unable to cross the placental barrier but are present in high concentration in the colostrum. Haemolytic anaemia and jaundice develop in the foal following ingestion of colostral antibodies which are absorbed from the small intestine.

In addition to its role as an organ of physiological exchange, the placenta is an important source of endocrine secretions. To establish and maintain pregnancy, a synergistic equilibrium has to exist between maternal endocrine secretions and those of placental origin. The placenta produces oestrogen, progesterone and a variety of gonadotrophins. In cattle, pigs and rabbits, placental secretions may prolong the functioning of the corpus luteum, supplementing the luteotrophic effect of the maternal adenohypophysis. Removal of the ovaries is followed by abortion in these species. In some species, including humans, horses, sheep and cats, the ovaries may be removed at a certain stage of pregnancy without causing abortion as the placenta secretes sufficient progesterone to maintain pregnancy (Table 10.3).

Passive immunity refers to the transfer of antibodies from an actively immune animal to a susceptible animal. Without passive immunity, which occurs naturally when neonatal animals ingest colostrum, newborn animals would be susceptible to a wide range of respiratory and enteric pathogens. In some species, transfer of passive immunity from dam to offspring may occur *in utero* (Table 10.4). In other species, antibodies produced by the dam and secreted in colostrum passively protect newborn animals against infectious agents. Placental transfer of passive immunity occurs in humans and other primates, rabbits and guinea-pigs. Ingestion of colostral antibodies by the young of these species provides additional protection against enteric pathogens during the first weeks of life.

Table 10.3 Days of pregnancy in particular species after which ovaries can be removed without inducing abortion.

Species	Days of pregnancy
Cats	30
Horses	100
Humans	40 to 60
Sheep	50

Table 10.4 Transmission of passive immunity from dam to offspring.

Species	*In utero*	Colostrum
Horses	–	+++
Pigs	–	+++
Ruminants	–	+++
Dogs and cats	+	++
Mice	++	++
Rats	+	++
Humans	+++	+
Rabbits	+++	+
Guinea-pigs	+++	+
Birds	*In ovo*	–

–, no transmission; +++, maximum transmission.

As the placentae of a number of domestic animals are not permeable to immunoglobulins, foals, calves, lambs, piglets and kids are born agammaglobulinaemic and acquire passive immunity only through colostrum. Maternal antibodies secreted in colostrum are absorbed most effectively from the small intestine in the hours immediately after birth. As the ability to absorb intact immunoglobulin molecules from the small intestine is transitory and persists for less than 48 hours post-natally, early feeding of colostrum to newborn animals is essential to achieve optimal passive protection.

Although some passive transfer of immunoglobulins may occur *in utero* in domestic carnivores, most of the passive immunity acquired by pups and kittens is colostral in origin. Post-natal transmission of immunoglobulins, which is not confined to colostrum, may continue for weeks in the milk secreted by the dam. Antibodies passively acquired initially from colostrum and later through milk play an important role in protecting neonatal and young animals against bacterial and viral pathogens with an affinity for the alimentary tract.

In birds, passive immunity protects newborn chicks against a wide range of infectious agents. While the developing ovum is still in the ovary, serum immunoglobulins, mostly IgG, are transferred from the hen's circulation to the yolk. As the ovum passes down the oviduct, IgM and IgA antibodies are incorporated into the albumen. Antibodies present in yolk are gradually absorbed into the circulation as the embryo develops. The newly hatched chick continues to absorb antibodies from the yolk sac which is retracted into the abdominal

cavity shortly before hatching. Because albumen mixes with amniotic fluid and both are swallowed by the developing embryo, IgM and IgA antibodies may be present in the intestine at the time of hatching. An additional source of passive protection derives from antibodies incorporated into the albumen as the ovum moves through the oviduct. Mixing of albumen, containing maternal antibodies, with amniotic fluid which is swallowed by the developing chick, facilitates absorption of immunoglobulins from the alimentary tract.

Immunological aspects of foetal–maternal relationships

An unexplained aspect of pregnancy is that the foetus, which expresses histocompatibility antigens different from the mother, is not rejected by the dam as an allograft. Despite species diversity at the placental level, some common means of avoiding rejection of an allogenic conceptus may exist. It is evident that the embryo must be provided with appropriate maternal endocrine support to ensure a suitable *in utero* environment for implantation and development. In order to ensure continued maternal support, the embryo and, later, the foetus must maintain a low antigenic profile to avoid immunological recognition by the dam and the risk of rejection as an allograft.

Up to the time of implantation, the blastocyst makes minimal contact with the endometrium. In domestic animals, the placenta provides an unbroken outer layer of trophoblastic cells which establish contact with the endometrium in different forms in different species. The trophoblast and extra-embryonic membranes therefore constitute a defined line of separation between mother and foetus. Despite the close anatomical relationship between maternal and foetal tissues, the two circulatory systems remain entirely separate throughout gestation. In humans and some domestic animals, if foetal red blood cells or platelets enter the mother's circulation, as sometimes occurs at birth, antibodies are produced against them. There is evidence that human trophoblastic cells which come into direct contact with maternal tissue do not express polymorphic major histocompatibility complex (MHC) class I or class II molecules. In the human syncytiotrophoblast, it is reported that the class Ib MHC antigens, HLA-G and HLA-E are present in the extra-villous cytotrophoblast in a low or non-polymorphic form, thus avoiding presentation of paternally-inherited antigens to the maternal immune system. It is also reported that the HLA-G molecule can bind to the killer cell inhibitory receptors on maternal natural killer (NK) cells, thereby inhibiting destruction of foetal cells by maternal NK cells. Although there have been suggestions that the foetus is not recognised as foreign by the mother, there is clear evidence in the human population that women who have had multiple pregnancies have antibodies to the father's MHC antigens. In most instances, these antibodies are not damaging to the foetus or they are not accompanied by cytotoxic T lymphocyte responses against the foetal or placental tissue. Some maternal antibodies may actually inhibit the destruction of foetal cells by coating paternal MHC antigens, thereby avoiding destructive cell-mediated responses against foetal tissue by cytotoxic maternal lymphocytes.

Formerly, much emphasis was placed on the role of cytokines, especially T_H2 cell-regulating factors such as interleukin-10 (IL-10), on the control of maternal immune responses to pregnancy. Both uterine epithelium and the trophoblast secrete transforming growth factor, and also IL-4 and IL-10. This cytokine pattern tends to promote T_H2 responses and suppress T_H1 responses. Injection or induction of interferon-γ and IL-12, which promote T_H1 responses, can predispose to foetal resorption in experimental animals. The role of particular cytokines in the continuation of normal pregnancy, however, is now being questioned as many other soluble factors including hormones, protein and glycoprotein molecules may have an immunomodulatory effect on the maternal immune response. In ruminants, interferon-τ, produced by the trophoblast, is reported to inhibit maternal lymphocyte proliferation. Immunosuppressive phospholipids, present in moderate concentrations in amniotic fluid, may exert their effect at many levels. Some isoforms of α-fetoprotein, a protein synthesised in the yolk sac and foetal liver, also have immunosuppressive properties.

There is clinical evidence that pregnant cows, sensitised to tuberculin through infection with *Mycobacterium bovis*, exhibit immunosuppression as a consequence of pregnancy. Such animals show marked decrease in their responses in the tuberculin test, which is based on a cell-mediated hypersensitivity reaction. The increase in *Demodex canis* numbers in pregnant and lactating bitches, which facilitates transmission of the mites to pups, is also taken as evidence of immunosuppression related to pregnancy.

Despite many years of investigation, the basis of maternal immunological tolerance to foetal antigens is not well understood. Two important attributes of the conceptus, however, may account for the lack of strong maternal response: the nature of the tissue barrier surrounding the foetus and a degree of maternal immunosuppression induced by foetal and placental factors. The weakly antigenic or non-antigenic tissue barrier surrounding the foetus probably plays a central role in the avoidance of rejection. Production of a range of immunosuppressive factors by foetal and placental tissue, which depress both humoral and cell-mediated maternal responses, is likely to further diminish deleterious maternal responses against foetal tissue.

Further reading

Allen, W.R. (2004) Development and functions of the equine placenta. In *Proceedings of a Workshop on the Equine Placenta.* Maxwell H. Gluck Equine Research Center, Lexington, Ky, pp. 20–32.

Allen, W.R., Hamilton, D.W. and Moor, R.M. (1973) The origin of equine endometrial cups. II: Invasion of the endometrium by the trophoblast. *Anatomical Record* **177**, 485–502.

Amoroso, E.C. (1952) Placentation. In *Marshall's Physiology of Reproduction*, 3rd edn, Vol. II. Ed. A.S. Parkes. Longmans Green, London, pp. 127–311.

Anderson, J.W. (1969) Ultrasound of the placenta and fetal membranes of the dog. The placental labyrinth. *Anatomical Record* **165**, 15–36.

Barrau, M.D., Abel, J.H., Torbit, C.A. and Tietz, W.J. (1975) Development of the implantation chamber in the pregnant bitch. *American Journal of Anatomy* **143**, 115–130.

Betteridge, K.J. (1989) The structure and function of the equine capsule in relation to embryo manipulation and transfer. *Equine Veterinary Journal* Suppl., **8**, 92–104.

Burton, G.J. (1982) Review article. Placental uptake of maternal erythrocytes: a comparative study. *Placenta* **3**, 407–434.

Carter, A.M. (2004) Evolutionary aspects of placentation. In *Proceedings of a Workshop on the Equine Placenta.* Maxwell H. Gluck Equine Center, Lexington, Ky, pp. 12–15.

Dantzer, V. (1985) Electron microscopy of the initial stages of placentation in the pig. *Anatomy and Embryology* **172**, 281–293.

Dantzer, V. (1999a) Endotheliochorial placentation. In *Encyclopedia of Reproduction*, Vol. 1. Eds. E. Knobil and J.D. Neill. Academic Press, San Diego, pp. 1077–1084.

Dantzer, V. (1999b) Epitheliochorial placentation. In *Encyclopedia of Reproduction*, Vol. 2. Eds. E. Knobil and J.D. O'Neill. Academic Press, San Diego, pp. 18–28.

Denker, H.W., Eng, L.W. and Hamner, C.E. (1978) Studies on the early development and implantation in the cat. Implantation process. *Anatomy and Embryology* **54**, 39–54.

Engelhardt, H. (2004) Immunological adaptations to pregnancy in the pig. In *Proceedings of a Workshop on the Equine Placenta.* Maxwell H. Gluck Equine Center, Lexington, Ky, pp. 49–53.

Ford, S.P. (1999) Cotyledonary placenta. In *Encyclopedia of Reproduction*, Vol. 1. Eds. E. Knobil and J.D. Neill. Academic Press, San Diego, pp. 730–738.

Hamilton, D.W., Allen, W.R. and Moor, R.M. (1973) The origin of equine endometrial cups. III: Light and electron microscopic study of fully developed equine endometrial cups. *Anatomical Record* **177**, 503–518.

Imakawa, K., Chang, K.-T. and Christenson, R.K. (2004) Pre-implantation conceptus and maternal uterine communications: molecular events leading to successful implantation. *Journal of Reproduction and Development* **50**, 155–169.

Keys, J.L. and King, C.J. (1990) Microscopic examination of porcine conceptus–maternal interface between days 10 and 19 of pregnancy. *American Journal of Anatomy* **188**, 221–228.

King, C.J., Atkinson, B.A. and Robertson, H.A. (1979) Development of the bovine placentome during the second month of gestation. *Journal of Reproduction and Fertility* **55**, 173–180.

King, C.J., Atkinson, B.A. and Robertson, H.A. (1981) Development of the intercaruncular areas during early gestation and establishment of the bovine placenta. *Journal of Reproduction and Fertility* **61**, 469–474.

Leiser, R. and Enders, A.C. (1980a) Light and electron microscopy study of the near term paraplacenta of the domestic cat. 1. Polar zone and paraplacental functional areas. *Acta Anatomica* **106**, 293–311.

Leiser, R. and Enders, A.C. (1980b) Light and electron microscopy study of the near term paraplacenta of the domestic cat. 2. Paraplacental hematoma. *Acta Anatomica* **106**, 312–326.

Mossman, H.W. (1987) *Vertebrate Fetal Membranes.* Rutgers University Press, New Brunswick, New Jersey.

Père, M-C. (2003) Materno-foetal exchanges and utilisation of nutrients by the foetus: comparison between species. *Reproduction Nutrition Development* **43**, 1–15.

Renfree, M.B. and Shaw, G. (2000) Embryonic diapause in animals. *Annual Review of Physiology* **62**, 353–375.

Sharp, D.C., McDowell, K.J., Weithenauer, J. and Thatcher, W.W. (1989) The continuum of events leading to maternal recognition of pregnancy in mares. *Journal of Reproduction and Fertility*, Suppl., **37**, 101–107.

Steven, D.H., ed. (1975) *Comparative Placentation.* Academic Press, New York.

Vejlsted, M., Avery, B., Schmidt, M., Greve, T., Alexopoulos, N. and Maddox-Hyttel, P. (2005) Ultrastructural and immunohistochemical characterization of the bovine epiblast. *Biology of Reproduction* **72**, 678–686.

Wooding, F.B.P. (1992) The synepitheliochorial placenta of ruminants: binucleate cell fusions and hormone production. *Placenta* **13**, 101–113.

Wooding, F.B.P. and Flint, A.P.F. (1994) Placentation. In *Marshall's Physiology of Reproduction*, vol. III 4th edn. Ed. G.E. Lamming. Chapman and Hall, London, pp. 233–460.

11 Cardiovascular System

In the early stages of embryological development, the respiratory, excretory and nutritional requirements of the embryo are provided through simple diffusion. As the mammalian embryo increases in size, diffusion is inadequate for its nutritional, respiratory and excretory needs. Because of its increasing size and complexity, the developing embryo requires a system for delivering oxygen and nutrients to its tissues, and for transporting its waste products. These requirements are supplied by the cardiovascular system. As one of the first functional systems to develop in the embryo, the cardiovascular system consists of a central cardiac pumping organ linked to a network of arteries which convey blood to the tissues. Another system of vessels, veins, carry blood from the tissues back to the heart. An auxiliary system, the lymphatic system, assists in the return of extra-cellular fluids to the vascular system.

Blood vessel formation occurs in two sequential steps, vasculogenesis and angiogenesis. Vasculogenesis, the formation of blood vessels from blood islands, commences during the third week of gestation in domestic mammals, first in the yolk sac and later in the allantois. A number of factors including fibroblast growth factor 2 (Fgf-2), vascular endothelial growth factor (Vegf) and the angiopoietin proteins are considered to have an initiating role in vasculogenesis. Fibroblast growth factor induces splanchnic mesodermal cells to form haemangioblasts in the yolk sac. Vascular endothelial growth factor, which is expressed at high levels in areas proximal to active blood vessel formation, acts on tyrosine kinase receptors such as Flk1 present on haemangioblasts and angioblasts and promotes the differentiation of angioblasts into endothelial vessels.

The contribution of haemangioblasts to the formation of blood vessels and to haematopoiesis is outlined in Fig. 11.1.

Angiopoietins promote the interaction between endothelial cells and smooth muscle cells which eventually surround some developing blood vessels. Development of blood vessels involves a complex series of events during which endothelial cells differentiate, proliferate, migrate and become organised into an orderly vascular network. Splanchnic mesodermal cells lining the yolk sac form clusters, referred to as blood islands. With the formation of extra-embryonic vascular channels, a primitive circulatory system becomes established. Angiogenesis describes budding and sprouting of new vessels

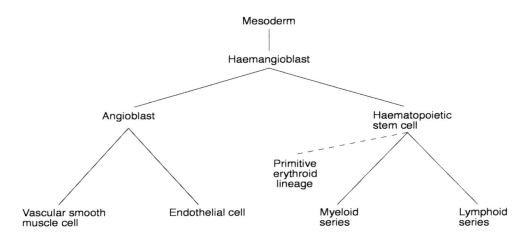

Figure 11.1 Outline of the origin and differentiation of angioblasts and haematopoietic stem cells from a common mesodermal precursor, the haemangioblast. The haematopoietic stem cell initially gives rise to a primitive erythroid lineage but, as maturation proceeds, definitive erythrocytes and myeloid cells are produced along with cells from which the lymphoid lineage develops.

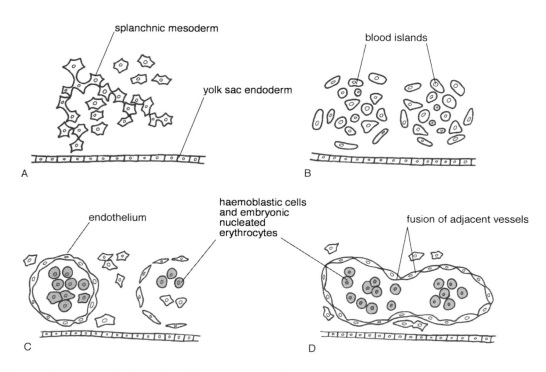

Figure 11.2 Sequential stages in the formation of blood vessels and blood cells from blood islands in the yolk sac.

from existing vessels. This process, a fundamental requirement for embryological development, continues post-natally. Vegf produced by the mesenchymal cells acts on the endothelial cells, at points where new vessel formation commences. Angiopoietin 1 subsequently interacts with receptor Tie-2 on endothelial cells at sites where sprouting occurs. At these points, endothelial cells can proliferate and form new vessels. In response to the angiopoietin 1–Tie-2 interactions, which occur during angiogenesis, endothelial cells release the signalling molecule platelet-derived growth factor (Pgdf) which stimulates migration of mesenchymal cells towards the vascular endothelium. In response to the release of other growth factors by endothelial cells, differentiation of mesenchymal cells into vascular smooth muscle cells occurs. Other mechanisms of angiogenesis include remodelling of existing vessels through anastomosis and branching or by an increase in luminal diameter.

At first, the haematopoietic islands are compact structures. Later, cells at the periphery of the blood islands change their shape under the influence of growth factors and become squamous, enclosing the centrally-located cells. The squamous cells form the endothelial lining of the emerging vascular system and the rounded centrally-located cells become the haemoblastic cells or embryonic nucleated erythrocytes (Fig. 11.2).

Vascular development occurs under the influence of specific growth factors. Basic fibroblast growth factor, which binds to receptors on splanchnic mesodermal cells, induces them to form haemangioblasts. Vascular

endothelial growth factor promotes the differentiation of peripheral haemangioblasts in blood islands into angioblasts which, in turn, differentiate into endothelial cells and form blood vessels. Maturation of the capillary network is influenced by platelet-derived growth factor and transforming growth factor-β. Development of individual channels in the network depends on the volume and direction of blood flow. The channels which convey the greatest volume of blood increase in diameter and acquire additional tissue layers from the surrounding mesoderm, becoming thick-walled vessels, referred to as arteries; the other vessels, veins, remain thin-walled. Blood vessels which develop in the foetal membranes, referred to as extra-embryonic vessels, consist of paired vitelline (yolk sac) and umbilical (allantoic) arteries and veins. Intra-embryonic formation of blood vessels, which proceeds in a similar manner to extra-embryonic vasculogenesis, commences soon after blood vessel formation begins in the extra-embryonic membranes. Subsequently, the extra-embryonic and intra-embryonic vessels anastomose, completing the rudimentary circulatory system of the conceptus (Fig. 11.3).

Development of the cardiac tubes

During the third week of gestation, the embryo has a pear-shaped outline and consists of three layers, namely, a dorsal layer of ectoderm, a ventral endodermal layer and a middle mesodermal layer. Small discrete spaces in the left and right lateral mesoderm enlarge and coalesce, forming a left and a right intra-embryonic coelom, thereby splitting the lateral mesoderm into parietal and

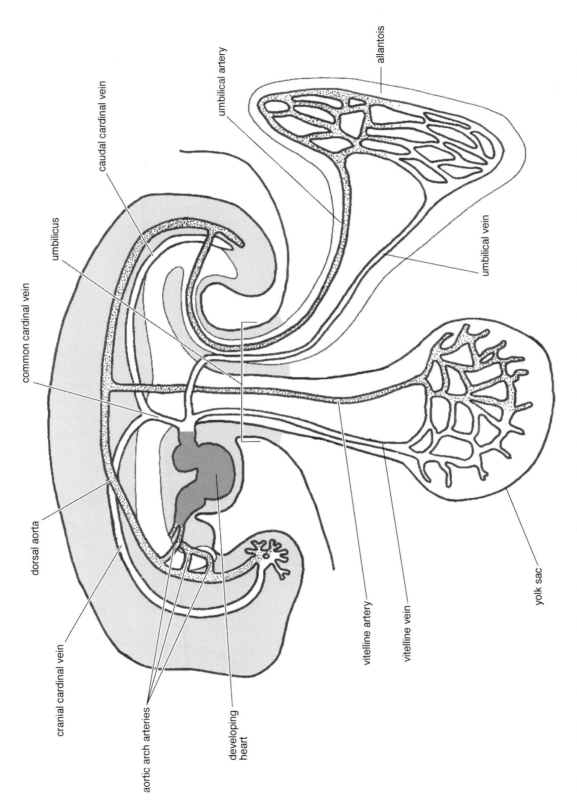

Figure 11.3 The rudimentary cardiovascular system of a mammalian embryo showing the intra-embryonic and extra-embryonic blood vessels on the left side.

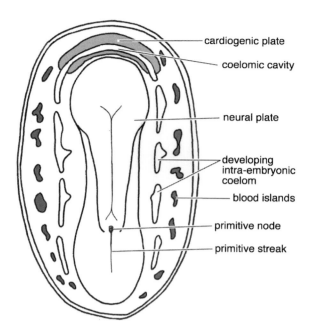

Figure 11.4 Development of the cardiac tube and the coelomic cavity at the embryonic disc stage.

splanchnic layers. Later, the coelom on the right and the coelom on the left fuse cranial to the developing neural plate, forming an enlarged horseshoe-shaped coelomic cavity (Fig. 11.4). Ventral to the coelom, groups of cells in the splanchnic mesoderm form the cardiogenic plate which is also horseshoe-shaped. Within the cardiogenic plate, angiogenic cell clusters give rise to a horseshoe-

shaped structure, the endocardial tube. The lateral limbs of the horseshoe-shaped vessel form the left and right endocardial tubes. Splanchnic mesodermal cells, which migrate towards and surround the endocardial tubes, form the myoepicardial mantle. At first, this mantle does not attach to the endothelium of the tubes. The intervening space contains a loose, gelatinous reticulum referred to as cardiac jelly. Many of the major intra-embryonic blood vessels, including the dorsal aortae, which develop in the dorsal mesenchyme of the embryonic disc, are formed contemporaneously with the endocardial tubes and extra-embryonic vessels. Mesodermal cells proliferate in a position anterior to the cardiogenic plate and form the septum transversum. The developing embryonic disc undergoes cranial–caudal and lateral folding. As a consequence of folding of the cranial portion of the embryo, the endocardial tubes and coelom and the septum transversum rotate through an angle of 180° on a lateral axis. Thus, the endocardial tubes are dorsal to the coelom, ventral to the foregut and caudal to the oropharyngeal membrane (Fig. 11.5). The caudal rotation of the developing heart is accompanied by rapid growth of the brain in an anterior direction so that it extends over the cardiac area. As a consequence of the rotation, the convex segment of the fused endocardial tubes, which initially occupied a position at the anterior margin of the embryonic disc, becomes positioned caudal to the brain. In this position, the convex segment of the fused endocardial tubes anastomoses with the vitelline veins from the yolk sac (Fig. 11.6). As a

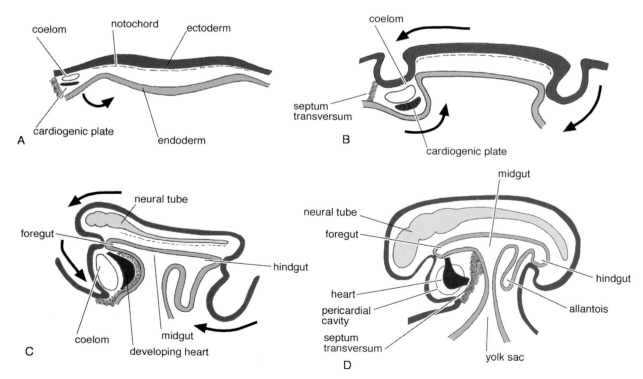

Figure 11.5 Sequential stages in the cranial–caudal folding of the embryo showing the changed relationship of the developing heart to other embryonic structures. Arrows indicate the direction of cranial and caudal folding.

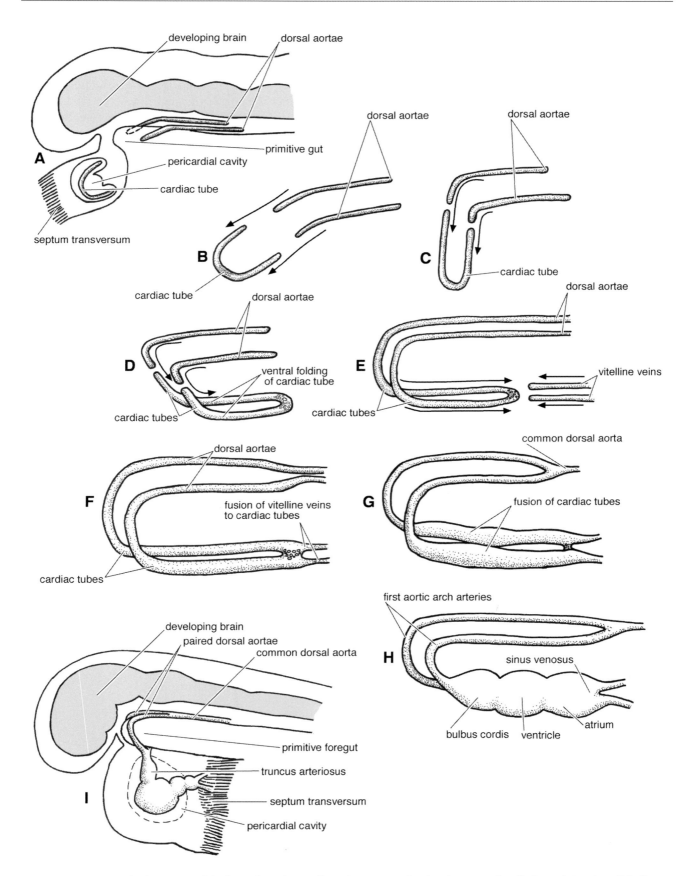

Figure 11.6 Stages in the formation of the heart from the cardiac tube stage to the development of an S-shaped structure (A to I).

result of the folding of the cranial portion of the embryo, the septum transversum occupies a position caudal to the heart where, at a later stage, it gives rise to the tendinous part of the diaphragm. Before joining the convex segment of the endocardial tube, the vitelline and umbilical veins pass through the septum transversum. The cranial portions of the dorsal aortae, which are drawn ventrally, form dorso-ventral loops. These loops, the first aortic arch arteries, fuse with the endocardial tubes (Fig. 11.6). With lateral folding of the embryo, the left and right endocardial tubes, surrounded by their muscular layers, gradually approach each other. Fusion of the medial walls of the endocardial tubes first occurs midway along their length. Later, fusion extends cranially and caudally until a single cardiac tube is formed (Figs. 11.6 and 11.7). However,

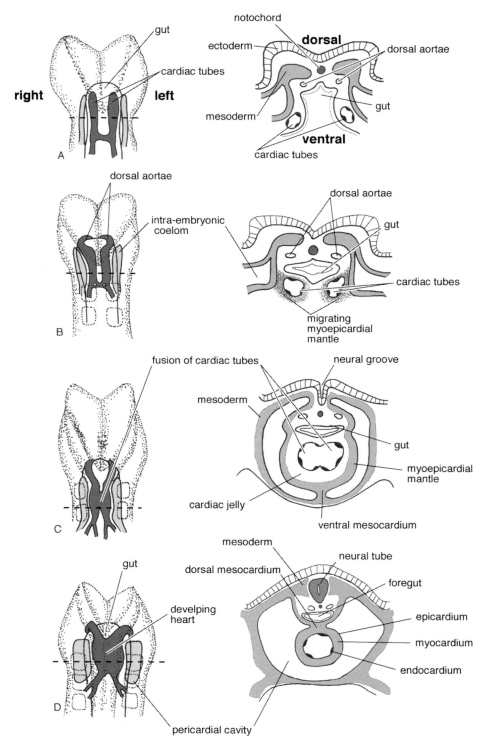

Figure 11.7 Ventral views of the developing cardiac tubes and coelom with corresponding cross-sections.

as fusion does not extend along the entire length of the endocardial tubes, the cranial and caudal ends remain separated. The endothelial lining of the single cardiac tube becomes the endocardium, the myoepicardial layer forms the myocardium, and from the visceral layer lining the pericardial cavity the epicardium is formed.

The cardiac tube, which is located in the pericardial cavity, is initially suspended by a dorsal mesocardium and anchored by a ventral mesocardium (Fig. 11.7). This cardiac tube undergoes differential growth along its length, which results in expanded portions separated by non-expanded portions. Listed in sequential order from the cranial end, these expanded portions are the truncus arteriosus, the bulbus cordis, the ventricle, the atrium and the sinus venosus (Fig. 11.8). The caudal end of the sinus venosus remains bifurcated. The ventral mesocardium persists for a short period only, unlike the dorsal mesocardium which persists for a longer time. The dorsal mesocardium gradually breaks down leaving the primitive heart unattached, apart from its points of attachment to the pericardium at the truncus arteriosus and ventricle. At first, the atrium and sinus venosus are located outside the pericardial cavity in the septum transversum. Because the primitive heart increases in size faster than the pericardial cavity, especially in the bulbo-ventricular region, a U-shaped bend, the bulbo-ventricular loop, forms. As a consequence of this development the atrium and sinus venosus become drawn into the cavity (Fig. 11.8). The loop occupies a ventral position in the pericardial cavity, to the right of the medial plane. Further growth of the developing heart causes the atrium to occupy a position dorsal to the bulbus cordis and ventricle, where it expands towards the truncus arteriosus. The sinus venosus is drawn into the pericardial cavity, and at this stage the developing heart becomes S-shaped (Fig. 11.8).

A number of transcription factors have been implicated in the process of bulbo-ventricular loop formation. These include Hand-1 and Hand-2 transcription factors which are regulated by Nkx-2.5. As heart development proceeds, Hand-1 expression becomes confined to the developing left ventricle and Hand-2 to the developing right ventricle. Deletion of genes which encode Hand-1 or Hand-2 factors results in hypoplasia of the ventricle in which they are normally expressed. The T box factors, Tbf-5 and Tbf-20, together with Bmp-4, also influence the formation of the bulbo-ventricular loop. Differential contraction of the actin cytoskeleton has been proposed as a determining factor in the formation of the bulbo-ventricular loop.

During cardiac morphogenesis, blood vessel formation continues within the embryo. Two major blood vessels which form ventral to the neural tube become the left

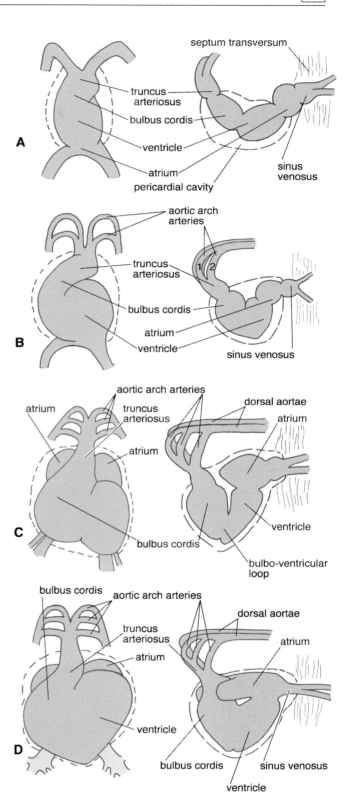

Figure 11.8 Dorso-ventral and left lateral views of sequential stages in the differentiation of the cardiac tube, from the bulbo-ventricular loop stage to the expansion of the bulbo-ventricular loop ventrally, and the common atrium dorsally.

and right dorsal aortae. Cranially, they fuse with the left and right limbs of the endocardial tubes. Associated with the lateral folding of the embryo, the dorsal aortae caudal to the developing heart fuse, forming a common aorta. In the mesenchyme adjacent to the truncus arteriosus, an additional series of paired aortic arch arteries develop which join the dilated end of the truncus arteriosus with the dorsal aortae (Fig. 11.8). Branches of the dorsal aortae, the intersegmental arteries, supply the developing somites. Additional branches supply the yolk sac through the vitelline arteries, and the umbilical arteries supply the allantois. Following the formation of the vitelline veins which drain the yolk sac, the umbilical veins which drain the allantois, the cranial cardinal veins draining the head and the caudal cardinal veins conveying blood from the body wall, venous blood is returned to the caudal end of the primitive heart, the sinus venosus (Fig. 11.3). On each side of the developing embryo, the cranial and caudal cardinal veins fuse, forming the common cardinal veins which enter the sinus venosus. At this precise stage of morphogenesis, the developing mammalian cardiovascular system bears a strong resemblance, both morphologically and functionally, to that of the fully formed circulatory system of fish.

Molecular aspects of cardiac development

The transcription factor Nkx-2.5 is central to the initial induction of splanchnic mesodermal cells which ultimately contribute to cardiogenic mesoderm formation. This transcription factor is up-regulated under the influence of Bmp and Fgf factors. Nkx-2.5 activates the synthesis of other transcription factors such as members of the GATA-4 and Mef-2 families. These transcription factors up-regulate the expression of cardiac-specific proteins, including cardiac actin and α-myosin. Left–right patterning proteins such as Nodal and Lefty-2 influence the pattern of asymmetry, a feature of heart formation. The transcription factor Pitx-2, which is up-regulated by Nodal, is critical for normal heart morphogenesis.

Formation of the cardiac chambers

Partitions which form in the primordial mammalian heart gradually convert the single pulsating cardiac tube into a complex four-chambered organ. Although formation of cardiac septa takes place at approximately the same time, for descriptive purposes their formation is described as if they were separate events. The foetal heart continues to function effectively as these ongoing major structural changes occur.

Partitioning of the atrio-ventricular canal

In the region of the atrio-ventricular canal, two masses of cardiac mesenchymal tissue known as endocardial cushions, which are located between the endocardium and the myocardium, extend towards each other and fuse. The fused endocardial cushions form the septum intermedium, which divides the common atrio-ventricular canal into left and right atrio-ventricular openings (Fig. 11.9).

Partitioning of the common foetal atrium

During proliferation of the endocardial cushions, a crescent-shaped fold, the septum primum, arises from the dorsal wall of the common foetal atrium and extends towards the endocardial cushions. The septum primum gradually divides the common atrium into a left and a right atrium (Fig. 11.10). As the septum primum grows towards the endocardial cushions, an opening, the foramen primum, persists between the left and right foetal atria. This foramen gradually decreases in size and, when the septum primum reaches the cushions, it eventually closes. Before closure of the foramen primum, however, programmed cell death in the central part of the septum primum results in the formation of a new communication channel between the left and right atria, the foramen secundum (Fig. 11.10). A second membrane, the septum secundum, arises from the dorsal wall of the right atrium, to the right of the septum primum, and extends towards the septum intermedium. The central portion of the septum secundum overlaps the foramen secundum, but does not extend as far as the septum intermedium. The opening which persists between the free edge of the septum secundum and the foramen secundum is known as the foramen ovale. The upper part of the septum primum fuses with the septum secundum while the remaining portion becomes a valve-like structure for the foramen ovale. The lower margin of the septum secundum divides the blood flow returning to the heart via the caudal vena cava into two streams. The greater amount is directed through the foramen ovale into the left atrium, while a lesser amount is directed through the right atrio-ventricular opening into the right ventricle. Due to its functional role, the lower margin of the septum secundum is appropriately named the crista dividens. At birth, the valve-like structure of the foramen ovale closes, completing the separation of the left and right atria.

Final form of the right atrium

In the early stages of cardiac morphogenesis, blood returning from the left side of the embryo enters the left horn of the sinus venosus. Blood from the right side of the embryo enters the right horn of the sinus. The venous blood entering the sinus venosus enters the embryonic atrium through the sino-atrial opening, which is regulated by the sino-atrial valve composed of left and right components. Development of venous shunts between the left and right systemic venous

Figure 11.9 Stages in the division of the common atrio-ventricular canal into left and right atrio-ventricular openings, resulting from the fusion of the endocardial cushions and the formation of the septum intermedium at the level of the endocardial cushions. Arrows in A and B indicate direction of growth of endocardial cushions; arrows in C indicate direction of blood flow.

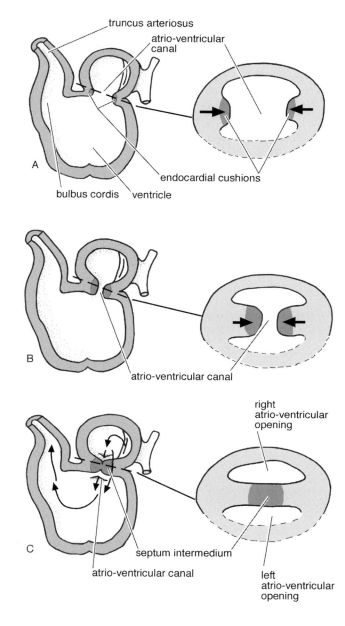

systems leads to the preferential direction of flow to the right side, resulting in enlargement of the right horn of the sinus venosus while the left horn decreases in size. As partitioning of the atrium proceeds, the sino-atrial opening occupies a position in the right half of the foetal atrium. Gradually, the right horn of the sinus venosus becomes incorporated into the right foetal atrium. In its final form, the right atrium consists of the right foetal atrium which becomes the muscular right auricle, while the right horn of the sinus venosus becomes the thin-walled sinus venarum into which the venous return from the body enters the heart (Fig. 11.11). During morphological adaptation, the left portion of the sino-atrial valve fuses with the septum secundum, while part of the right portion forms an internal ridge, the demarcation between the auricle and the sinus venarum, termed the crista terminalis. On the external surface a depression, the sulcus terminalis, marks this division. The remainder

of the right portion of the sino-atrial valve contributes to the formation of the valves of the caudal vena cava and coronary sinus. The regressing left horn of the sinus venosus contributes to the formation of the coronary venous sinus which opens into the right atrium.

Final form of the left atrium

The embryonic pulmonary vein develops as an outgrowth of the left foetal atrium, to the left of the septum primum. The vein divides into left and right branches which supply the developing bronchial buds. Later, the left and right branches subdivide. In a manner similar to the incorporation of the right horn of the sinus venosus into the right atrium, the enlarged pulmonary vein and its branches become incorporated into the left atrium. Thus, four pulmonary veins are incorporated into the fully formed left atrium, two from each lung. The left

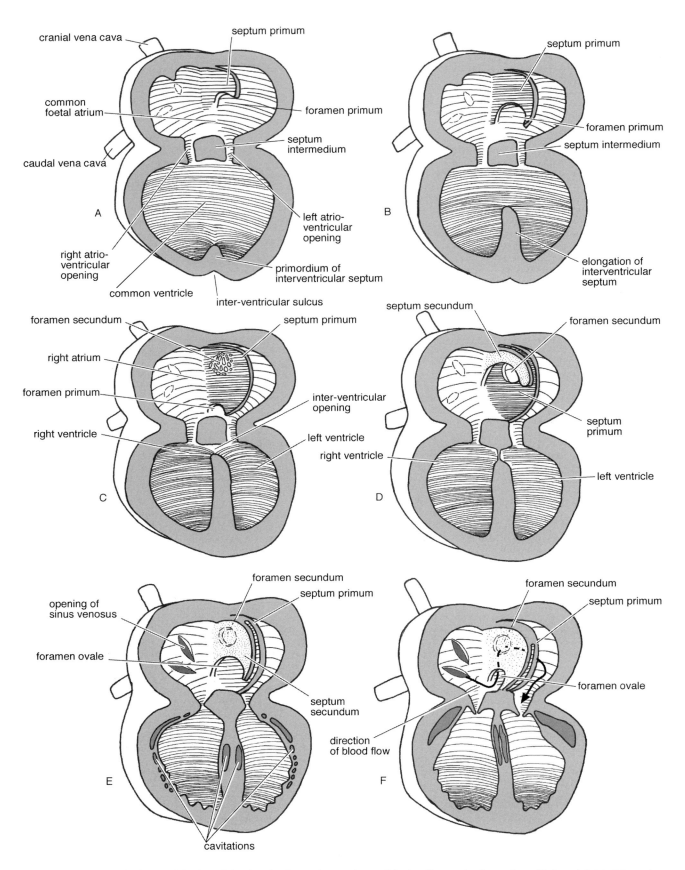

cranial vena cava
septum primum
common foetal atrium
foramen primum
septum intermedium
caudal vena cava
A
right atrio-ventricular opening
left atrio-ventricular opening
common ventricle
primordium of interventricular septum
inter-ventricular sulcus

septum primum
foramen primum
septum intermedium
B
elongation of interventricular septum

foramen secundum
septum primum
right atrium
foramen primum
inter-ventricular opening
right ventricle
left ventricle
C

septum secundum
foramen secundum
septum primum
right ventricle
left ventricle
D

foramen secundum
septum primum
opening of sinus venosus
foramen ovale
septum secundum
E
cavitations

foramen secundum
septum primum
foramen ovale
direction of blood flow
F

Figure 11.10 Stages in the partitioning of the developing atrium and ventricle, leading to the formation of left and right atria and ventricles (A to F). The arrow in F indicates the direction of blood flow through the foramen ovale.

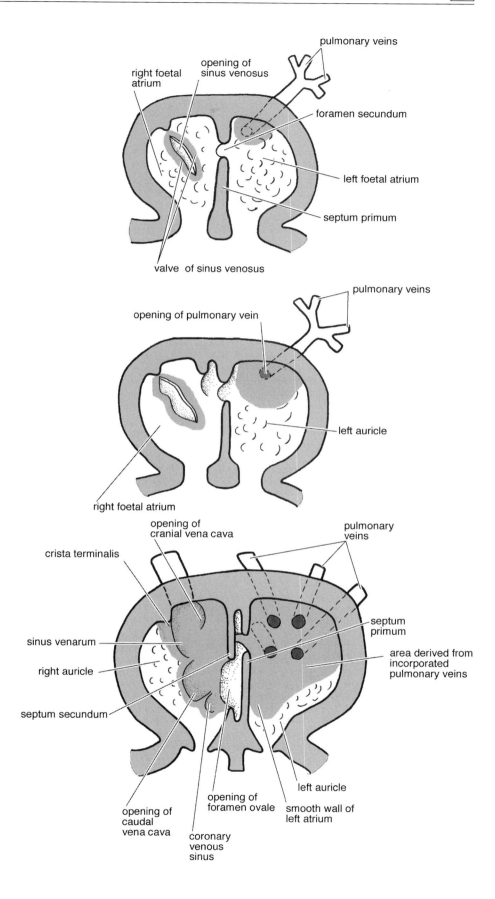

Figure 11.11 Incorporation of the sinus venosus into the right foetal atrium and incorporation of the pulmonary veins into the left foetal atrium.

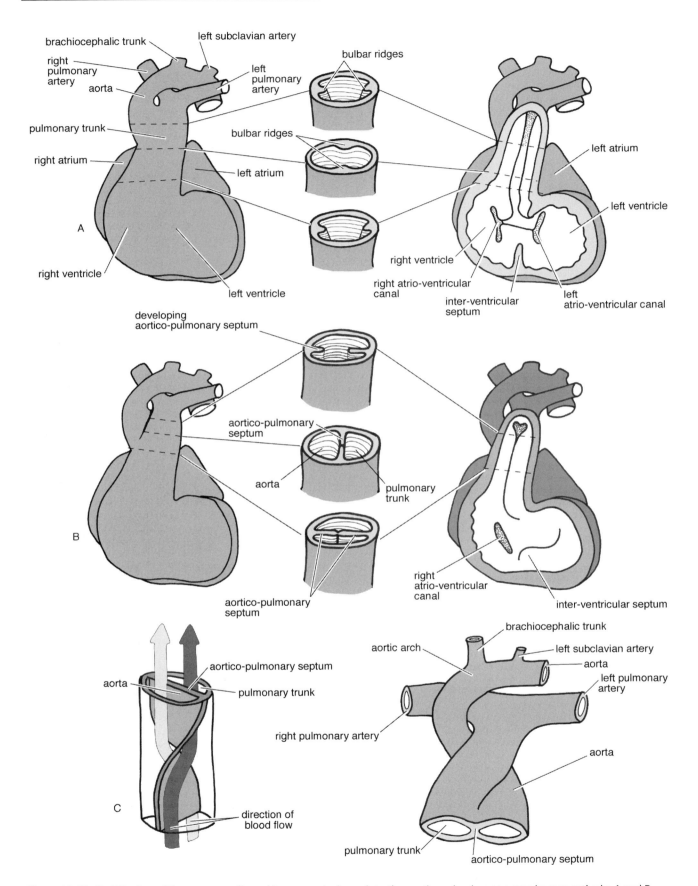

Figure 11.12 Partitioning of the conus cordis and truncus arteriosus into the aortic and pulmonary trunks respectively, A and B. The spiral arrangement of the aortico-pulmonary septum and the final relationship of the aortic and pulmonary trunks is also illustrated, C.

atrium therefore comprises the left foetal atrium, which becomes the left auricle, and the integrated pulmonary veins, which form the smooth portion of the wall of this chamber (Fig. 11.11).

Formation of the left and right ventricles

Following its differential growth, the bulbus cordis consists of a dilated portion adjacent to the ventricle and a non-dilated portion referred to as the conus cordis, which is continuous with the truncus arteriosus. The dilated portion of the bulbus cordis and the embryonic ventricle form a common chamber. Externally, the division between the bulbus cordis and ventricle is marked by a groove, the inter-ventricular sulcus, and internally by a muscular fold, the primordial inter-ventricular septum (Fig. 11.10). As the walls of the ventricle and bulbus cordis increase in thickness, diverticulation of their inner surfaces imparts a trabecular appearance to the myocardium. At this stage, the embryonic ventricle can be considered as the primitive left ventricle and the dilated bulbus cordis as the primitive right ventricle. The ventricles enlarge by peripheral growth which is closely followed by increased diverticulation and trabeculation of their inner walls. As the inter-ventricular sulcus deepens and the walls of the expanding ventricles meet medially at the sulcus, the walls become apposed and fuse, contributing to the elongation of the inter-ventricular septum. Continued peripheral growth of the myocardial tissue of each ventricle accounts for the progressive increase in length of the inter-ventricular septum. At this stage, the septum does not completely separate the two ventricles, which communicate through the inter-ventricular foramen. Later, as a consequence of differential cellular proliferation, the inter-ventricular foramen closes (Fig. 11.10).

Partitioning of the conus cordis and truncus arteriosus

Two sub-endocardial thickenings, the bulbar ridges, which fuse forming the aortico-pulmonary septum, divide the conus cordis and truncus arteriosus into an aortic trunk and a pulmonary trunk (Fig. 11.12). The spiral form of the aortico-pulmonary septum ensures that the aortic trunk becomes continuous with the fourth aortic arch arteries and that the pulmonary trunk communicates with the sixth aortic arch arteries. Mesenchymal cells of neural crest origin, which migrate from the cranial region, contribute to the formation of the aortico-pulmonary septum.

Closure of the inter-ventricular foramen

The developmental changes which lead to the closure of the inter-ventricular foramen are complex. The membranous portion of the inter-ventricular septum, which causes closure of the inter-ventricular foramen, is formed from proliferation of tissues derived from the bulbar ridges of the aortico-pulmonary septum, the septum intermedium, and the muscular inter-ventricular septum (Fig. 11.13). Following closure, the pulmonary trunk carries blood from the right ventricle and the aortic trunk conveys blood from the left ventricle.

Formation of cardiac valves

The aortic and pulmonary valves, which are necessary for prevention of backflow of blood into the left and right ventricles, arise from three swellings of sub-endothelial mesenchymal tissue at the origins of the aortic and pulmonary trunks. Mesenchymal tissue of neural crest origin contributes to the formation of these valves. As a consequence of hollowing out, these ridges become re-modelled forming three thin-walled cusps, composed of folded endothelial tissue with connective tissue cores (Fig. 11.14).

As the endocardial cushions fuse and divide the common atrio-ventricular opening into left and right openings, the left and right atrio-ventricular valves form at these openings. The left atrio-ventricular valve is composed of two cusps and is referred to as bicuspid, while the right atrio-ventricular valve is composed of three cusps and is referred to as tricuspid. Mesenchymal tissue proliferates around the rim of each orifice. Cavitation of the muscular layer immediately beneath the mesenchymal thickening, and re-modelling of the associated tissue, contribute to the formation of the cusps of the atrio-ventricular valves (Fig. 11.15). Because the valves are partially derived from mesenchymal tissue which was originally attached directly to the myocardium at the orifices, the valves remain anchored by muscular strands to the ventricular walls. With diverticulation and resultant thinning of the ventricular walls, muscular strands remain attached along the ventricular surface of the valve cusps. These thin muscular structures are gradually replaced by dense connective tissue, the chordae tendineae, which connect the valve cusps to muscular projections of the ventricular walls referred to as papillary muscles (Fig. 11.15).

Conducting system of the heart

Specialised myocardial cells responsible for the initiation and conduction of the electrical impulses which regulate the rate of cardiac contractions, develop in myocardial tissue. These cells form structures referred to as pacemakers. The first pacemaker is located in the caudal part of the left cardiac tube. Subsequently, a site in the right horn of the sinus venosus assumes this role. When the right horn of the sinus becomes incorporated into the definitive right atrium, the specialised tissue is referred to as the sino-atrial node.

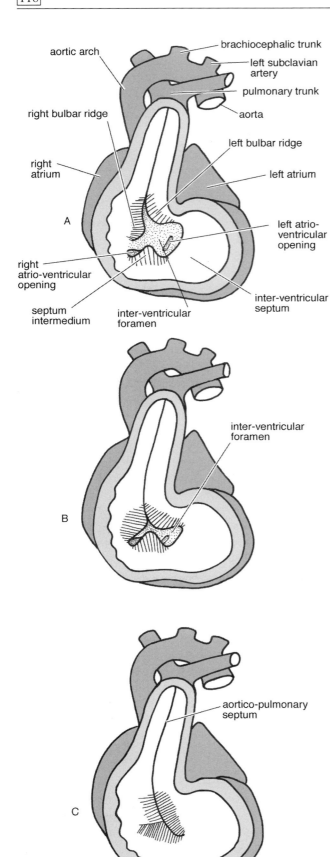

Figure 11.13 Stages in the closure of the inter-ventricular foramen.

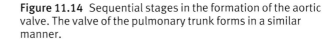

Figure 11.14 Sequential stages in the formation of the aortic valve. The valve of the pulmonary trunk forms in a similar manner.

At a stage early in cardiac development, prior to the formation of separate cardiac chambers, the myocardium surrounding the entire cardiac tube contracts as a unit. As the chambers of the heart develop, a band of connective tissue, derived from the epicardium, separates the musculature of the atria from the musculature of the ventricles. Specialised atypical muscle fibres, Purkinje

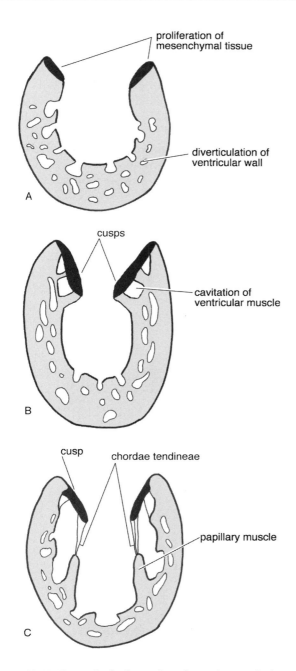

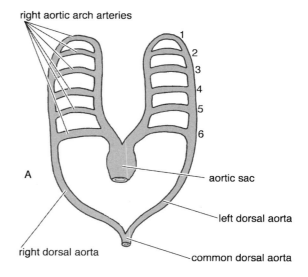

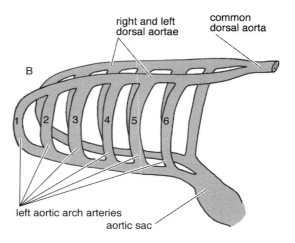

Figure 11.15 Stages in the formation of an atrio-ventricular valve, showing diverticulation of the ventricular musculature, formation of papillary muscles and attachment of chordae tendineae to valve cusps.

Figure 11.16 Illustration showing a ventral view, A, and a left lateral view, B, of the six pairs of aortic arch arteries. Although they develop sequentially, the illustration represents them as if they were present contemporaneously.

fibres, form the atrio-ventricular bundle which conducts impulses from the musculature of the atria to the musculature of the ventricles. These fibres, which extend from a node of special muscle cells, the atrio-ventricular node located in the septum intermedium, continue through the band of connective tissue to the ventricular walls.

Development of the arterial system

The intra-embryonic blood vessels develop in a manner similar to that described for the extra-embryonic vessels.

The dorsal aortae, which are the first major vessels to develop, fuse with the endocardial tubes. As a result of the cranial-caudal body folding, the cranial portions of the dorsal aortae form arches which are lateral to the foregut and are surrounded by the mesenchyme which forms the first pharyngeal arches. These segments of the dorsal aortae are referred to as the first aortic arch arteries. The junction of the aortic arch arteries with the truncus arteriosus, which becomes dilated, is called the aortic sac. As subsequent pharyngeal arches develop, pairs of arch arteries, which arise from the aortic sac, pass through the arches before joining the dorsal aortae. A total of six pairs of aortic arch arteries are formed, and from them other major vascular structures arise (Fig. 11.16).

Although it is usual to represent the paired arch arteries diagrammatically as if they were all present simultaneously, in reality they develop sequentially. At the stage of development when the first and second arch arteries are formed, the fourth and sixth arteries have not yet developed. By the time the sixth pair of arteries have formed, the first two pairs have largely atrophied.

Derivatives of the aortic arch arteries

Major developmental changes occur in the aortic arch arteries in dogs between the third and fourth weeks of gestation, and in humans and horses, between the third and seventh weeks of gestation. These changes take place contemporaneously with the establishment of separate venous and arterial circulations. The dorsal aortae caudal to the heart fuse forming the single caudal aorta; cranial to the heart they remain paired. Apart from the portions which persist as the small left and right maxillary arteries, the first pair of aortic arch arteries atrophy (Fig. 11.17). Small remnants of the second pair of aortic arch arteries persist as branches to the left and right middle ears, the stapedial arteries. The left and right third aortic arch arteries form the common carotid

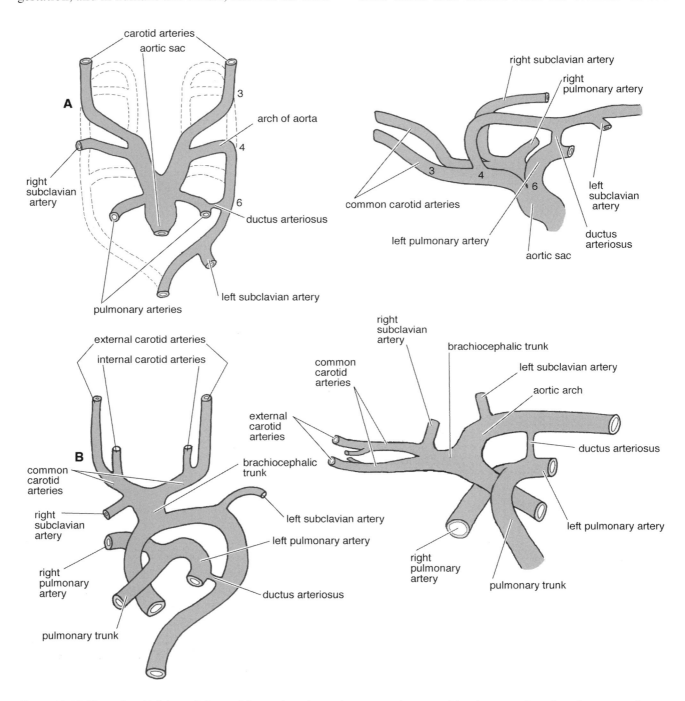

Figure 11.17 Ventral and left lateral views of the aortic arch arteries at an early stage of development, A, and at a late stage of development, B. Dotted lines represent vessels undergoing atrophy.

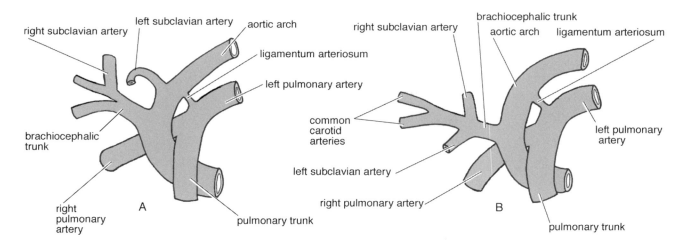

Figure 11.18 Post-natal arrangement of the major blood vessels which arise from the arch of the aorta and the pulmonary trunk of domestic carnivores, A, and of horses and ruminants, B.

arteries and contribute to the formation of the internal carotid arteries. The cranial portions of the dorsal aortae form the remainder of the internal carotid arteries. The portions of the dorsal aortae between the third and fourth arch arteries atrophy (Fig. 11.17). The external carotid arteries form as outgrowths of the third aortic arch arteries. The fate of the fourth pair of aortic arch arteries is different on the right and on the left sides. The left fourth aortic arch artery forms part of the arch of the aorta. The remainder of the arch of the aorta derives in part from the aortic sac and the left dorsal aorta. The right fourth aortic arch artery forms the proximal segment of the right subclavian artery. The remainder of the subclavian artery derives from the right dorsal aorta and the right seventh dorsal intersegmental artery. The segment of the right dorsal aorta between the origin of the right subclavian artery and the common caudal aorta atrophies. In common with the fifth pharyngeal arches, the fifth pair of aortic arch arteries are usually rudimentary and subsequently atrophy. The sixth pair of aortic arch arteries supply branches to the developing lungs. On the left side, the proximal segment of the sixth aortic arch artery, between the pulmonary branch and the aortic sac, persists as the proximal part of the left pulmonary artery. The distal segment persists as a shunt, the ductus arteriosus, which links the pulmonary artery with the dorsal aorta. The proximal part of the right sixth aortic arch artery becomes the proximal part of the right pulmonary artery, while the distal segment atrophies.

The brachiocephalic trunk develops from remodelling of the aortic sac and its fusion with portions of the left and right third and fourth aortic arch arteries. In its definitive form, this trunk arises from the aortic arch. In dogs, the brachiocephalic trunk gives off the left common carotid artery, and at its point of bifurcation forms the right common carotid artery and right subclavian

artery (Fig. 11.18). In horses, cattle and pigs, the left and right common carotid arteries arise from bifurcation of a single branch from the brachiocephalic trunk. The seventh dorsal intersegmental artery, which arises from the left dorsal aorta at the level of the seventh somite, contributes to the formation of the left subclavian artery. During remodelling of the aortic arch arteries, the seventh intersegmental artery migrates cranially from a position caudal to the ductus arteriosus to a location close to the aortic arch. In pigs and dogs, the left subclavian artery arises directly from the aortic arch, distal to the origin of the brachiocephalic trunk, while in horses and cattle the left subclavian artery, which migrates to a more cranial position, arises directly from the brachiocephalic trunk (Fig. 11.18B).

The recurrent laryngeal branch of the vagus nerve on either side, which passes caudal to the developing sixth aortic arch artery, innervates the musculature of the sixth pharyngeal arch. When the heart and associated vessels move into the thoracic cavity, the recurrent laryngeal nerves are drawn caudally. Because the distal part of the right sixth aortic arch artery and the entire fifth aortic arch artery atrophy, the right recurrent laryngeal nerve becomes hooked around the right subclavian artery which accounts for its more cranial position in comparison with the left recurrent laryngeal nerve. On the left side, the recurrent laryngeal nerve remains hooked around the sixth aortic arch artery, the blood vessel which subsequently gives rise to the ductus arteriosus (Fig. 11.19). After birth, as the ductus arteriosus persists as the ligamentum arteriosum, the left recurrent laryngeal nerve remains hooked around the ligamentum arteriosum and the aortic arch.

The close relationship of the left recurrent laryngeal nerve to the aortic arch has been proposed as a factor in the aetiology of paralysis of the left side of the larynx in

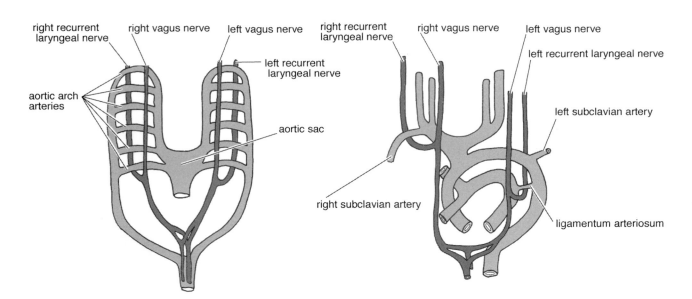

Figure 11.19 The initial relationships of the recurrent laryngeal nerves to the aortic arch arteries and their subsequent relationships to the blood vessels which arise from the aortic arch arteries.

horses. It has been suggested that the functioning of the nerve becomes impaired by the pulsations of the arch of the aorta. Another possible factor, especially in long-necked horses, may be that the nerve is prevented from moving by the aortic arch and can be damaged by stretching when the horse's neck is fully extended to the right. Because the right subclavian artery is less rigidly fixed than the aortic arch, the right recurrent laryngeal nerve, which is hooked around the right subclavian artery, is less likely to become damaged by stretching. Accordingly, paralysis of the right side of the larynx is uncommon in horses.

Branches of the aorta

Dorsal, lateral and ventral branches arise from the paired dorsal aortae. Following fusion of the aortae, paired dorsal inter-segmental arteries which pass between the somites arise along the length of the fused vessel. These inter-segmental arteries give off dorsal branches to the developing spinal cord and the epaxial musculature, and ventral branches to the hypaxial musculature. The seventh inter-segmental arteries supply the developing forelimb buds. A series of longitudinal anastomoses develop between the inter-segmental arteries. In the cervical region, the first six inter-segmental arteries between the longitudinal anastomoses and the dorsal aortae atrophy. The artery formed from these anastomoses, the vertebral artery, arises from the seventh inter-segmental artery. In the thoracic region, the anastomoses form the internal thoracic artery, and the inter-segmental arteries persist as the intercostal arteries (Fig. 11.20). The inter-segmental arteries in the lumbar region form the lumbar arteries. The most caudal lumbar

inter-segmental arteries supply the pelvic limb buds and form the external iliac arteries. The umbilical arteries, which arise directly from the paired dorsal aortae, supply the allantois. With the formation of the common aorta and the inter-segmental arteries, the umbilical arteries appear as branches of the internal iliac arteries.

The paired lateral branches of the aorta give rise to renal, phrenico-abdominal, adrenal, gonadal and deep circumflex arteries on either side. The unpaired ventral aortic branches, which supply the splanchnopleure of the thoracic and abdominal cavities, give rise to the broncho-oesophageal, coeliac, cranial mesenteric and caudal mesenteric arteries. Endothelial sprouts, which arise near the commencement of the aorta and anastomose with a plexus of vessels in the sub-epicardial layer of the developing heart, form the coronary vessels, the principal blood supply to the heart.

Development of the venous system

The venous system develops under the influence of specific growth factors in a manner similar to the development of the arterial system. Early in embryological development, three pairs of major veins are formed, vitelline veins, umbilical veins and cardinal veins (Fig. 11.3).

Arterial and venous differentiation

While endothelial cells possess the inherent capability of ultimately developing along the venous pathway, exposure to Vegf and Notch signalling can promote arterial formation. The membranes of the endothelial cells of the developing arterial system possess the transmembrane

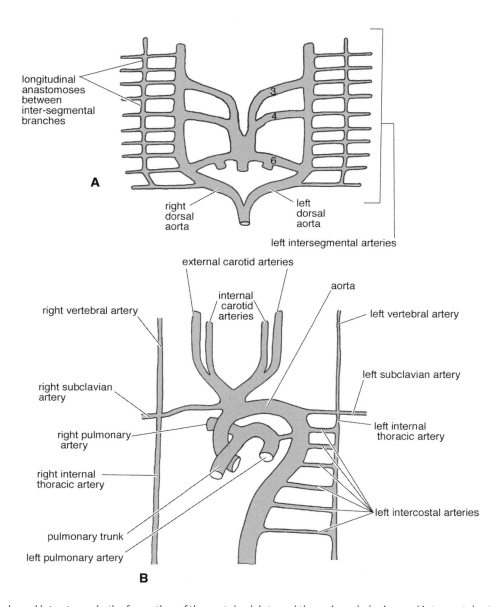

Figure 11.20 Early and late stages in the formation of the vertebral, internal thoracic, subclavian and intercostal arteries. Vessels in A labelled 3, 4 and 6 are the aortic arch arteries which persist and from which definitive arteries arise, B.

protein ephrin-B2, while the endothelial cells of the venous system contain a receptor for ephrin-B2 called Eph-B4 on their surface membranes (Fig. 11.21). During angiogenesis, interaction between ephrin-B2 and Eph-B4 at the points of anastomosis of the arterial and venous systems, ensures that end-to-end fusion can occur only between arterial and venous capillaries, while lateral fusion between arterial and venous capillaries is prevented.

Vitelline veins

The paired vitelline veins, which convey blood from the yolk sac to the heart, pass through the umbilicus into the embryo and run cranially, one on either side of the foregut, through the septum transversum and enter the sinus venosus (Fig. 11.22). Cells of the developing liver cords extend into the septum transversum leading to the formation of a venous plexus which arises from the middle segments of the vitelline vessels. This vascular network becomes incorporated into the developing liver forming the hepatic sinusoids. The fate of the cranial segments of the left and right parts of the vitelline veins, located between the developing liver and the sinus venosus, differs. The left cranial segment of the vitelline vein, which enters the left horn of the sinus venosus, atrophies. The right cranial segment of the vitelline vein persists and becomes that segment of the caudal vena cava which conveys blood from the liver into the right horn of the sinus venosus. Two anastomoses, one cranial and one caudal, form between the caudal segments of the left and right vitelline veins. The cranial anastomosis is located dorsal to the midgut, while the caudal anastomosis is located ventral to the midgut. Following

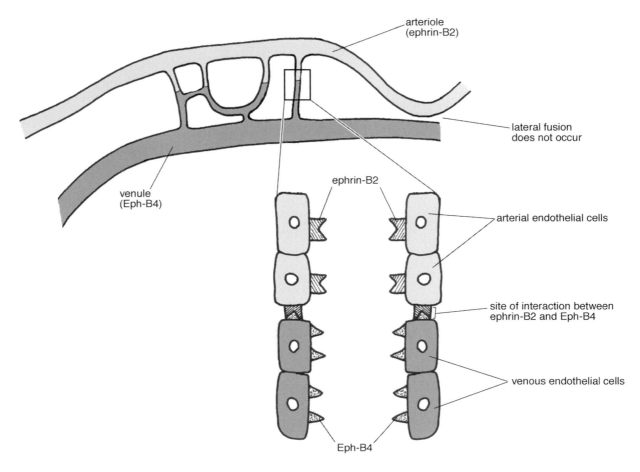

Figure 11.21 The role of receptor–ligand interactions in fusion of arterial and venous endothelial cells.

rotation of the stomach and a gradual alteration in the patency of segments of the left and right vitelline veins, re-direction of blood flow occurs. The portal vein is formed from the patent segments of the left and right vitelline veins and their anastomoses. The non-patent segments of the left and right vitelline veins atrophy.

Umbilical veins

Paired umbilical veins, which convey blood from the allantois through the umbilical cord, pass through the septum transversum and enter the sinus venosus (Fig. 11.22). As a consequence of the enlargement of the developing liver, the umbilical veins become subdivided into cranial, middle and caudal segments, each with a different developmental fate. As the liver expands later-ally, the middle portions of the umbilical veins become incorporated into the hepatic tissue and contribute to the formation of the liver sinusoids. The cranial seg-ments of the left and right umbilical veins atrophy. At the umbilicus, fusion of the left and right umbilical veins occurs. Subsequently, the caudal segment of the right umbilical vein atrophies and, as a consequence, the caudal segment of the left umbilical vein enlarges

and conveys oxygenated blood from the placenta to the embryonic liver. Initially, blood flows through the hepatic sinusoids to reach the right horn of the sinus venosus. Most of the blood follows a more direct course with the development of a venous shunt between the left umbilical vein and the cranial segment of the right vitelline vein. This venous shunt is referred to as the ductus venosus. The ductus venosus persists up to birth in carnivores and ruminants but atrophies during gestation in horses and pigs. As a consequence, in both equine and porcine foetuses, blood from the umbilical vein passes through the sinusoids of the liver. The remnant of the left umbilical vein which persists and is present in the adult as the round ligament of the liver, is contained within the falciform ligament

Cardinal veins

The paired cranial cardinal veins drain blood from the head and neck region while the paired caudal cardinal veins drain the body wall. These cranial and caudal cardinal veins on the left and right sides fuse forming the left and right common cardinal veins which open into the sinus venosus (Fig. 11.23). As the venous system

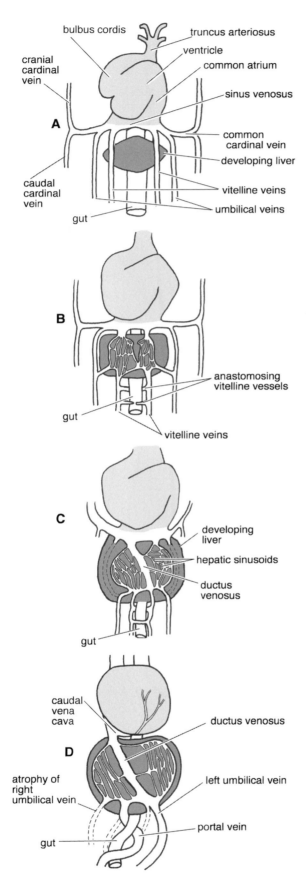

Figure 11.22 Sequential stages in the differentiation of the vitelline and umbilical veins. During this differentiation, the hepatic sinusoids and the portal vein are formed.

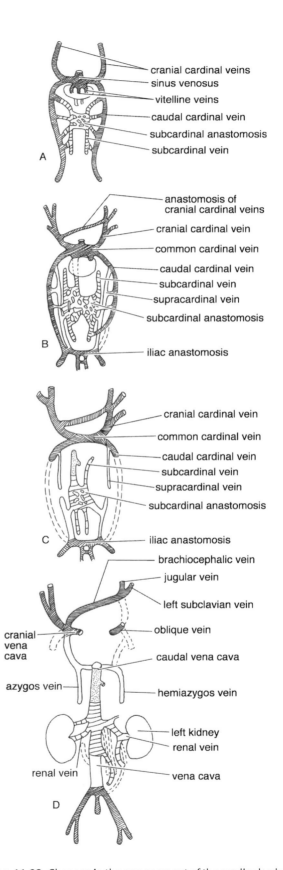

Figure 11.23 Changes in the arrangement of the cardinal veins and their branches leading to the formation of the cranial vena cava and the caudal vena cava and their associated veins.

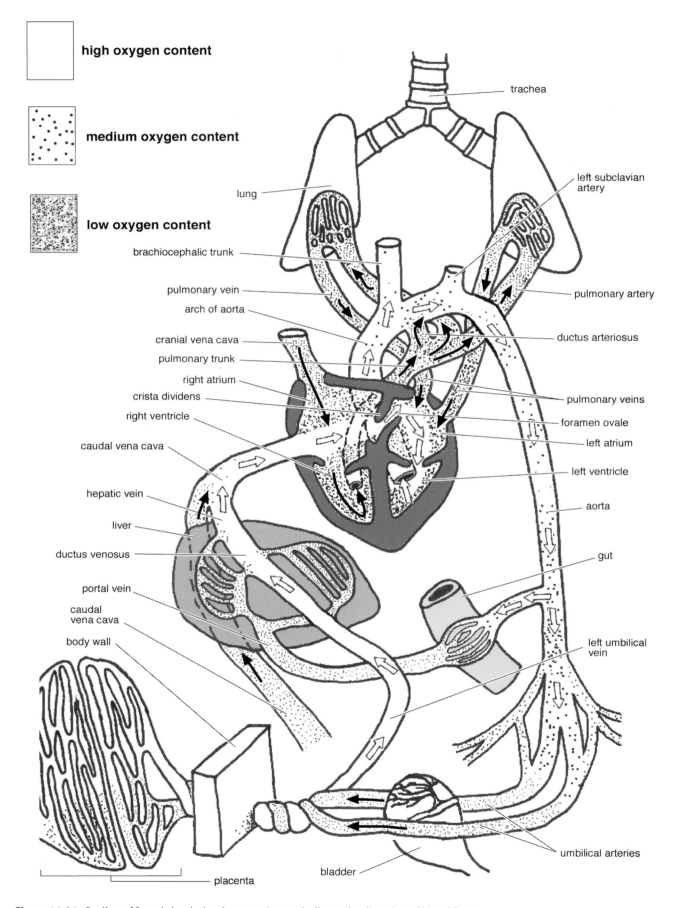

high oxygen content

medium oxygen content

low oxygen content

trachea

lung

left subclavian artery

brachiocephalic trunk

pulmonary vein

arch of aorta

cranial vena cava

pulmonary trunk

right atrium

crista dividens

right ventricle

caudal vena cava

hepatic vein

liver

ductus venosus

portal vein

caudal vena cava

body wall

pulmonary artery

ductus arteriosus

pulmonary veins

foramen ovale

left atrium

left ventricle

aorta

gut

left umbilical vein

umbilical arteries

placenta

bladder

Figure 11.24 Outline of foetal circulation *in utero*. Arrows indicate the direction of blood flow.

continues to develop, the cranial cardinal veins give rise to the internal and external jugular veins, brachiocephalic veins and the cranial vena cava. Two sets of paired veins arise from the caudal cardinal veins. The subcardinal veins drain the developing mesonephros, and the supracardinal veins drain the dorsal region of the body wall. The caudal vena cava arises from a combination of atrophy and anastomosis of the right vitelline vein, the caudal cardinal veins and the supracardinal veins. The azygos veins arise from atrophy and anastomosis of the supracardinal veins.

The circulation before birth and after birth

The placenta, acting as an organ of gaseous exchange, supplies oxygenated blood to the developing embryo. The oxygenated blood travels from the placenta via the left umbilical vein to the liver where most of it bypasses the hepatic sinusoids by way of the ductus venosus and enters the caudal vena cava (Fig. 11.24). A small volume of blood from the left umbilical vein passes through the hepatic sinusoids and mixes with the de-oxygenated blood from the portal vein. This blood also enters the vena cava. The blood in the caudal vena cava and hepatic veins, which has a decreased oxygen concentration, mixes with blood from the ductus venosus. Thus, the degree of oxygenation of blood entering the right atrium is reduced relative to the oxygen tension in the umbilical vein. The lower border of the septum secundum, the crista dividens, directs most of the blood entering the right atrium through the foramen ovale into the left atrium where it mixes with a small volume of blood of lower oxygen concentration, returning from the non-functioning foetal lungs through the pulmonary veins. This blood enters the left ventricle and is pumped throughout the body via the aortic arch. As the coronary arteries and the brachiocephalic trunk are the first branches given off by the aorta, the cardiac musculature and the brain receive highly oxygenated blood. Some of the blood from the caudal vena cava, which enters the right atrium, is directed into the right ventricle and mixes with de-oxygenated blood returning from the head via the cranial vena cava and from the myocardium via the coronary veins. The blood from the right ventricle is pumped to the pulmonary trunk where, due to the resistance of the pulmonary vessels, the greater volume passes through the ductus arteriosus to the caudal aorta. Most of the blood in the aorta is returned to the placenta for oxygenation through the umbilical arteries. Branches from the caudal aorta supply the thoracic and abdominal organs.

Circulatory changes at birth

Due to the replacement of the placenta as an organ of respiratory exchange by the functioning lungs of the newborn animal, important circulatory changes occur at birth (Fig. 11.25). As a result of compression of the thorax during birth, amniotic fluid in the bronchial tree is expelled and replaced by air as the lungs expand.

A number of important events occur in the cardiovascular system at birth:

(1) Immediately prior to birth, the umbilical arteries contract, preventing passage of blood to the placenta. After rupture of the cord, contraction of the smooth muscle and recoil of the elastic fibres in the tunica media seal the lumina of the arteries preventing haemorrhage.

(2) Contraction of the umbilical veins forces blood from the placenta into the circulation of the neonatal animal. The placental blood can contribute up to 30% of the total blood volume of the newborn animal. It is important that blood flow through the ductus venosus is halted by contraction of the muscle in its wall. Closure of the ductus venosus becomes permanent after two to three weeks. At delivery, the umbilical cord should not be immediately clamped or cut so that as much placental blood as possible is transferred to the newborn animal.

(3) Immediately after birth, contraction of the musculature of the wall of the ductus arteriosus closes this foetal shunt. As a consequence of this physiological closure, all blood in the pulmonary arteries is directed to the functioning lungs. With physiological closure, a temporary reverse flow may occur, giving rise to a transient cardiac murmur in foals, calves and pigs. Complete anatomical closure, which takes up to 2 months, is produced by infolding of the endothelium and proliferation of the subintimal connective tissue layer. Factors which may contribute to the physiological closure of the ductus arteriosus include the increased oxygen content of the blood passing through it and the production of the vasoactive amine, bradykinin, which causes smooth muscle contraction.

(4) Prior to birth, most of the blood from the caudal vena cava is directed by the crista dividens through the foramen ovale into the left atrium. The valve-like structure of the septum primum is kept open by the higher pressure of blood in the right atrium than in the left atrium. At birth the blood pressure in the right atrium decreases due in part to cessation of blood flow from the placenta, while pressure in the left atrium increases, due to increased pulmonary flow. As a result, the valve-like flap of the septum primum presses against the septum secundum closing the foramen ovale. Although functional closure occurs quickly, anatomical closure occurs gradually during the first year of life in most species of domestic animals.

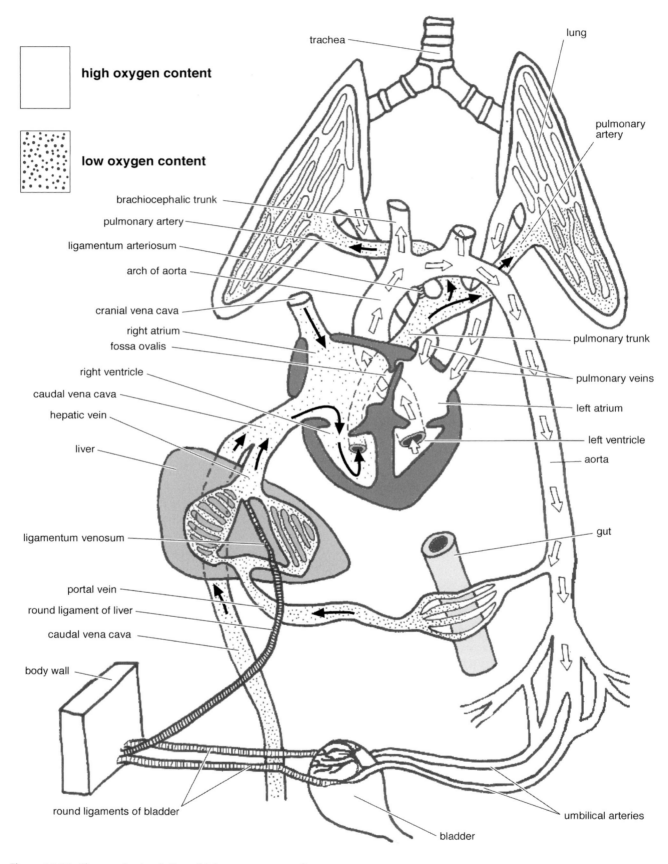

Figure 11.25 Changes in circulation which occur post-natally.

Lymphatic vessels and lymph nodes

In common with arteries and veins, lymphatic vessels arise from mesoderm by vasculogenesis and angiogenesis. Shortly after the establishment of the cardiovascular system, lymphatic vessels develop in a manner similar to that described for blood vessels. Initially, six primary lymph sacs develop in the late embryonic period. Paired jugular sacs develop lateral to the internal jugular veins, followed by a single retroperitoneal sac close to the root of the mesentery. An additional sac, the cisterna chyli, develops dorsal to the retroperitoneal sac. A pair of iliac sacs also develop at the junction of the iliac veins. Lymphatic vessels draining the head, neck and fore-

limbs arise from the jugular sacs. Drainage of lymph from the pelvic region and hind limbs is through the iliac sacs, while the retroperitoneal sac and cisterna chyli drain the viscera. Each jugular sac is connected to the cysterna chyli by a large lymphatic vessel. Anastomoses between these two vessels gives rise to a plexus of lymphatic vessels. From the combination of fusion, atrophy and remodelling of these vessels, the thoracic duct is formed. At a later stage of lymphatic development, the lymphatic sacs become interconnected by a series of lymphatic vessels and a lymphatic drainage system becomes established (Fig. 11.26). The plexus between the jugular sacs and the cisterna chyli gives rise to the thoracic duct which opens into the jugular vein. Other

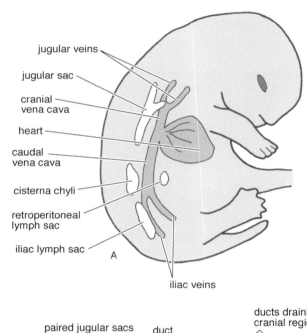

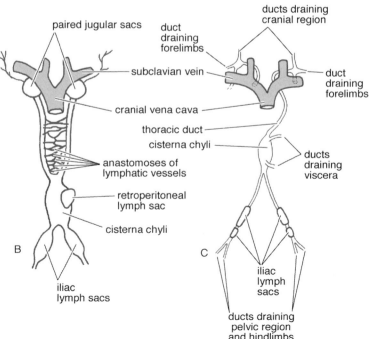

Figure 11.26 Outline of the developing lymphatic system and its drainage into the venous system.

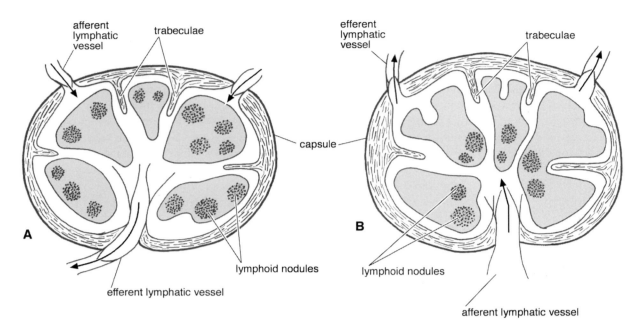

Figure 11.27 Comparative structural features of a typical mammalian lymph node, A, and a porcine lymph node, B, illustrating the distribution of lymph nodules and the direction of lymph flow (arrows).

connections between the lymphatic system and the venous system atrophy.

Development of lymph nodes

Apart from the cisterna chyli, the lymph sacs become converted into lymph nodes by aggregation of lymphoid tissue around the sacs. Mesenchymal cells which surround the sacs infiltrate these structures and convert them into a network of lymph channels. Later in development, additional lymph nodes develop along the course of the lymphatic vessels throughout the body. Lymph nodes are encapsulated structures composed of a meshwork of reticular cells containing numerous lymphocytes. The capsule and connective tissue framework of lymph nodes is also mesenchymal in origin. Developing lymph nodes become seeded by differentiated lymphocytes from the thymus and bone marrow which give rise to the nodular lymphoid masses. A typical mammalian lymph node consists of a cortical region and a medullary region (Fig. 11.27A). The cortical parenchyma at the periphery contains lymph nodules while the central medullary region contains anastomosing cords of lymphoid tissue. In most species the direction of lymphatic drainage is from the cortical region through the medulla to the hilus. The structure of the porcine lymph node differs from other domestic animals in that the lymph nodules are centrally located with the cords at the periphery (Fig. 11.27B). The flow of lymph in the porcine lymph node is in the opposite direction to that in other domestic animals, with lymph entering at the hilus and leaving from the cortex.

Adult derivatives of foetal blood vessels and associated structures

(1) The remnant of the intra-abdominal portion of the left umbilical vein persists in the adult animal as the round ligament of the liver.
(2) The ductus venosus becomes the ligamentum venosum.
(3) After anatomical closure, the foramen ovale is represented by a depression known as the fossa ovalis.
(4) The intra-abdominal portions of the umbilical arteries form the round ligaments of the bladder which are located in the lateral ligaments of the bladder (Fig. 11.25). The remains of the urachus is present in the medial ligament of the bladder.
(5) The ductus arteriosus becomes the ligamentum arteriosum.

Developmental anomalies of the cardiovascular system

In view of the complexity of the processes involved in the development of the heart and the major blood vessels, and the dramatic circulatory changes which occur at birth, it is not surprising that congenital anomalies occur occasionally in mammals. The prevalence of congenital cardiovascular anomalies in dogs is approximately 1% with a higher incidence in pedigree animals than in mixed breeds. Although patent ductus arteriosus, pulmonary stenosis, aortic stenosis, vascular ring anomalies, tetralogy of Fallot, ventricular defects and atrial defects are reported periodically in many dog breeds, the frequency of their occurrence is not constant worldwide. The frequency of cardiovascular anomalies in horses is 0.2%, in cattle 0.17% and in pigs up to 4%. In horses, cattle and pigs, ventricular septal defects and aortic stenosis are the most common cardiovascular anomalies reported. The lower recorded frequency of cardiovascular anomalies in food-producing animals may be attributed to the fact that many are usually slaughtered before clinical signs become evident.

Patent ductus arteriosus

If the ductus arteriosus remains patent after birth, rising pressure in the aorta and left ventricle forces blood from the aorta into the pulmonary artery and occasionally into the right ventricle (Fig. 11.28B). In order to maintain adequate systemic circulation for normal function, the cardiac output must be increased. The condition may be suspected by the presence of a machine-like or continuous murmur on auscultation over the region of the aortic and pulmonary valves. Patent ductus arteriosus may be hereditary in some breeds of dogs such as poodles, collies and German shepherds and occurs more commonly in bitches than in male dogs.

Pulmonary stenosis

Narrowing of the pulmonary artery or pulmonary valves impedes the normal flow of blood from the right ventricle to the lungs, a condition referred to as pulmonary stenosis (Fig. 11.28C and D). The valvular form of the condition occurs more frequently than the arterial form. The condition is reported more frequently in bulldogs, fox terriers, beagles and keeshounds than in other breeds of dogs. Clinical signs may not be detected in pups, but evidence of right heart failure can become obvious between six months and three years of age, characterised by weakness, fatigue, shortness of breath, syncope and venous congestion. In this condition, a systolic murmur can be heard on auscultation over the region of the pulmonary valve.

Aortic stenosis

Narrowing of the aorta or aortic valves impedes normal aortic outflow from the left ventricle, a condition referred to as aortic stenosis. It occurs most commonly in Newfoundland dogs, Rottweilers, boxers and German shepherds. The condition is usually caused by a sub-valvular proliferation of fibro-muscular tissue or by defective valve formation which leads to left ventricular dilatation and hypertrophy. A systolic murmur may be heard on auscultation in the region of the fourth left intercostal space of dogs with this condition (Fig. 11.28E).

Tetralogy of Fallot

Congenital malformation of the aortico-pulmonary septum, resulting in the unequal division of the truncus arteriosus, associated with a ventricular septal defect gives rise to a condition known as tetralogy of Fallot (Fig. 11.28F). The condition is characterised by an inter-ventricular septal defect, pulmonary stenosis and an enlarged aorta which is partially positioned over the right ventricle thereby allowing de-oxygenated blood from the right ventricle to enter the aorta. This anomalous development, which results in right ventricular hypertrophy, a compensatory response to pulmonary stenosis, occurs occasionally in domestic animals. Signs of this defect, which become evident early in life, include stunted growth and cyanosis following limited exercise.

Inter-atrial septal defects

Conditions involving the inter-atrial septum may arise due to failure of the foramen ovale to close leaving a permanent opening, defective development of either the foramen primum or secundum, or failure of the development of both septa resulting in the persistence of a common atrium (Fig. 11.29A).

Inter-ventricular septal defects

Defects, which are usually observed in the membranous part of the inter-ventricular septum, may occur in isolation, but are more often observed in association with other developmental anomalies. A small defect is usually of little consequence but large inter-ventricular defects result in increased pressure on the right ventricle, a consequence of increased blood volume received directly from the left ventricle (Fig. 11.29B).

Abnormalities of the position of the heart

An abnormal position of the heart may be due to interference with its normal descent into the thoracic cavity. Ectopic hearts, usually located in the neck, are observed more frequently in cattle than in other species. The condition is compatible with normal growth and development, and cows with ectopic hearts can become pregnant and give birth to normal calves.

Other cardiovascular anomalies include transposition of the great vessels, persistent truncus arteriosus and a persistent common atrio-ventricular canal.

Congenital venous shunts

Anomalies which arise due to persistence of anastomoses between the portal vein and the caudal vena cava, resulting in venous blood from the intestine bypassing

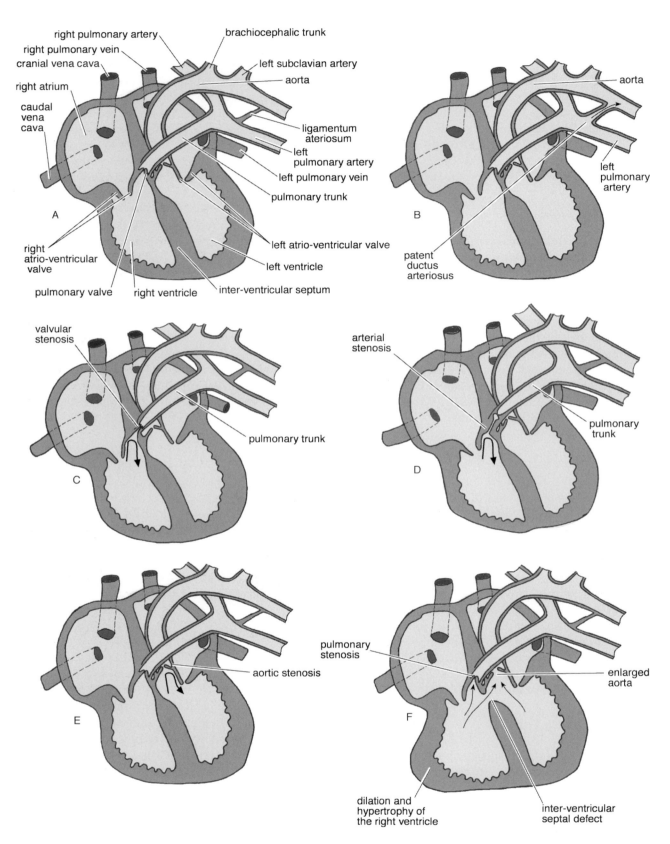

Figure 11.28 Sections through the heart showing normal anatomical arrangement, A. B, Patent ductus arteriosus. C and D, Pulmonary stenosis. E, Aortic stenosis. F, Tetralogy of Fallot. Arrows indicate direction of blood flow.

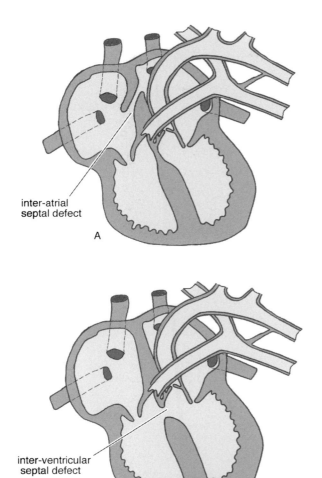

inter-atrial
septal defect

A

inter-ventricular
septal defect

B

Figure 11.29 Sections through the heart showing an inter-atrial defect, A, and an inter-ventricular defect, B.

the hepatic circulation, are referred to as congenital venous shunts. Persistence of the ductus venosus, which allows blood from the portal vein to bypass the liver and enter the caudal vena cava, is an example of an intra-hepatic venous shunt. Failure of blood to circulate through the liver results in the accumulation of toxic substances such as ammonia in the blood, which can lead to neurological dysfunction. Intra-hepatic venous shunts, which are encountered in dogs and cats, occur more frequently in retrievers, Irish setters and Irish wolfhounds than in other dog breeds. Extra-hepatic venous shunts, which arise from anastomosis between the portal and azygos veins, have been reported in small dog breeds.

Vascular ring anomalies

Anomalies in the development of the aortic arch arteries can lead to partial or complete vascular rings around the oesophagus and trachea at the base of the heart. Vascular rings may be formed from a persistent right

aortic arch derived from the right fourth aortic arch artery combined with a left ductus arteriosus, an aberrant subclavian artery, or a double aortic arch.

Persistent right aortic arch combined with left ductus arteriosus

Most vascular ring anomalies are associated with a persistent right aortic arch. If, during differentiation of the aortic arch arteries, the right fourth aortic arch forms the arch of the aorta and the right sixth aortic arch artery gives rise to the ductus arteriosus while the left segment of the dorsal aorta atrophies, a mirror image of the normal vascular arrangements occurs which is compatible with normal physiological functioning. However, if the aortic arch develops from the right fourth aortic arch artery and the ductus arteriosus arises from the left sixth aortic arch artery and the left segment of the dorsal aorta persists, a vascular ring is formed by the left ductus arteriosus and the segment of left dorsal aorta around the oesophagus and trachea (Fig. 11.30). This condition has been described in all domestic animals.

Aberrant right subclavian artery

During normal development, the right subclavian artery arises from the fourth aortic arch artery and the right seventh intersegmental artery. The segment of the right dorsal aorta between the origin of the right seventh intersegmental artery and the common aorta atrophies. If the segment of the right dorsal aorta between the right seventh intersegmental artery and the common aorta persists, and the right fourth aortic arch artery atrophies, then the right subclavian artery arises from the caudal segment of the aorta (Fig. 11.31). The artery runs cranially from its origin passing to the right of the oesophagus and coursing around the first rib. This aberrant course of the right subclavian artery can result in the formation of a partial vascular ring around the oesophagus.

Double aortic arch

Failure of the right dorsal aorta to atrophy leads to a vascular ring involving the left and right fourth aortic arch arteries and left and right dorsal aortae. This condition, which is rare, has been reported in humans and dogs.

Clinical manifestations of vascular ring anomalies

Clinical signs of vascular ring anomalies include evidence of oesophageal constriction which prevents the passage of solid food but permits fluid to pass into the stomach. Signs become evident when the animal is weaned and fed on solid food. Soon after eating,

CARDIOVASCULAR SYSTEM 11

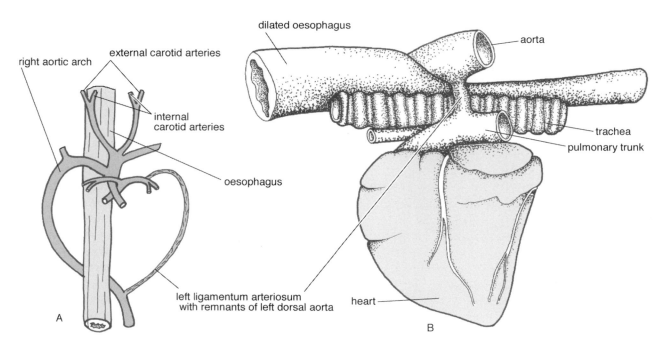

Figure 11.30 Ventral view of persistent right aortic arch with left ligamentum arteriosum, A. Left lateral view of the constriction of the oesophagus caused by left ligamentum arteriosum, B; anterior to the constriction the oesophagus is dilated.

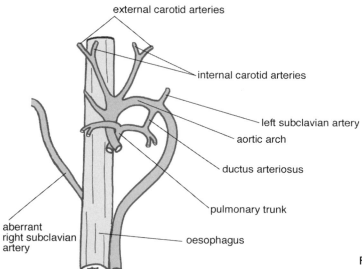

Figure 11.31 Ventral view of aberrant right subclavian artery.

regurgitation occurs. Additional complications include aspiration of food into the lungs and dyspnoea. Oesophageal dilatation, which occurs cranial to the constriction, can be detected radiographically.

Further reading

Adams, R.H. (2003) Molecular control of arterial venous blood vessel identity. *Journal of Anatomy* **202**, 105–112.

Bishop, S.P. (1998) Embryologic development: the heart and great vessels. In *Canine and Feline Cardiology*. Eds. P.R. Fox, D. Sisson and N.S. Moise. Saunders, Philadelphia, PA, pp. 3–12.

Brand, T. (2003) Heart development: molecular insights into cardiac specification and early morphogenesis. *Developmental Biology* **258**, 1–19.

Cottrill, C.M., Yenho, S. and O'Connor, W.N. (1997) Embryological development of the equine heart. *Equine Veterinary Journal*, Suppl. **24**, 14–18.

Coulter, C.B. (1909) The early development of the aortic arch arteries of the cat, with special reference to the presence of a fifth arch. *Anatomical Record* **3**, 578–592.

Field, E.J. (1946) The early development of the sheep heart. *Journal of Anatomy* **80**, 75–88.

Grimes, M.R., Greenstein, J.S. and Foley, R.C. (1958) Observations on the early development of the heart in bovine embryos with six to twenty somites. *American Journal of Veterinary Research* **19**, 591–599.

Harvey, N.L. and Oliver, G. (2004) Choose your fate: artery, vein or lymphatic vessel. *Current Opinion in Genetics and Development* **14**, 499–505.

Hiruma, T., Nakajama, Y. and Nakamura, H. (2002) Development of the pharyngeal arch arteries in the early mouse embryo. *Journal of Anatomy* **201**, 15–29.

Kienle, R.D. and Kittleson, M.D. (1998) Cardiac embryology and anatomy. In *Small Animal Cardiovascular Medicine*. Mosby, St. Louis, MO, pp. 1–10.

Lohse, C.L. and Suter, P.F. (1977) Functional closure of the ductus venosus during postnatal life of the dog. *American Journal of Veterinary Research* **38**, 839–844.

Martin, E.W. (1960) The development of the vascular system in five to twenty-one somite dog embryos. *Anatomical Record* **137**, 378.

Risau, W. (1997) Mechanisms of angiogenesis. *Nature* **386**, 671–674.

Risau, W. and Flamme, I. (1995) Vasculogenesis. *Annual Review of Cellular and Developmental Biology* **11**, 73–91.

Robinson, W.F. and Maxie, M.G. (1993) The cardiovascular system. In *Pathology of Domestic Animals*, Vol. 3, 4th edn. Eds. K.V.F. Jubb, P.C. Kennedy and N. Palmer. Academic Press, San Diego, pp. 1–100.

Schwarz, R. (1987) The fusion of the cardiac anlages and the formation of cardiac loop in the cat (*Felis domestica*). *American Journal of Anatomy* **20**, 45–72.

Van Mierop, L.H.S. (1969) Embryology, Vol. 5, Heart. In *Ciba Collection of Medical Illustrations*. Ed. F.F. Yonkman. Ciba Foundation, New York.

Vitums, A. (1969) Development and transformation of the aortic arches in the equine embryo with special attention to the formation of the definitive arch of the aorta and common brachiocephalic trunk. *Zeitschrift für Anatomie und Entwicklungsgeschichte* **128**, 243–270.

Vitums, A. (1981) The embryonic development of the equine heart. *Anatomia, histologia, embryologia* **10**, 193–211.

Weinstein, B.M. (1999) What guides early embryonic blood vessel formation? *Developmental Dynamics* **215**, 2–11.

White, R.N. and Burton, C.A. (2000) Anatomy of the patent ductus venosus. *The Veterinary Record* **146**, 425–429.

12 | Embryological and Post-natal Features of Haematopoiesis

Although blood cells have a finite life span in normal animals, the number of each cell type in the circulation is usually maintained at a relatively constant level by a process of carefully controlled production of mature cells balanced with the rate at which blood cells leave the circulation. In the absence of infectious diseases which can damage both red blood cells and white blood cells and lead to their premature removal, normal levels of cellular blood components are carefully controlled by the removal of ageing cells and their replacement by cells produced either in the bone marrow or by cells arising from the bone marrow and maturing in lymphoid organs. Sustained abnormal elevations of blood cell numbers occur in neoplastic conditions which affect the bone marrow or lymphoid tissue. At an early stage in embryological development, blood islands which form in the splanchnic mesoderm of the yolk sac contain pluripotent stem cells which can differentiate into myeloid or lymphoid progenitor cells.

A remarkable feature of haematopoiesis, the production of blood cells, is that every functionally specialised mature blood cell and a number of other cell types not present in the circulation, such as macrophages and mast cells, are derived from the same pluripotent mesodermal stem cells. Post-natally, haematopoietic cells develop and mature in the bone marrow on a meshwork of non-haematopoietic support cells, referred to as stromal cells, which include endothelial cells, fibroblasts and cells of the monocyte-macrophage series. By providing an appropriate microenvironment, stromal cells influence the growth and differentiation of haematopoietic stem cells. A range of growth factors, including colony-stimulating factors, induce the formation of distinct haematopoietic cell lines. The times at which these pluripotent stem cells move to other sites and the differentiation factors which influence their migratory routes have not yet been established with certainty. Differentiation of myeloid and lymphoid cells in the bone marrow and maturation of specialised lymphocytes in organs such as the thymus in domestic mammals, and in the cloacal bursa (bursa of Fabricius) in birds, are influenced by locally-secreted differentiation factors together with substances produced in developing tissues. Bone marrow haematopoietic stem cells lasting for the lifetime of the animal are capable of giving rise to all blood cell lineages.

Many tissues in mature animals are formed from cells which have a defined life span and are not replaced. In contrast, cells of other tissues such as epithelial cells and red blood cells undergo constant replacement when the former are sloughed and the latter are removed from the circulation by the spleen at predetermined times related to membrane alterations associated with ageing. Haematopoiesis is a complex, highly regulated process which ultimately relies on bone marrow stem cells for its continuation. Defining characteristics of embryonic stem cells include the ability to be passaged continuously, chromosome stability, the ability to form clones and the expression of a wide range of molecular, biochemical and antigenic markers. The ability to differentiate into various types of tissue sets embryonic stem cells apart from other cells in the developing embryo. Post-natally, stem cells produce populations which give rise not only to more stem cells, but also to cells capable of undergoing further development and differentiation as committed cells. From these committed stem cells, progenitor cells capable of differentiating into myeloid and lymphoid lineages arise. In haematopoiesis, therefore, haematopoietic stem cells can produce progenitors of all the myeloid and lymphoid cells required by the animal. Among these cells, red blood cells are concerned with oxygen transportation and binding of carbon dioxide for excretion by the lungs, the granulocyte-macrophage series contribute to innate immune responses, and cells of the lymphoid series participate in specific cell-mediated and humoral responses to infectious agents.

Embryological aspects of haematopoiesis

Haematopoiesis in vertebrates occurs in two successive stages and in two different anatomical sites in the developing embryo. A transient extra-embryonic phase, which

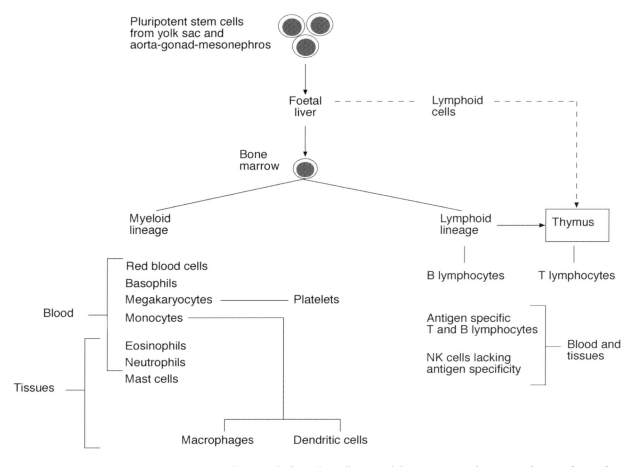

Figure 12.1 Outline of the origin and migration of stem cells from the yolk sac and the aorta–gonad–mesonephros region to the bone marrow in mammals. In the bone marrow, cells of the myeloid lineage differentiate into red blood cells, leukocytes, mast cells and megakaryocytes. Further differentiation can occur after some leukocytes are released into the bloodstream. Cells belonging to the lymphoid lineage include antigen-specific T and B lymphocytes and NK cells which lack antigen specificity. Following appropriate antigenic stimulation, B cells differentiate into plasma cells which secrete antibody. The distribution of cell types in blood and in tissues is indicated.

commences in the splanchnic mesoderm of the yolk sac with the formation of blood islands, is followed by a definitive intra-embryonic phase at a site in the vicinity of the dorsal aorta, referred to as the aorta–gonad–mesonephros (AGM) (Fig. 12.1). The murine embryo has been used extensively to elucidate haematopoiesis in mammals and much of the research data referred to in this chapter derive from the murine model.

Haematopoietic and vascular development within the yolk sac and subsequently in the embryo are closely related events. Once a circulatory system becomes established, haematopoietic stem cells (HSCs) present in the yolk sac produce primitive nucleated red blood cells which enter the embryonic circulation as a response to its increasing oxygen demands. Angioblasts and haematopoietic stem cells arise from a common splanchnic mesodermal precursor, the haemangioblast. Emergence of haematopoietic precursor cells during murine embryogenesis occurs at approximately seven days after fertilisation, as the extra-embryonic mesodermal cells

in association with the endoderm form blood islands. The outer cells of these blood islands differentiate into endothelial cells and the inner cells become primitive erythroblasts. Subsequently, the first primitive erythroid and macrophage precursors can be recognised morphologically and expression of genes characteristic of the haematopoietic cell lineage can be detected. The close relationship between haemangioblasts and HSCs is confirmed by the fact that they share various markers including vascular endothelial growth factor receptor, a receptor for foetal liver kinase (Flk-1) and expression of transcription factors for stem cell leukaemia (SCL), LMO2 and GATA-2. Despite advances in the recognition of HSCs through the identification of various markers, the only conclusive assay is assessment of their ability to give rise to myeloid and lymphoid lineages in a lethally irradiated host following transplantation.

As the first site of haematopoiesis, the yolk sac blood vessels contain mainly erythrocytes, macrophages and megakaryocytes. These cells differ in a number of ways from cells produced by mammals after birth: embryonic erythrocytes contain nuclei, macrophages bypass the monocyte stage and synthesise a different range of enzymes from the macrophages that arise from the myeloid stem cell, and the megakaryocytes produce platelets at an accelerated rate. A second wave of haematopoietic development occurs in the AGM. The dorsal aorta is considered by many investigators to be the principal site of HSC formation early in gestation in all vertebrates. In this site, cells progress to an early stem cell phase but do not differentiate into erythrocytes and do not express the transcription factor GATA-1 expressed by cells of the myeloid–erythroid lineage. It is suggested that cells derived from the AGM enter the circulation and become distributed to the foetal liver, to bone marrow and, perhaps, to other organs. Alternatively, it is possible that cells from the AGM may migrate directly through the tissues to these sites of haematopoiesis.

The *GATA-1* gene is expressed in cells of the myeloid–erythroid lineage but is required only for the maturation of erythroid progenitor cells beyond the proerythroblast stage. During murine embryogenesis, primitive nucleated red blood cells enter the circulation from the yolk sac at about the ninth day of gestation and the role of the yolk sac as a site of haematopoiesis probably declines after this time. Unresolved questions remain regarding multipotent cells of yolk sac origin. There is evidence that multipotent cells derived from the yolk sac at the ninth day of gestation are capable of generating myeloid cells that can give rise to erythroid cells, macrophages, granulocytes, mast cells, megakaryocytes and, in addition, B-lymphoid cells. It is probable, therefore, that the AGM cells support definitive development of HSCs of yolk sac origin and may later replace these progenitor cells as embryogenesis proceeds. Whether or not definitive haematopoiesis begins in an extra-embryonic location in the yolk sac, and is gradually replaced by HSCs produced in the AGM, remains unresolved and awaits further experimental investigation.

Reliable identification of cells during embryogenesis is a prerequisite for establishment, beyond reasonable doubt, of the origins of HSCs. The juxtaposition and parallel development of the endothelial and haematopoietic lineages as observed in the yolk sac and AGM have led to the concept of a common precursor – the haemangioblast – for the endothelial and the haematopoietic lineage (Fig. 11.1). The close relationship between these two lineages includes the observation that genes encoding receptor tyrosine kinases, such as Flk-1, are directly involved in endothelial cell proliferation and angiogenesis.

Haematopoietic progenitor cells have been identified in the para-aortic splanchnopleure/AGM region of murine

embryos at the ninth day of gestation. At the tenth day of gestation, cells from the AGM of a donor are capable of long-term repopulation of irradiated recipients with multi-lineage cell populations. By the thirteenth day of gestation, this haematopoietic activity of transplanted AGM cells cannot be detected. This implies that the AGM is no longer associated with haematopoietic activity and its role is probably replaced by the foetal liver after this time. Haematopoietic cells within the AGM region express genes encoding transcriptional regulators associated with HSC formation. These include *SCL, Runx-1, c-Myb, LMO-2* in addition to genes encoding the cell surface marker CD34 and the receptor molecule c-KIT. The proto-oncogene *c-Myb* selectively affects definitive haematopoiesis and haematopoietic cells in the para-aortic splanchnopleure–AGM region. The transmembrane proteins CD34 and c-KIT are recognised as important stem cell markers in the bone marrow, not only in mice, but also in other vertebrates.

Haematopoietic activity extends from the yolk sac and AGM to the liver, spleen and finally to the bone marrow as embryogenesis proceeds. The foetal liver, however, does not produce its own haematopoietic cells but acquires its blood-forming capacity from cells originating in the yolk sac or AGM. In mice, the liver primordium is recognisable as an endodermal outgrowth from the foregut beneath the pericardial cavity at the tenth day of gestation. Colonisation of the murine foetal liver begins after the tenth day of gestation and, by the 12th day, non-nucleated erythroid cells are found in the circulation and the population of primitive erythrocytes declines as definitive haematopoiesis commences. Although a range of myeloid and lymphoid progenitor cells are present in the developing liver, erythropoiesis is the principal activity of the foetal liver. By day 14, maturing erythroid cells form erythroblastic islands, but as hepatic haematopoietic activity declines, the size of these islands decreases. Haematopoiesis in the liver decreases after birth and the erythroblastic islands gradually disappear.

Towards the end of foetal life, the spleen is primarily an erythropoietic organ which aids in the transfer of haematopoiesis from the foetal liver to the bone marrow. Although the splenic rudiment which forms as a mesenchymal thickening in the dorsal mesogastrium is colonised by HSCs at the 12th day of gestation in the mouse, it does not become a haematopoietic site until the 16th day when both immature erythroid cells and small lymphocytes can be recognised in splenic tissue. Despite inconclusive supporting evidence for the presence of HSCs in the murine bone marrow by the 18th day, it is likely that they are present, as B cell precursors have been demonstrated by the 15th day with lymphopoiesis occurring by the 17th day. The murine bone marrow remains the main site of haematopoiesis throughout adult life. An outline of the origin, differentiation and maturation of blood cells and related cells produced during haematopoiesis in mammals is shown in Fig. 12.2.

Avian haematopoiesis has some common features with the murine model but also has some different developmental stages. Extra-embryonic mesodermal cells of the yolk sac differentiate into primitive red blood cells after 36 hours of incubation and the embryonic circulation begins by the second day, once the vascular network has developed. In the avian embryonic system, primitive red blood cells are of yolk sac origin. Whereas all definitive haematopoietic cells arise from an intra-embryonic location, there is evidence that haematopoietic activity arises in the avian bone marrow independent of HSCs of AGM origin. Unlike haematopoiesis in mammals, blood cell formation in the chick embryo does not include a hepatic stage.

Two regions in the avian AGM exhibit haematopoietic activity, the intra-aortic clusters and the para-aortic foci. Between the third and the fourth days of incubation, the intra-aortic clusters are closely associated with the endothelium within the dorsal aorta and express genes encoding c-Myb and the cell surface molecule CD45. The para-aortic foci arise between the sixth and the eighth days in the ventral wall of the aorta and display diffuse haematopoietic activity which corresponds with the colonisation of the splenic, thymic and bursal rudiments. Haematopoietic activity in the para-aortic foci ceases two days before blood formation commences in the bone marrow. It has been suggested that HSCs may derive from the allantois, as it is capable of producing haematopoietic cells which can seed the bone marrow. Before hatching, the bone marrow becomes the primary source of haematopoietic cells and it continues to produce blood cells throughout the lifetime of the bird.

Although there is limited information on human haematopoiesis, the data available suggest that the human and murine embryos have many common developmental features both in the sequential progression of haematopoiesis in different sites and in the embryonic tissues involved. In the human embryo, the CD34 glycoprotein is a marker for both vascular endothelial cells and the earliest multipotent haematopoietic stem cells. The pan-leukocyte surface molecule CD45 can be used to distinguish the two populations of CD34+ cells as it is present only on haematopoietic cells. After the 18th day of gestation, primitive erythroblasts and CD34+ haematopoietic cells can be identified in the human yolk sac, confirming that haematopoiesis has begun. At the 22nd day of gestation, the heart begins to beat, and subsequently erythroid cells are present in the embryonic circulation. After the 24th day of gestation, the yolk sac ceases to be a source of HSCs.

Between the 24th and the 34th days of gestation haematopoietic cells with both lymphoid and myeloid capability have been detected in the para-aortic splanchnopleure and the aorta. On the 26th day of gestation, CD34+ haematopoietic cells are present in the mesenchyme surrounding the dorsal aorta and cells with the same characteristics are present in the endothelium of the dorsal aorta shortly afterwards.

The primordial human liver, which is present on the 23rd day of gestation, becomes colonised by CD45+ and CD34+ haematopoietic cells about seven days after its formation. The CD34+ cell population in hepatic tissue increases up to the 42nd day and, at this stage, the liver is the main haematopoietic organ in the developing embryo. Erythroid cells, which are the major cell type present in the embryonic liver, are located extra-vascularly. Although scattered erythroid precursor cells may be present in the livers of some neonatal babies, haematopoiesis in hepatic tissue usually ceases at birth. After the tenth week of gestation, small numbers of CD34+ haematopoietic cells can be detected in the bone marrow and haematopoiesis continues in the bone marrow throughout life.

Cell differentiation and maturation during haematopoiesis

HSCs are attracted to the bone marrow microenvironment, a process referred to as homing. The mechanisms which regulate homing may be active processes or, alternatively, may be merely attraction of HSCs to particular sites by locally-secreted chemotactic factors with subsequent binding of adhesion proteins on the surface of HSCs to extra-cellular matrix at those particular sites. The events which initiate and regulate homing of HSCs are not yet defined.

Within the bone marrow, stem cells and their derivatives are intimately associated with connective tissue cells, termed bone marrow stromal cells. The developmental pathway of pluripotent stem cell descendants is greatly influenced by microenvironmental factors in the bone marrow, especially by haematopoietic growth factors and other cytokines (Fig. 12.3).

Bone morphogenic protein 4 (Bmp-4) acting on splanchnic mesoderm promotes haematopoietic development. This factor is critical in the formation of blood islands in mammalian extra-embryonic mesoderm. The haemangioblast expresses both Flk-1 and SCL, the former promoting endothelial development and the latter promoting haematopoietic commitment.

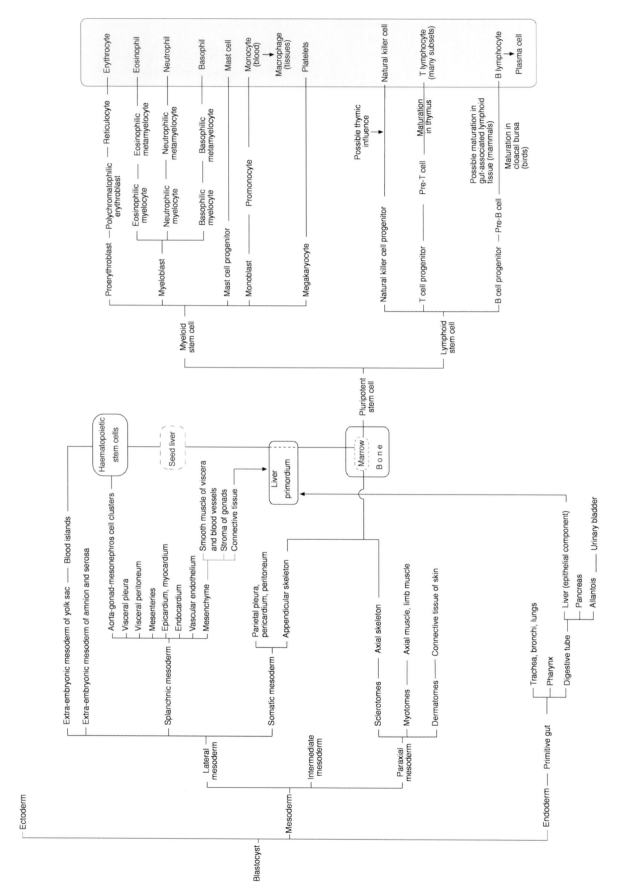

Figure 12.2 Outline of the origin of pluripotent stem cells in the bone marrow and their derivatives.

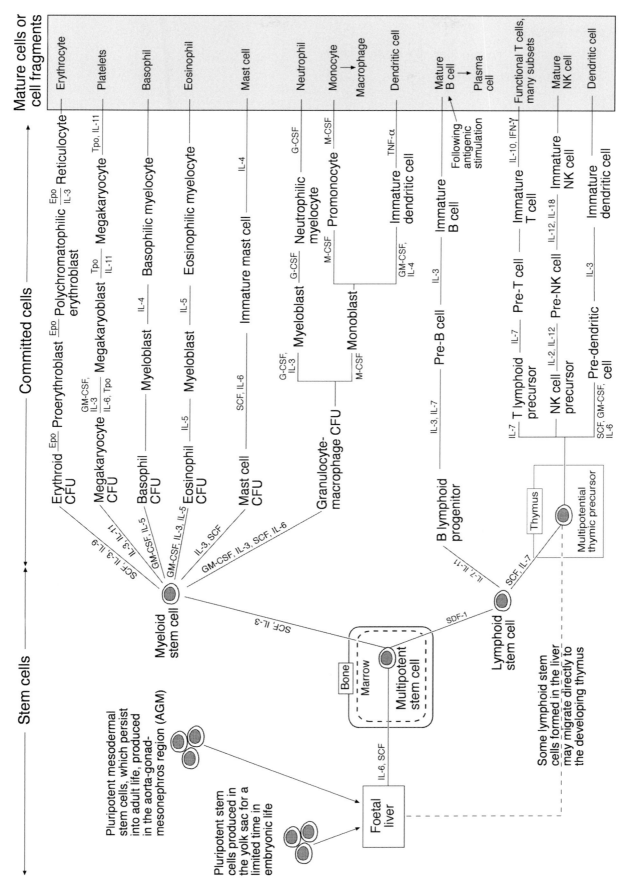

Figure 12.3 Proposed scheme for the origin, differentiation and maturation of blood cells and related cells which are produced during haematopoiesis in mammals. The precise origin, site of differentiation and maturation of some cell types awaits supporting experimental evidence. Extra-cellular growth factors and differentiation factors play a major role in determining the lineage of haematopoietic cells.

Epo: Erythropoietin

CFU: Colony forming unit

GM-CSF: Granulocyte–monocyte colony-stimulating factor

G-CSF: Granulocyte colony-stimulating factor

IL: Interleukin

IFN-γ : Interferon-γ

M-CSF: Monocyte colony-stimulating factor

SCF: Stem cell factor

SDF-1: Stromal-derived factor-1

TNF-α: Tumour necrosis factor-α

Tpo: Thrombopoietin

Figure 12.3 (*continued*)

Flk-1 is a cell surface receptor for vascular endothelial growth factor exclusively expressed on endothelial cells. Haematopoiesis can be considered as a process of cellular development and differentiation largely controlled by a hierarchical array of transcription factors, many with overlapping patterns of activity. Some of these factors are expressed only in immature cells while others have lineage specificity. The basic transcription factor SCL is expressed in all embryonic haemogenic sites and is absolutely required for haematopoiesis. The genetic regulator Runx-1 is strongly expressed at all haemogenic sites after the eighth day of gestation in murine embryos, and mutation of *Runx1* blocks definitive but not primitive haematopoiesis leading to embryonic death by the 12th day. Two transcription factors, GATA-1 and GATA-2, are associated with the myeloid lineage; the former is required for erythrocyte differentiation and the latter is present in all myeloid precursor cells. Hox genes are expressed in dynamic patterns during blood cell maturation throughout the life of an animal. Among these genes, expression of *HoxB-4* is critical for the self-renewal of HSCs in adult animals and expression of this gene in yolk sac HSCs enables these cells to repopulate the bone marrow in adult animals. Stem cell homeostasis in adult animals may be strongly influenced by microenvironmental factors such as bone morphogenic proteins which regulate early embryogenesis; Hedgehog signalling may promote stem cell differentiation through modulation of the bone morphogenic protein pathway. Stromal factors such as c-Kit and Flt-3 ligands, which act on their respective tyrosine kinase receptors, have their principal effects at the progenitor cell level.

More than 20 extra-cellular proteins, referred to as haematopoietic growth factors, affect cell proliferation and differentiation at various stages during haematopoiesis. Colony assays have been used to investigate growth factor requirements of differentiating cells from the mesoderm to committed lineage development. Activin A and Bmp-4 are able to induce mesoderm formation using *in vitro* models. The ability of Bmp-4 to direct haematopoietic activity in splanchnic mesoderm has been demonstrated and synergism between Bmp-4 and vascular endothelial growth factor in the generation of colony-forming cells indicates a possible role for Bmp-4 in the promotion of haemangioblast development. In addition to its role in the regulation of megakaryocyte differentiation and proliferation and in the regulation of platelet production, thrombopoietin has recently been shown to play an important role in the maintenance of HSC proliferation and in yolk sac haematopoiesis. Growth factors associated with myeloid lineage development include granulocyte–macrophage colony-stimulating factor (GM-CSF), macrophage colony-stimulating factor (M-CSF) and granulocyte colony-stimulating factor (G-CSF). For the development of most myeloid cells from their earliest progenitors, GM-CSF is usually required. The combination of GM-CSF and G-CSF tends to stimulate neutrophil formation from the common granulocyte-macrophage progenitor cell whereas M-CSF in combination with GM-CSF stimulates differentiation of the monocyte-macrophage lineage from the same progenitor cell. It is evident that growth and differentiation factors do not have strict specificity for one target cell as their effect on individual cells is influenced by the associated action of other factors acting on cells of that lineage. There is still debate as to whether cells in the haematopoietic series are genetically committed to a particular lineage or whether soluble factors determine lineage selection. However, it seems probable that exposure to soluble factors may not be a requirement for stem cell differentiation and that these factors have a facilitating rather than an inductive role. Stages in the maturation of lymphoid and myeloid cells are shown in Figs. 12.4 and 12.5 respectively. A summary of the important features of blood cells and associated cells is presented in Table 12.1.

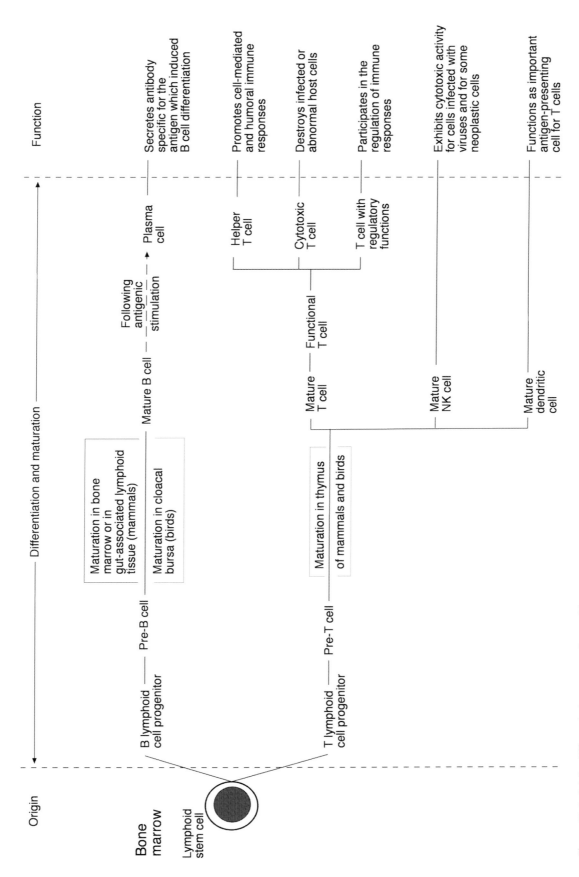

Figure 12.4 Origin, differentiation, maturation and functional activity of lymphoid cells.

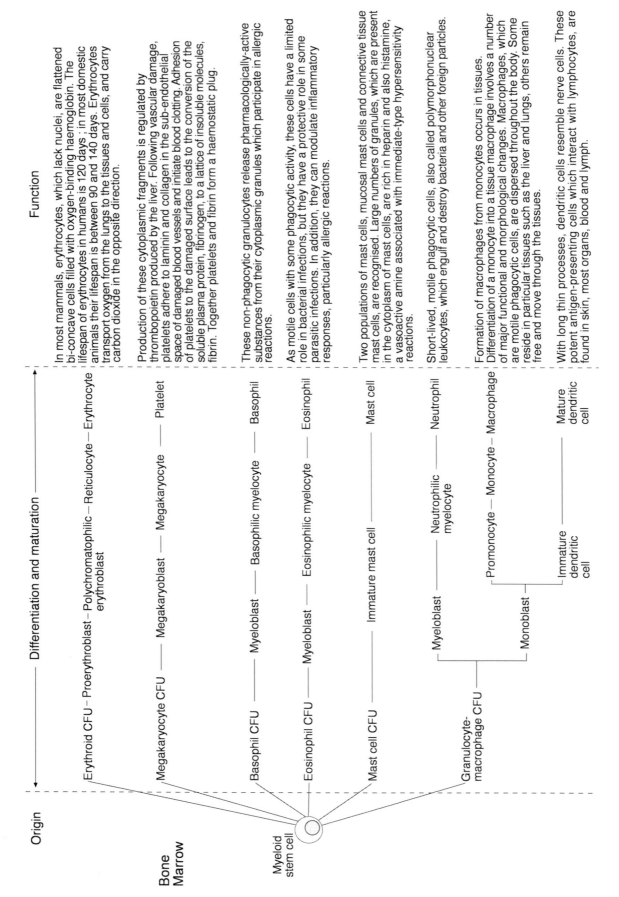

Figure 12.5 Origin, differentiation, maturation and functional activity of cells and formed elements which derive from myeloid stem cells.

Table 12.1 Origin, lineage, distribution and other attributes of cells or formed elements produced during haematopoiesis or derived from blood cells.

Cells or formed elements	Origin	Lineage	Morphology	Distribution	Comments
Basophils	Bone marrow	Myeloid	Lobed nuclei, with large metachromatic cytoplasmic granules	Blood	Non-phagocytic granulocytes, which constitute less than 1% of circulating white blood cells. Their granules, which stain deeply with basic dyes, contain pharmacologically active substances which participate in allergic reactions.
B lymphocytes	Bone marrow	Lymphoid	Round or slightly indented condensed nuclei	Blood and tissues	All lymphocytes arise from a common stem cell in the bone marrow and, unlike T lymphocytes, which mature in the thymus, B lymphocytes of mammals mature either in the bone marrow or in gut-associated lymphoid tissue. The site of maturation of B lymphocytes in birds is the bursa of Fabricius. When stimulated by antigen for which they have receptors, B cells differentiate into plasma cells which produce specific antibody. Following antigenic stimulation, some B cells, known as memory cells, persist and these cells are responsible for immunological memory.
Dendritic cells	Bone marrow	Some arise from myeloid stem cells; others may derive from lymphoid stem cells	Large mononuclear cells with long thin processes resembling dendrites of nerve cells	Found in skin, most organs, lymphoid tissue, blood and lymph	These important antigen-presenting cells for T lymphocytes are assigned names associated with their location: Langerhans cells in the epidermis, interstitial dendritic cells in most organs, interdigitating dendritic cells in T cell areas of secondary lymphoid tissue, and circulating dendritic cells in blood and lymph.
Eosinophils	Bone marrow	Myeloid	Bi-lobed nuclei with large cytoplasmic granules which have an affinity for acidic dyes	Blood and tissues	Motile cells with some phagocytic ability, which have a protective role against metazoan parasites. They also have a role in the modulation of inflammatory responses, particularly hypersensitivity reactions.
Erythrocytes	Bone marrow	Myeloid	Non-nucleated flattened, bi-concave cells	Blood	The rate of erythrocyte production is controlled by the hormone erythropoietin which is produced by cortical and medullary kidney cells. Production of erythropoietin is regulated by oxygen tension; under conditions of low oxygen tension, the level of circulating erythropoietin increases. Erythrocytes, which are the most abundant cells in the blood, have a life span of 120 days in humans and between 90 and 140 days in domestic animals. They transport oxygen from the lungs to the tissues and carry carbon dioxide in the opposite direction.
Macrophages	Bone marrow	Myeloid	Large mononuclear cells; the nuclei have irregular outlines	Present in tissues throughout the body. Some reside in particular organs, others move through the tissues	Formation of macrophages from monocytes occurs in the tissues. Resident macrophages which occur in the tissues and organs are named according to their location: alveolar macrophages in the lung, Kupffer cells in the liver, microglial cells in the brain, mesangial cells in the kidney. Macrophages are motile, long-lived phagocytic cells involved in destruction of microbial pathogens and antigen presentation to T lymphocytes. Activated macrophages secrete a range of cytokines and actively participate in both non-specific and specific immunity.
Mast cells	Bone marrow	Myeloid	Mononuclear cells with metachromatic cytoplasmic granules	Connective tissue near blood vessels and nerves, the lamina propria of mucosal tissue	The membrane-bound granules of mast cells are rich in histamine and heparin. These cells also synthesise lipid mediators and cytokines. Histamine and lipid mediators are involved in immediate-type hypersensitivity reactions. Membrane receptors for IgE on mast cells bind these immunoglobulins which, when cross-linked by antigen, trigger degranulation of mast cells and release of mediators.

Table 12.1 (*continued*)

Cells or formed elements	Origin	Lineage	Morphology	Distribution	Comments
Monocytes	Bone marrow	Myeloid	Large mononuclear cells with kidney-shaped nuclei	Blood	Motile phagocytic cells, present for hours in the circulation. On entry into tissues, they differentiate into macrophages and dendritic cells.
Natural killer cells	Bone marrow	Lymphoid	Large granular mononuclear cells	Blood and peripheral tissues	These large granular lymphocyte-like cells, which lack antigen-specific receptors, play a role in the early stages of non-specific immunity. They can bind directly and non-specifically to virus-infected cells and tumour cells, and kill these target cells. Because natural killer cells have receptors for the Fc portion of IgG molecules, they can participate in antibody-dependent cell-mediated cytotoxicity with the destruction of target cells with antibody bound to their surfaces.
Neutrophils	Bone marrow	Myeloid	Multi-lobed nuclei with pale pink cytoplasmic granules	Blood; migrate into tissues in response to chemotactic stimuli	Short-lived, motile phagocytic cells, also called polymorphonuclear leukocytes, which engulf and destroy many common bacteria and other foreign particles. Their primary granules contain elastase and myeloperoxidase, and their secondary granules contain proteases and also lysozyme, an important antibacterial substance.
Plasma cells	Bone marrow	Lymphoid	Basophilic cells with prominent Golgi apparatus and endoplasmic reticulum and eccentric cartwheel-shaped nuclei	Connective tissue and secondary lymphoid organs including the spleen, lymphoid aggregates and lymph nodes	Following antigenic stimulation of B cells, these lymphocytes differentiate into antibody-secreting plasma cells. The interaction of antigen with surface membrane-bound IgM or IgD on B cells, often with the participation of antigen-presenting cells and helper T cells, selectively induces activation and differentiation of B cell clones of corresponding specificity. Plasma cells, which are terminally differentiated cells, have a life span of up to 2 weeks.
Platelets	Bone marrow, from megakaryoctes	Myeloid	Cytoplasmic fragments	Blood	Platelets are small cytoplasmic fragments produced by megakaryocytes under the influence of thrombopoietin. Adhesion of platelets to the sub-endothelium of damaged blood vessels initiates blood clotting.
T lymphocytes	Arise from lymphoid stem cells in the bone marrow which mature in the thymus	Lymphoid	Round or slightly indented condensed nuclei	Blood and tissues	Two major functional subsets, termed cytotoxic T cells and helper T cells, can be distinguished by the expression of membrane glycoprotein molecules. Cytotoxic T cells have CD8 molecules, and helper T cells have CD4 molecules. All T cell sub-populations express the T cell receptor which cannot combine with antigen unless the antigen is complexed with particular cell membrane proteins called major histocompatibility complex proteins. Cytotoxic T cells can kill infected or abnormal host cells; helper T cells can promote cell-mediated and humoral immune responses.

Stem cells in human adults and mature animals

In recent years, stem cells in adults, capable of maintaining, generating and replacing terminally differentiated cells within their own committed line of differentiation, have been described and characterised. Examples of such stem cells in human adults include haematopoietic stem cells capable of producing bone marrow, lymphoid and myeloid cells, neural stem cells with the ability to differentiate into neurons, astrocytes and oligodendrocytes, and pancreatic stem cells capable of producing beta cells. A surprising finding from *in vitro* studies using marked, unselected cells of bone marrow origin transplanted into suitably prepared animals was the ability of the transferred cells to form non-lymphoid, non-myeloid tissue such as muscle fibres, hepatocytes, microglia and astroglia, and neuronal tissue. Further evidence that haematopoietic stem cells are capable of multifunctional differentiation has been provided by *in vitro* transfer of single cells which differentiated into mature haematopoietic cells and also into epithelial cells of the skin, lungs and gastrointestinal tract. The differentiation of stem cells derived from bone marrow into organ-specific, non-myeloid, non-lymphoid cells raises many fundamental questions about the inherent pluripotentiality of stem cells and their ability to produce lineage-restricted tissue in some defined microenvironments and, in other circumstances, to evade the lineage barrier and produce an unexpected range of tissues and cells, a phenomenon referred to as trans-differentiation. Mechanisms suggested for the generation of solid-organ tissue cells through differentiation of bone marrow-derived and circulating stem cells from adults include trans-differentiation of lineage-restricted stem cells, and de-differentiation of mature cells followed by re-differentiation. A number of scientific reports, however, strongly support the plasticity of lineages within the haematopoietic system and extending also to non-haematopoietic lineages. It has been suggested that migration of HSCs throughout the circulatory system and the influence of signalling factors such as vascular endothelial growth factor or cytokines such as granulocyte colony-stimulating factor may be responsible for many organs becoming HSC reservoirs. It has also been suggested that the heterogeneity of stem cells rather than trans-differentiation or de-differentiation may account for the apparent plasticity of HSCs *in vivo*. This latter proposal implies that many stem cell types may be distributed in various sites throughout the developing embryo or that they may migrate subsequently to the bone marrow where they may coexist. A spectrum of stem-like cells representing a continuum of mesoderm, haemangioblasts and HSCs may be maintained in the bone marrow throughout life. Irrespective of the underlying mechanisms, it appears that haematopoietic stem cells may, in some instances, be lineage-restricted, and in other circumstances these pluripotent cells may not be subject to lineage restriction.

Immunodeficiency

Protection against infectious agents is a fundamental requirement for survival. An optimally functioning immune system comprising naturally-occurring soluble antimicrobial factors such as lysozyme and complement, and phagocytic cells of the myeloid series together with B and T lymphocytes, are required to ensure protection against opportunistic infection of environmental origin or the more serious threat arising from infection with pathogenic microorganisms (Fig. 12.6). Any defect in the cells or secretions which cooperatively contribute to protection against infection renders animals, especially newborn animals, vulnerable to tissue invasion by

microbial pathogens. Immunodeficiency, a failure in non-specific immunity or specific immunity, may be either primary or secondary in origin. As the principal consequence of immunodeficiency is an increased susceptibility to infection, animals with immunodeficiencies are prone to a range of infections with bacteria, viruses, fungi and protozoa. They are also prone to certain types of tumours caused by oncogenic viruses.

Primary or congenital immunodeficiency is a result of developmental failure of lymphoid stem cells, intrinsic defects in T cells, B cells, phagocytic cells or NK cells or a deficiency in complement components. Sites at which defects leading to primary immunodeficiency can occur are shown in Fig. 12.7. Secondary immunodeficiency, unlike primary immunodeficiency, is not due to a failure or intrinsic defect in B or T lymphocytes or in cells of the myeloid series. The factors which contribute to the occurrence of secondary immunodeficiency include infectious and neoplastic conditions, exposure to ionising radiation, malnutrition, administration of cytotoxic drugs, and consumption of toxic substances in food, such as mycotoxins. These deleterious factors can interfere with the normal production of B and T lymphocytes in the bone marrow and thymus. Damage to stem cells in the bone marrow can also adversely affect production of myeloid cells associated with non-specific immunity, particularly neutrophils and macrophages. Humans and animals with secondary immunodeficiencies become susceptible to infection with opportunistic microorganisms to which they would normally be resistant.

Primary immunodeficiency syndromes

Reticular dysgenesis

The most severe primary immunodeficiency in humans results from a defect at the level of the haematopoietic multipotent stem cell in the bone marrow. This condition, which has an autosomal recessive mode of inheritance, leads to developmental failure of B cells, T cells and granulocytes. Reticular dysgenesis leads to early death of affected babies.

Severe combined immunodeficiency disease

In this heterogeneous group of diseases, both cell-mediated immunity and antibody production are defective. Severe combined immunodeficiency diseases are due to developmental defects at the level of the lymphoid stem cell in the bone marrow, and in humans about half of these are X-linked and affect only male children. In general, there is lymphopoenia with deficiency of B and T lymphocytes. The thymus, which is usually hypoplastic, contains few or no lymphocytes. Blood lymphocyte numbers and antibody titres are

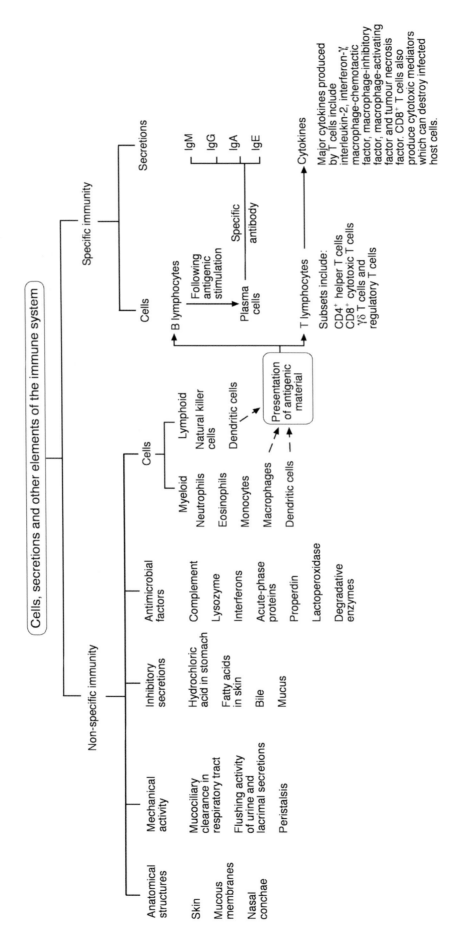

Figure 12.6 Anatomical structures, physiological activities, cells and their secretions which cooperatively contribute to protection against infection.

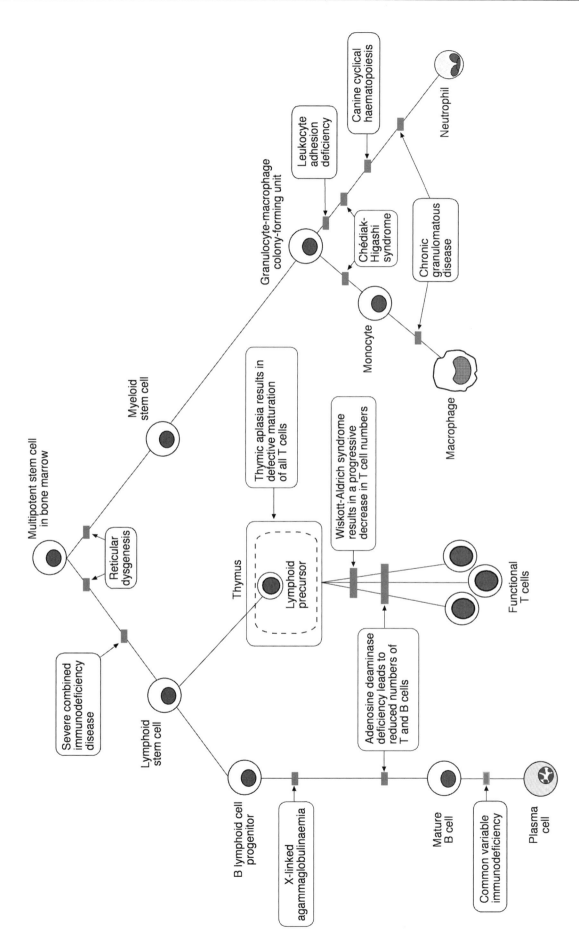

Figure 12.7 Sites at which defects in the development or maturation of lymphoid and myeloid cells lead to primary immunodeficiencies in humans and in some animals.

markedly reduced. Affected babies are highly suscept-ible to infection and rarely survive more than a few months. About 50% of the autosomal recessive form of severe combined immunodeficiency diseases are due to deficiency of an enzyme called adenosine deaminase which catalyses the deamination of adenosine and deoxyadenosine, producing inosine and deoxyinosine respectively. The enzyme, which is widely distributed in cells, is particularly abundant in lymphocytes. When adenosine deaminase deficiency occurs, accumulation of deoxyadenosine and deoxyadenosine triphosphate occurs in many cells, particularly B and T lymphocytes. These metabolites, by inhibiting ribonucleotide reduc-tase activity, block DNA synthesis. As a consequence of adenosine deaminase deficiency, reduced numbers of B and T lymphocytes are produced. In contrast to other forms of severe combined immunodeficiency diseases, children with adenosine deaminase deficiency have Hassal's corpuscles in their thymic glands.

Severe combined immunodeficiency is the most import-ant congenital immunodeficiency recognised in Arabian horses. Affected foals fail to produce functional B or T lymphocytes and few circulating lymphocytes are pre-sent in their blood. Neutrophil and monocyte function is usually normal in affected foals. Maternal antibodies, acquired through ingestion of colostrum, usually confer passive protection for up to three months. Once these passively transferred immunoglobulins are catabolised, affected foals are unable to produce antibodies of their own and they become agammaglobulinaemic; most die before six months of age from infections caused by opportunistic pathogens. On post-mortem examination, the spleens of affected animals lack lymphoid follicles and germinal centres, lymph nodes lack germinal centres, and cellular depletion is evident in their paracortical regions. Thymus development is so limited that thymic tissue may be difficult to find in affected animals. As severe combined immunodeficiency is inherited in an autoso-mal recessive manner, its occurrence indicates that both parents carry the mutation and this can be confirmed by DNA analysis. Arabian foals homozygous for the trait are clinically affected. Genetic analysis has shown that more than 8% of Arabian horses carry the gene.

An autosomal recessive mutation which arose in an inbred strain of CB mice resulted in severe combined immunodeficiency. In homozygous mice with this defect, referred to as SCID mice, both B and T cells are absent. Affected mice have no serum immunoglobulins and are unable to produce cell-mediated immune responses. The defects in SCID mice result from an inability to express antigen-specific receptors on their lymphocytes due to an absence of DNA recombinase required for rearrange-ment of T cell receptors and immunoglobulin genes. In this mutation, development of B cells ceases before

expression of cytoplasmic or cell-membrane immuno-globulins. Likewise, T cell development is arrested at an early stage before antigen-specific receptors are expressed. Thus, no functional B or T lymphocytes are produced.

Thymic aplasia or hypoplasia

This condition, referred to as the DiGeorge syndrome in humans, occurs when the immune system is deprived of thymic influence due to defective development of the third and fourth pharyngeal pouches. Failure of neural crest cell migration to the third and fourth pharyngeal pouches results in cardiac abnormalities and also in failure of normal thymus and parathyroid development. In addition to defects in cell-mediated immunity, hypo-calcaemia and associated tetany are commonly observed in DiGeorge syndrome. Few or no mature T cells are present in the blood, lymph nodes or spleen. In periph-eral blood, both the number of B cells and immuno-globulin levels are usually normal. Affected children have an increased susceptibility to infection with viruses, intracellular bacteria, fungi and protozoa. DiGeorge syndrome, which is not hereditary, occurs sporadically and is associated with translocations involving chromo-some 22.

An important animal model of T cell immunodeficiency is the nude mouse. This mouse strain has an inherited defect of epithelial cells in the skin leading to hairless-ness, and also in the lining of the third and fourth pha-ryngeal pouches, resulting in a non-functional thymus. The condition is due to a recessive gene on chromosome 11 and, accordingly, occurs in homozygous animals only. As affected mice have rudimentary thymic glands, T cell maturation does not occur and there are few or no mature T lymphocytes in peripheral lymphoid tissue. Nude mice do not exhibit typical cell-mediated immune responses, yet they can clear infections with intracellular bacteria. This surprising finding is attributed to normal or even increased numbers of NK cells in these animals. As NK cells can produce interferon-γ which activates macrophages, intracellular bacteria can be eliminated by these phagocytic cells.

X-linked agammaglobulinaemia

Agammaglobulinaemia which is inherited in an X-linked manner and is characterised by an absence of immuno-globulins in the serum is called X-linked agamma-globulinaemia or Bruton-type agammaglobulinaemia. Although pre-B cells are present at normal levels, they fail to develop into mature B cells. The genetic defect in affected children relates to mutation of Bruton's tyro-sine kinase gene which is normally expressed at all stages of B cell differentiation. Without this gene, terminal dif-ferentiation of B cells does not take place. It is possible that Bruton's tyrosine kinase is involved in signalling events which are essential for light chain gene expression. A mutant mouse strain called CBA/N has an X-linked defect in B cell development which is a consequence of a point mutation in the tyrosine kinase gene.

Wiskott–Aldrich syndrome

An uncommon X-linked immunodeficiency, referred to as the Wiskott–Aldrich syndrome, is characterised by eczema, thrombocytopenia and immunodeficiency. Although first described as a blood-clotting disorder, this syndrome is also associated with immunodeficiency due to reduced T cell numbers, impaired T cell function and a failure of antibody responses to encapsulated bacteria. This syndrome is caused by a defective gene on the X chromosome encoding a protein called Wiskott–Aldrich syndrome protein (WASP). This protein is known to regulate the organisation of the actin cytoskeleton and to be important for the effective interaction of B and T lymphocytes. In patients with this condition and in mice whose *WASP* gene has been knocked out, cytotoxic T cell responses are impaired and T cell support for B cell responses to polysaccharide antigens is lacking. As *WASP* is expressed in haematopoietic cell lineages, it is likely to be important in regulation of lymphocyte and platelet development and function.

Inherited defects in natural immunity

Natural or innate immunity is mediated principally by phagocytic cells and complement. Through their phagocytic activity, polymorphonuclear leukocytes, monocytes and macrophages play an important part in natural immunity. Phagocytic defects are well recognised in humans and domestic animals.

Chronic granulomatous disease

In chronic granulomatous disease, the final step in killing of engulfed microorganisms is defective. The intra-cellular survival of bacteria leads to granuloma formation. More than 60% of cases of chronic granulomatous diseases show an X-linked pattern of inheritance. In this disease, phagocytes cannot produce the superoxide radical and their antibacterial activity is thereby greatly impaired.

When neutrophils and macrophages engulf bacteria and fungi, they rapidly consume oxygen and liberate superoxide which is a precursor of the reactive oxygen intermediates involved in the intra-cellular killing of microbial pathogens. Superoxide generation is mediated by an enzyme, nicotinamide adenine dinucleotide phosphate oxidase (NADPH-oxidase). Several different genetic defects affecting any one of the four constituent proteins of the NADPH-oxidase system can lead to failure of intra-cellular killing of bacteria. The most common form is due to mutation of a gene located on the X chromosome coding for cytochrome b.

Deficiencies in the enzymes glucose-6-phosphate dehydrogenase and myeloperoxidase also impair intra-cellular killing and lead to similar but less severe defects in affected children.

Chédiak–Higashi syndrome

The Chédiak–Higashi syndrome is an autosomal recessive disease characterised by abnormal giant granules and organelles in neutrophils, monocytes and NK cells, and defects in pigmentation and in platelet function. A defect in a gene encoding a protein involved in intra-cellular vesicle formation causes a failure of lysosomes to fuse properly with phagosomes. Because phagocytes in affected humans and animals have defective degranulation mechanisms, there is impaired fusion of lysosomes with phagosomes, and these phagocytic cells exhibit diminished ability to kill ingested microorganisms. Such phagocytic cells also have defective chemotactic responsiveness and reduced motility.

Chédiak–Higashi syndrome has been reported in humans, cattle, mink, Persian cats, white tigers, beige mice and killer whales. Some affected animals have ocular abnormalities and a tendency to bleed excessively after surgical procedures.

Leukocyte adhesion deficiency

Before neutrophils can leave blood vessels and migrate to sites of inflammation in tissues, they must first adhere to vascular endothelial cells. This is accomplished initially by slow rolling of the leukocytes along the endothelium through the interaction of selectins on the endothelium and selectin ligands on phagocytes. Chemoattractants then cause the cells to stop rolling and they adhere more firmly, followed by transendothelial migration. These latter steps involve the interaction of integrins on leukocytes with their ligands on endothelial cells. In the absence of integrins, neutrophils cannot adhere firmly to endothelial cells and migrate into tissues to combat bacterial infections.

Leukocyte adhesion deficiency, LAD, which has been described in animals and humans, is associated with recurring bacterial infections. In humans, two forms of this deficiency have been described, one in which the β chain of the integrin subunit on the phagocyte is missing (LAD I) and the other which involves a defect in selectin ligands on affected phagocytes for the selectin molecules on endothelial cells (LAD II).

Leukocyte adhesion deficiency has been described in Irish setters and in Holstein calves. Affected animals usually die early in life from recurring bacterial infections.

Canine cyclical haematopoiesis

An autosomal recessive disease of collies, called canine cyclical haematopoiesis (grey collie syndrome), results in regular fluctuations in leukocyte numbers. Affected dogs have decreased skin pigmentation, eye lesions and silver grey hair. At intervals of approximately 12 days, a decrease in granulopoiesis occurs and lasts for about three days. During periods of leukopenia, affected animals are susceptible to bacterial infections. Although the nature of the disease is not clear, a defect in neutrophil maturation in the bone marrow is suspected.

Defective neutrophil function has been described in Doberman, Weimaraner and Rottweiler dogs, but the underlying causes of the defect have not been determined.

Further reading

Bellatuono, I. (2004) Haematopoietic stem cells. *International Journal of Biochemistry and Cell Biology* **36**, 607–620.

Benjamini, E., Coico, R. and Sunshine, G. (2000) Immunodeficiency and other disorders of the immune system. In *Immunology*, 4th edn. Wiley-Liss, New York, pp. 347–378.

Cruse, J.M. and Lewis, R.E. (1999) Immunodeficiencies: congenital and acquired. In *Atlas of Immunology*. CRC Press, Boca Raton, FL, pp. 325–343.

Fuchs, E. and Segre, J.A. (2000) Stem cells: a new lease of life. *Cell* **100**, 143–155.

Galloway, J.L. and Zon, L.I. (2003) Ontogeny of haematopoiesis: examining the emergence of haematopoietic cells in the vertebrate embryo. *Current Topics in Developmental Biology* **53**, 139–158.

Goldsby, R.A., Kindt, T.J. and Osborne, B.A. (2000) Cells and organs of the immune system. In *Kuby Immunology*, 4th edn. W.H. Freeman and Company, New York, pp. 27–58.

Körbling, M. and Estrov, Z. (2003) Adult stem cells for tissue repair – a new therapeutic concept? *New England Journal of Medicine* **349**, 570–582.

Kyba, M. and Daley, G.Q. (2003) Hematopoiesis from embryonic stem cells: lessons from and for ontogeny. *Experimental Hematology* **31**, 994–1006.

Lonza, R. and Rosenthal, N. (2004) The stem cell challenge. *Scientific American* **290**, 61–67.

Orkin, S.H. and Zon, L.I. (2002) Hematopoiesis and stem cells: plasticity *versus* developmental heterogeneity. *Nature Immunology* **3**, 323–328.

Tizard, I.R. (2004) Primary immunodeficiencies. In *Veterinary Immunology*, 7th edn. W.H. Saunders, Philadelphia, pp. 413–427.

Weissman, I.L. (2000) Stem cells: units of development, units of regulation and units of evolution. *Cell* **100**, 157–168.

13 Nervous System

Towards the end of the third week of embryological development in domestic animals, the notochord induces the overlying columnar ectodermal cells of the embryonic disc to become pseudostratified neuroepithelial cells and form a spoon-shaped thickening called the neural plate. The cranially expanded region of the neural plate forms the primordium of the brain, while the narrower region, caudal to the brain primordium, gives rise to the neural tube. The raised lateral edges of the neural plate form the neural folds, while the depressed midline region of the plate forms a groove, termed the neural groove (Fig. 13.1). Following progressive changes in the columnar neuroepithelium, folding of the neural plate occurs. The cells overlying the notochord become wedge-shaped, with their bases positioned on the basal lamina. These changes contribute to the neural plate becoming a V-shaped structure with a midline ventral axis. The neuroepithelial cells in contact with the surface ectodermal cells also become wedge-shaped with their apices positioned on the basal lamina. Cellular proliferation at the medial aspects of the neural folds causes these structures to gradually approach each other in the midline, meet

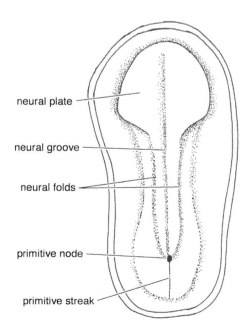

Figure 13.1 Dorsal view of a developing embryo at the stage when neurulation commences.

- neural plate
- neural groove
- neural folds
- primitive node
- primitive streak

and fuse, forming the neural tube which encloses a central neural canal (Fig. 13.2). Closure of the neural tube commences at the level of the fourth somite and, from this point, progresses cranially and caudally in a manner similar to the closure of a zip fastener. The cranial and caudal ends of the neural tube, which remain patent for a time, are termed the rostral and caudal neuropores. For a short time prior to closure of the neuropores, the neural canal communicates directly with the amniotic cavity. As the developing brain and spinal cord have a limited vascular supply at this stage in their development, it has been suggested that these structures receive their supply of nutrients from the amniotic fluid through the neuropores. The rostral neuropore closes midway through the embryonic period with closure of the caudal neuropore shortly afterwards. Subsequently, the neural tube loses its connection with the surface ectoderm and occupies a position ventral to the surface ectoderm. The process whereby the neural tube forms by folding, primary neurulation, extends from the rostral neuropore to the caudal neuropore.

Formation of the neural tube in the sacral and caudal regions of the developing embryo occurs through a process referred to as secondary neurulation. A solid column of mesenchymal cells, derived from the primitive streak in the caudal region of the developing embryo, fuses with the closed caudal end of the neural tube. A central canal in this cord of cells, formed by cavitation, becomes continuous with the neural canal formed during primary neurulation. The length of that region of the spinal cord which arises from secondary neurulation is closely related to the number of caudal vertebrae and, accordingly, is comparatively long in animals with long tails and short in higher primates.

Dorsal–ventral patterning of the neural tube

Once the neural plate has been induced to undergo neurulation by the underlying mesoderm, development of the neural tube commences. Two signalling centres, one located in the overlying ectoderm and the other in the notochord, influence the development and formation of the neural tube. The roof plate of the neural tube is exposed to Bmp-4 and Bmp-7 which arise from

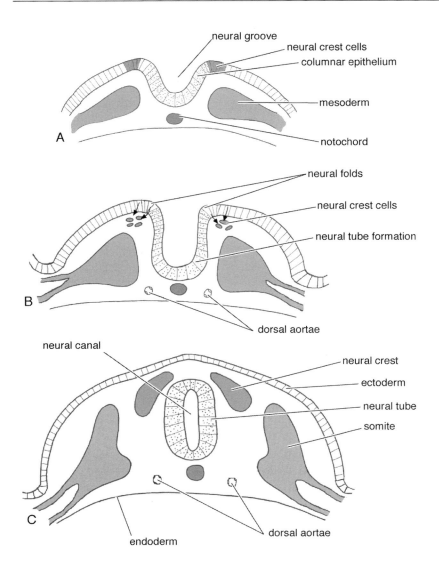

Figure 13.2 Sections through the embryo at sequential stages of primary neurulation. A, Formation of the neural groove and location of neural crest cells. B, Formation of neural folds. C, Formation of the neural tube.

surface ectoderm. The floor plate of the neural tube is influenced by Shh signals from the notochord. At a later stage of development, secondary signalling centres are established within the neural tube itself (Fig. 13.3). Bmp-4 is expressed and secreted by the roof plate cells and Shh is also expressed in the floor plate cells. Bmp-4 triggers a nested cascade of Tgf-β factors which diffuse ventrally into the neural tube, while Shh diffuses dorsally. The neural tube is exposed to gradients of these signalling molecules along the dorsal–ventral axis (Fig. 13.3). Depending on their position along the dorsal–ventral axis, cells are exposed to different concentrations of these signalling molecules which influence expression of transcription factors along this axis. Accordingly, cells located near the floor plate which are exposed to high concentrations of Shh and relatively low concentrations of Tgf-β signals synthesise Nkx6.1 and Nkx2.2 and become determined and differentiate into ventral neurons. Cells located in a dorsal position are exposed to low levels of Shh and high levels of Tgf-β, and hence different fate-determining transcription factors are expressed by these cells.

Neural crest

During fusion of the neural folds, a population of specialised cells derived from neuroepithelium develops along the lateral margins of the neural folds at the interface between the neural and surface ectoderm. These cells are specified by the bone morphogenic proteins produced at the boundary between the neural plate and surface ectoderm, together with Wnt-6 from the presumptive epidermis, to differentiate into neural crest cells. When induced by these factors, the neuroepithelial cells change their characteristics to those of mesenchyme-like cells and penetrate the basal lamina of the neural plate. In the presence of Wnt, Fgf proteins, Bmp-4 and Bmp-7, expression of Slug and RhoB is induced in these specialised cells. Both Slug and RhoB are believed to have a role in neural crest cell migration. It has also been suggested that the RhoB protein may be involved in cytoskeletal alterations which facilitate migration, and that Slug protein activates factors which dissociate tight junctions between adjacent cells. During neural crest cell migration, the cell adhesion protein, N-cadherin, is

Figure 13.3 Dorsal–ventral patterning of the neural tube.

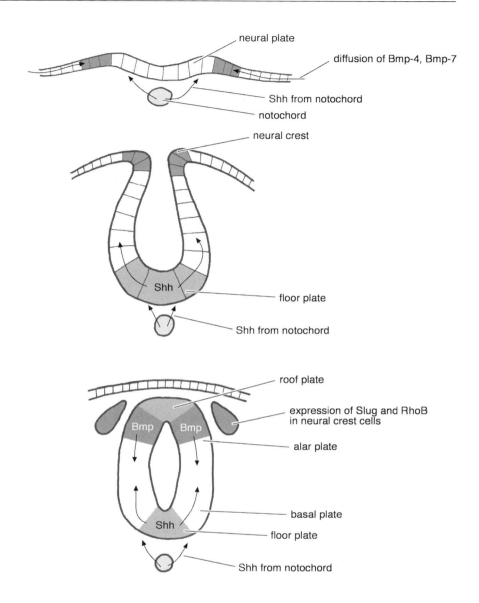

down-regulated. As neural crest cells migrate from the developing neural tube, they form segmental cellular aggregations in a dorsal position which extend along the length of the neural tube on either side. The micro-environment of the extra-cellular matrix influences migration of the neural crest cells. A number of proteins including fibronectin, laminin, tenascin and certain collagen molecules promote this migration, whereas ephrin proteins impede migration. Other factors, such as stem cell factor, allow the continued proliferation of the neural crest cells. A single pluripotent neural crest cell can differentiate into many cell types depending on its location within the early embryo. During neural crest cell migration, exposure to different concentrations of the Bmp and Wnt signalling factors can influence their determination in becoming defined cell types. Derivatives of cranial and spinal neural crest cells are shown in Fig. 13.4. Some derivatives of neural crest cells are not components of the nervous system. Neural components derived from neural crest cells include the

dorsal root ganglia, autonomic ganglia and the glial cells of the peripheral nervous system (Fig. 13.5).

Differentiation of the cellular components of the neural tube

The neural tube is initially lined with pseudostratified columnar neuroepithelial cells which give rise to two cell types, neuronal and glial progenitor cells (Fig. 13.6). Neuroblasts differentiate into the neurons of the central nervous system while gliablasts give rise to supporting cells. Following differentiation of neural epithelium, the neural tube consists of three distinct layers, an inner ependymal (ventricular) layer, a middle mantle (intermediate) layer and an outer marginal layer (Fig. 13.7A). Neuroblasts in the early stage of differentiation have characteristic large round nuclei with pale-staining nucleoplasm and prominent nucleoli. These cells, which migrate outwards from the ependymal layer, form the mantle layer. From this mantle layer, the grey matter of

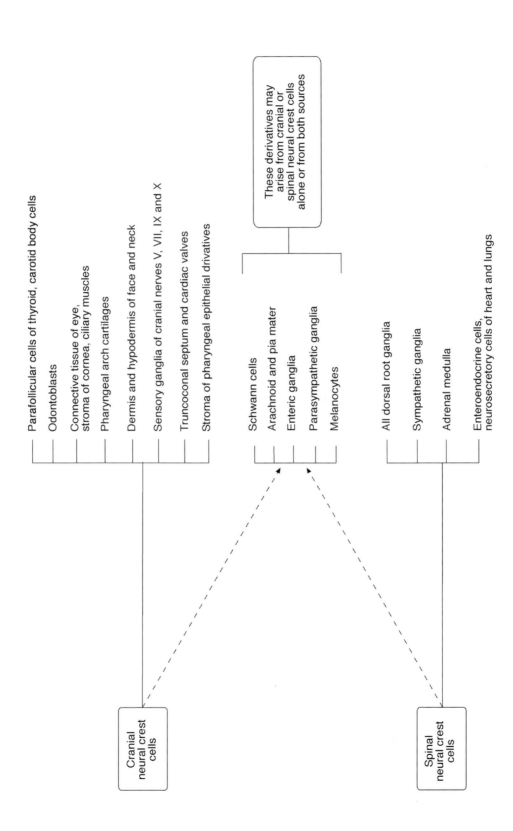

Figure 13.4 Derivatives of cranial and spinal neural crest cells.

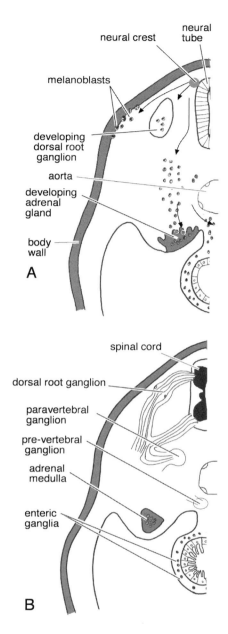

Figure 13.5 The origin and migratory pathways (arrows) of neural crest cells which arise from the thoraco-lumbar region of the developing embryo, A. In their final location in the tissues, derivatives of these cells give rise to specialised cells and tissues, B.

the spinal cord is formed. Cytoplasmic processes which extend laterally from the neuroblasts in the mantle layer contribute to the formation of the marginal layer of the neural tube. Gliablasts give rise to astrocytes, which are present in both the mantle and marginal layers, and oligodendroglia, which mainly populate the marginal layer. In addition to the production of neuroblasts and cells of glial lineage, the neuroepithelium differentiates into ependymal cells which form the lining of the brain

ventricles and the central canal of the spinal cord (Fig. 13.6). The third supporting cell type of the nervous system, microglial cells, which are of mesenchymal origin and are actively phagocytic, arrive in the central nervous system after it becomes vascularised. Neuroblasts in the dorsal and ventral regions of the mantle layer on either side of the midline proliferate rapidly, resulting in the formation of the left and the right dorsal and ventral thickenings. The dorsal thickenings, which form the alar plates, are populated by neuroblasts (Fig. 13.7B). Later, these neuroblasts become neurons, referred to as interneurons, which relay sensory impulses. The prominent ventral thickenings which form the basal plates are populated by neuroblasts which give rise to motor neurons. Left and right longitudinal grooves form along the inner wall of the central neural canal and each is referred to as a sulcus limitans. These grooves demarcate the boundary between the dorsal sensory alar plates and the ventral motor basal plates. The alar and basal plates expand due to accelerated cell division and the four plates fuse forming the characteristic butterfly-shaped grey area evident in a cross-section of the spinal cord (Fig. 13.7C). During this process, the sulci disappear and the original large central canal of the neural tube becomes reduced in diameter. Bilateral ventral bulging, as a consequence of mitosis and hypertrophy of the cells of the basal plates, results in a deep medial groove on the ventral surface of the spinal cord, referred to as the ventral fissure. A less prominent medial groove also develops dorsally. The dorsal roof plate and the ventral floor plate of the neural tube, which do not contain neuroblasts, serve as pathways for fibres crossing from one side of the spinal cord to the other. In dorso-lateral locations of the basal plate in the thoraco-lumbar region, a group of neuroblasts divide, forming enlargements referred to as lateral horns. These neuroblasts, which differentiate into motor neurons, form part of the sympathetic division of the autonomic nervous system. Cells from the neural crest, which are distributed segmentally along the dorso-lateral aspect of the left and right sides of the neural tube, give rise to the dorsal root ganglia, the sensory components of the peripheral nervous system.

Spinal nerves

Neuroblasts in the basal plates differentiate, develop cytoplasmic processes and become motor neurons. A number of short processes, known as dendrites, arise at one pole of the neuroblast and, at the opposite pole, a single long process referred to as an axon develops. A nerve cell with more than one dendritic process is referred to as a multipolar neuron. From each segment of the spinal cord, axons grow out through the marginal layer of the cord and enter the vertebral canal. The ventral roots leave the vertebral canal through the inter-

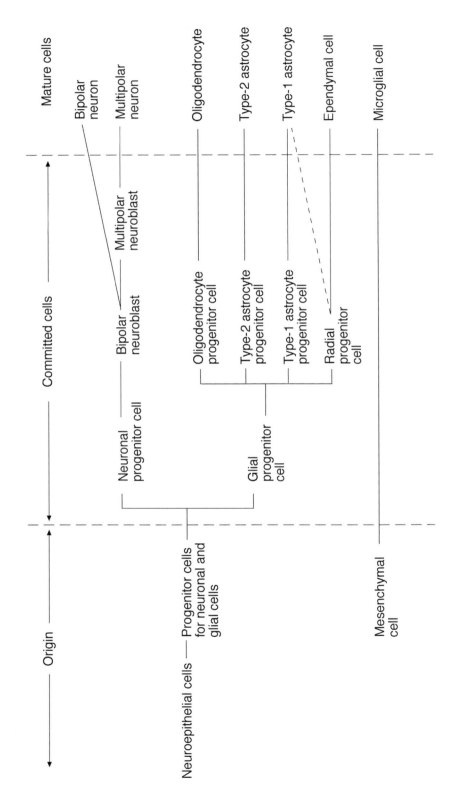

Figure 13.6 Origin, differentiation and maturation of neurons, different types of glial cells and ependymal cells of the central nervous system.

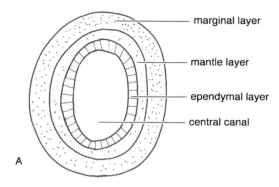

A

- marginal layer
- mantle layer
- ependymal layer
- central canal

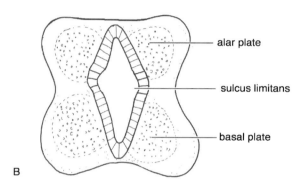

B

- alar plate
- sulcus limitans
- basal plate

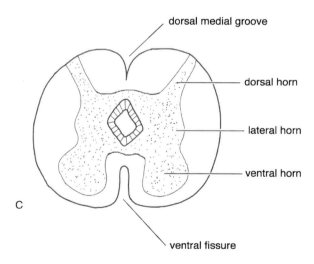

C

- dorsal medial groove
- dorsal horn
- lateral horn
- ventral horn
- ventral fissure

Figure 13.7 Transverse sections through the neural tube at different stages of formation of the spinal cord. A, The three layers of the neural tube. B, Formation of the alar and basal plates in the developing spinal cord. C, Fusion of the alar and basal plates which form the grey matter of the spinal cord, consisting of dorsal and ventral horns.

vertebral foramina on the side from which they derive and innervate effector organs. The sensory components of spinal nerves differentiate from neuroblasts in the dorsal root ganglia. Two cytoplasmic processes derive from each neuroblast in the dorsal root ganglia. One process extends into the dorsal horn of the spinal cord,

and the other process, which leaves the spinal canal by the intervertebral foramen, terminates in a sensory receptor in an organ such as the skin (Fig. 13.8). In most instances, the sensory nerve processes within the dorsal horn form synapses with interneurons in the grey matter of the dorsal horn. These interneurons may form synapses with either ipsilateral ventral motor neurons or they may synapse with motor neurons on the contralateral ventral horn, forming, in both instances, multi-synaptic reflex arcs. Occasionally, the processes from the dorsal root ganglia may form synapses directly with the motor neurons in the ventral horn of the cord and establish a mono-synaptic reflex arc. Axons derived from interneurons may penetrate the marginal layer of the cord and extend cranially forming synapses at higher levels within the cord. Alternatively, they may continue as nerve fibre tracts forming synapses in brain nuclei. Both mono-synaptic and multi-synaptic reflex arcs participate in what is referred to as the general somatic system of innervation. Spinal nerves contain general somatic afferent and general somatic efferent fibres. In the development of the general visceral efferent component of spinal nerves, axons of the visceral motor neurons, which emerge from the lateral horn of the spinal cord, leave the spinal canal via the vertebral foramina and form synapses with neurons in ganglia of the autonomic nervous system. Post-ganglionic autonomic fibres terminate in effector organs such as smooth muscle, cardiac muscle and glands. Thus, the visceral efferent system of a spinal nerve requires two neurons, in comparison with the somatic efferent system, which is a single-neuron system (Fig. 13.8).

Autonomic ganglia develop from neural crest cells. In the general visceral efferent system, the axons of autonomic neurons located in the lateral horn of the spinal cord are referred to as pre-ganglionic or pre-synaptic fibres. The axons, which derive from autonomic neurons located in ganglia, are referred to as post-ganglionic or post-synaptic fibres. A typical spinal nerve consists of a dorsal root comprising a large number of general somatic afferent fibres and general visceral afferent fibres, and a ventral root composed of general somatic efferent fibres and general visceral efferent fibres. Although dorsal afferent root fibres and ventral efferent root fibres intermingle at the intervertebral foramen forming a spinal nerve which contains the four functional groups of fibres, each group remains separate. On leaving the intervertebral foramen, a spinal nerve divides into a smaller dorsal and larger ventral branch. Each branch contains both somatic and visceral afferent and efferent fibres (Fig. 13.8). Ventral branches of spinal nerves, especially in the cervico-thoracic and lumbo-sacral regions, form plexuses associated with the developing limb buds. That portion of the spinal cord between the fifth and seventh cervical vertebrae increases in diameter

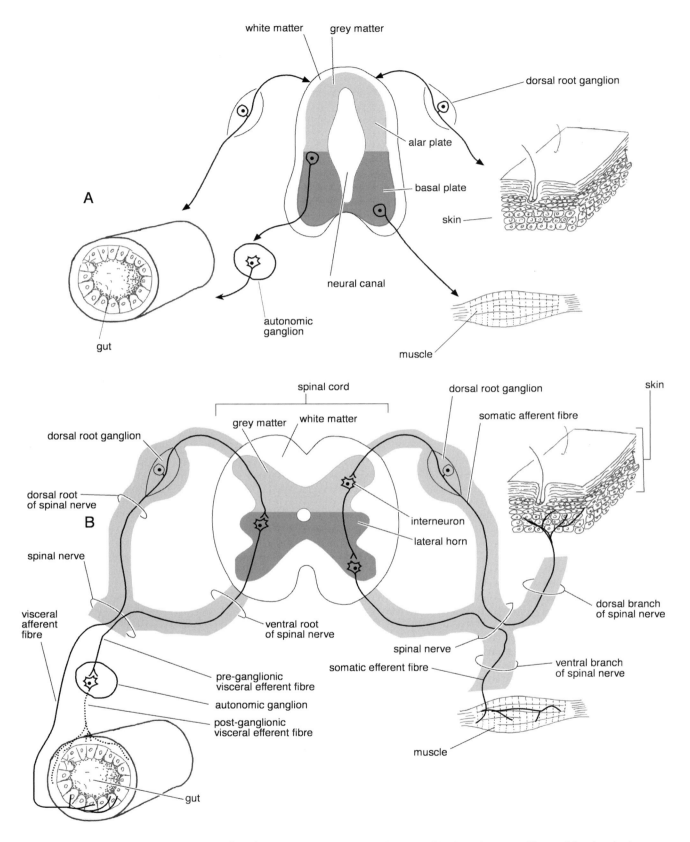

Figure 13.8 Formation of a spinal nerve. A (right), Motor axon growing out from a cell body in the ventral horn of the developing spinal cord innervating an effector organ. One process from a neuroblast in a dorsal root ganglion grows into the dorsal horn of the developing spinal cord while the other process terminates in a somatic sensory receptor. A (left), Motor axon growing out from a cell body in the lateral horn of the developing spinal cord towards an autonomic ganglion. Subsequently, axons grow out from the neuroblasts in the autonomic ganglion and terminate in effector organs. One process from a neuroblast in a dorsal root ganglion grows into the dorsal horn of the developing spinal cord while the other process terminates in a visceral sensory receptor. B, Elements which contribute to the functioning of a spinal nerve showing, on the left, visceral afferent and visceral efferent components and, on the right, somatic afferent and somatic efferent components.

almost filling the vertebral canal. This increase in size, referred to as the cervical intumescence, results from an increase in the number of neurons associated with innervation of the developing thoracic limbs. Similar enlargement in the lumbo-sacral region, the lumbar intumescence, is associated with innervation of the developing pelvic limbs.

Spinal nerves associated with the thoracic, lumbar, sacral and caudal regions of the vertebral column are assigned names related to the point at which they emerge from the vertebral canal through intervertebral foramina. The name assigned to a spinal nerve derives from the anatomical region of the vertebral column and the assigned number of the vertebra immediately cranial to the intervertebral foramen through which the spinal nerve passes. The first pair of thoracic nerves, which leave the intervertebral space caudal to the first thoracic vertebra, are designated the first thoracic spinal nerves (T1). Because there are eight spinal nerves in the cervical region and seven cervical vertebrae, this form of classification cannot be applied. The first pair of cervical spinal nerves pass through the lateral foramina of the atlas. The second pair of cervical spinal nerves pass through the first intervertebral foramina between the first and second cervical vertebrae. Accordingly, the eighth cervical spinal nerves pass caudal to the seventh cervical vertebra. That region of the spinal cord from which the dorsal and ventral roots of a spinal nerve arise is termed a segment of the cord. A spinal cord segment is assigned a number corresponding to the spinal nerves arising from that segment.

Myelination of peripheral nerve fibres

Schwann cells, neural crest-derived neurilemmal cells, participate in the myelination of peripheral nerve fibres. In this process, neurilemmal cells are described as wrapping themselves around axons, forming a myelin sheath. The degree to which the neurilemmal cell becomes wrapped around the neuronal process determines whether a nerve fibre is classified as a myelinated nerve fibre or as a non-myelinated nerve fibre. If the neurilemmal cell surrounds the nerve fibre and incorporates it into a deep invagination of the cell membrane, such a fibre is classified as non-myelinated. Through this process, a number of nerve fibres may be enclosed by a single neurilemmal cell. When a single nerve fibre becomes enveloped by a neurilemmal cell which sequentially wraps itself around the fibre a number of times so that the fibre is enclosed in concentric layers of neurilemmal cytoplasm and plasma membrane, such a fibre is referred to as a myelinated fibre. In the process of myelination, the neurilemmal cell cytoplasm is extruded and the layered plasma membrane of the neurilemmal cell fuses, forming the myelin sheath.

Changes in the relative positions of the spinal cord and the developing vertebral column

Towards the end of the embryonic period the spinal cord is the same length as the vertebral canal, and spinal nerves emerge from the vertebral column through the intervertebral foramina at levels corresponding to their points of origin. During the foetal period, however, the vertebral column grows at a faster rate than the spinal cord. Thus, in the late foetal period, the spinal cord is considerably shorter than the vertebral canal, and in different species of domestic animals terminates at different levels in the lumbo-sacral region. During this period of development, few if any neurons differentiate in the caudal end of the cord. Accordingly, the caudal extremity of the spinal cord tapers and forms a structure which is referred to as the conus medullaris. Caudal to the conus medullaris, the terminal portion of the spinal cord is composed of a cord-like strand of glial and ependymal cells, the filum terminale, which attaches the conus medullaris to the caudal vertebrae (Fig. 13.9). Due to the increased length of the vertebral canal relative to that of the spinal cord, the intervertebral foramina are positioned more caudally than the points of origin of the corresponding spinal nerves. As a result, the roots of the spinal nerves arising from the lumbar, sacral and caudal regions of the cord must pass caudally within the vertebral canal before emerging through the intervertebral foramina at points distant from their origins. Because of the anatomical appearance of the nerve roots, which extend in the vertebral canal caudally from their points of origin, they are collectively referred to as the cauda equina (Fig. 13.9).

Anomalies of the spinal cord

Failure of the neural tube to close may arise from faulty induction of the underlying notochord and from a range of teratogenic factors which adversely affect normal differentiation of the neuroepithelium. The defect may extend along the complete length of the neural tube or be restricted to a small region of the tube. Failure of neural tube closure adversely affects both the differentiation of the nervous system and development of the vertebral column.

Induction of the overlying vertebral arches is disrupted by failure of the neural tube to close. If the arches fail to fuse along the dorsal midline, the resulting open vertebral canal is referred to as spina bifida. While the term literally indicates a cleft in the spinal column, it can result in motor and sensory deficits and may predispose to a variety of severe clinical conditions including chronic infection. The defects associated with spina bifida range from minor anomalies of little clinical significance to more serious conditions which invariably lead

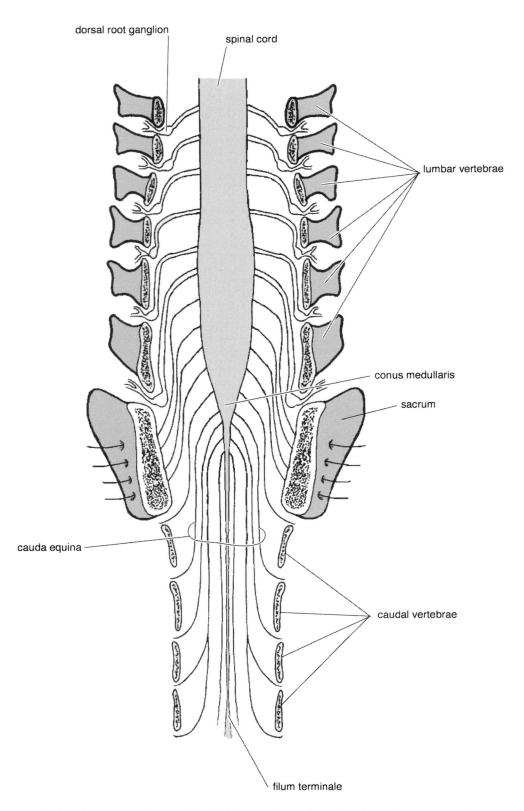

Figure 13.9 Longitudinal section through the caudal end of the vertebral column showing a dorsal view of the cauda equina and filum terminale.

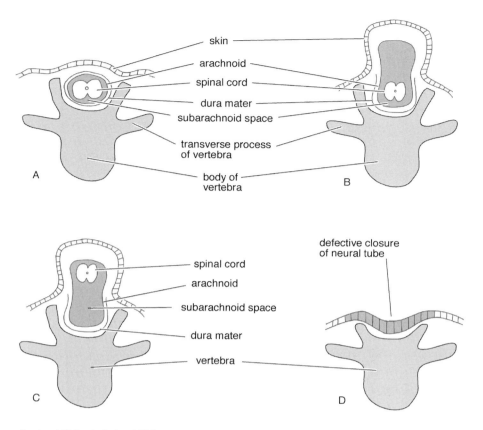

skin
arachnoid
spinal cord
dura mater
subarachnoid space
transverse process of vertebra
body of vertebra

A

B

spinal cord
arachnoid
subarachnoid space
dura mater
vertebra

C

defective closure of neural tube

vertebra

D

Figure 13.10 Forms of spina bifida. A, Spina bifida occulta. B, Meningocoele. C, Meningomyelocoele. D, Rachischisis results from failure of the neural tube to close and failure in the development of associated spinal structures.

to death of the affected animal (Fig. 13.10). One form of the defect, which usually occurs in the lumbo-sacral region, is called spina bifida occulta (Fig. 13.10A). This defect results from failure of the vertebral arch of one or two vertebrae to close and, as a consequence, the dura mater is located subcutaneously. The spinal cord and roots of spinal nerves develop normally and neurological symptoms are usually absent. In humans, the only sign of this defect may be a small tuft of hair over the affected region. If more than two vertebrae are involved, and especially if the dura mater ruptures, the meninges are inclined to herniate through the opening, resulting in a prominent subcutaneous bulge containing the arachnoid membrane and cerebrospinal fluid. If the spinal cord and roots of spinal nerves remain in position and only the meninges and fluid herniate, the anomaly is referred to as meningocoele (Fig. 13.10B). Minor neurological signs may be evident in meningocoele and the defect can be repaired surgically. When the spinal cord becomes displaced and occupies a position in the fluid-filled arachnoid protrusion, the condition is known as meningomyelocoele (Fig. 13.10C). Displacement of the spinal cord usually results in damage to the roots of the spinal nerves, causing neurological symptoms of varying severity. Complete failure of the neural tube to close, which is referred to as rachischisis, is invariably fatal (Fig. 13.10D).

In the human population, it is suggested that fertilisation of ova which are past the optimal time for fertilisation may lead to a higher incidence of neural tube anomalies. Prenatal diagnosis of spina bifida can be made by the detection of abnormally high levels of α-foetoprotein in the amniotic fluid or by ultrasonography.

Differentiation of the brain sub-divisions

The cranial expanded region of the neural plate gives rise to three dilatations, the primary brain vesicles, namely the prosencephalon (fore-brain), the mesencephalon (mid-brain) and the rhombencephalon (hind-brain) outlined in Fig. 13.11. In higher vertebrates, the compact nature of the brain and the relatively small space in which it develops are achieved through the formation of flexures and surface foldings as it is accommodated in the cranium. The ventral cranial flexure, which occurs in the mid-brain region, is known as the cephalic flexure. The flexure between the hind-brain and the spinal cord is termed the cervical flexure. The prosencephalon gives rise rostrally to the telencephalon and caudally to the diencephalon. The mesencephalon remains spinal-cord-like with a narrow central canal. The rhombencephalon forms two dilatations, the metencephalon and myelencephalon, both with dilated lumina (Table 13.1). A dorsal flexure, the pontine

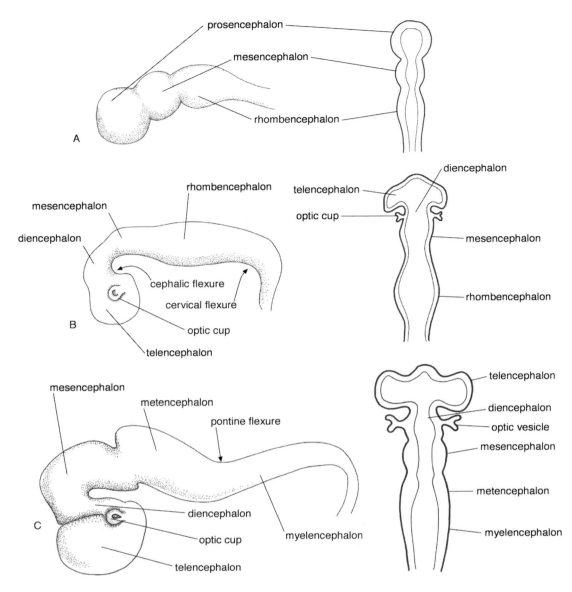

Figure 13.11 Left lateral views and sections through the developing brain. A, The three primary brain vesicles. B, Cephalic flexure and cervical flexure, and development of the telencephalon and diencephalon. C, Pontine flexure and development of the metencephalon and myelencephalon.

Table 13.1 Primary brain vesicles, brain sub-divisions and their major derivatives, and associated ventricles.

Primary brain vesicles	Brain subdivisions	Major derivatives	Associated ventricles
Prosencephalon (Fore-brain)	Telencephalon	Cerebral cortex Basal nuclei Limbic system	Lateral ventricles
	Diencephalon	Epithalamus Thalamus Hypothalamus	Third ventricle
Mesencephalon (Mid-brain)	Mesencephalon	Tectum Corpora quadrigemina Tegmentum Cerebral peduncles	Mesencephalic aqueduct
Rhombencephalon (Hind-brain)	Metencephalon	Pons Cerebellum	Rostral part of fourth ventricle
	Myelencephalon	Medulla oblongata	Caudal part of fourth ventricle

Figure 13.12 Cross-section through the myelencephalon showing the relative positions of columns of cranial nerve nuclei within alar and basal plates. Arrows indicate migration of cells from the alar plates to the olivary nuclei.

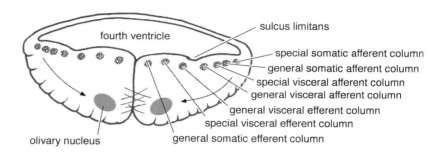

fourth ventricle

sulcus limitans

special somatic afferent column
general somatic afferent column
special visceral afferent column
general visceral afferent column
general visceral efferent column
special visceral efferent column
general somatic efferent column

olivary nucleus

flexure, occurs between the metencephalon and the myelencephalon (Fig. 13.11C). As the telencephalon expands dorsally and caudally, it overlies the diencephalon and mesencephalon, forming the cerebral hemispheres. Although there is no direct relationship between brain size and body size among non-primates, in general, the brains of large animals are small relative to their body size. The brains of humans and non-human primates are proportionately large relative to their body size.

Rhombencephalon

Soon after closure of the neuropores and as a consequence of the formation of the pontine flexure, the lateral walls of the rhombencephalon splay apart dorsally, stretching the roof plate into a thin rhomboid or diamond-shaped structure, overlying an enlarged central space referred to as the fourth ventricle. The region of the rhombencephalon rostral to the pontine flexure differentiates into the metencephalon, while that caudal to the flexure becomes the myelencephalon.

Myelencephalon

The myelencephalon is the most caudal subdivision of the brain. In many respects, the myelencephalon represents a structure which accommodates to the marked morphological differences between the brain and spinal cord, a structure with which it is continuous. It consists of lateral walls each with a dorsal alar and ventral basal plate separated by an intervening sulcus limitans, and also a roof and floor. The myelencephalon gives rise to the medulla oblongata, and the development of this structure is similar in most respects to the formation of the spinal cord. In the medulla oblongata, unlike the spinal cord, the walls splay laterally with the alar plates located lateral to the basal plates, whereas in the spinal cord the alar plates are dorsal to the basal plates. The roof plate of the myelencephalon consists of a single layer of ependymal cells covered by a vascular layer of mesenchymal cells which form the pia mater. The combined ependymal and vascular layers form the tela choroidea. Two projections of the vascular tela choroidea

invaginate into the fourth ventricle forming the choroid plexuses of the fourth ventricle which produce cerebrospinal fluid. In neurology, the term 'nucleus' is used to describe the collection of cell bodies from which a single cranial nerve derives. The basal plates contain three groups of motor nuclei: the medially-positioned general somatic efferent nuclei of cranial nerves VI and XII, the laterally-positioned general visceral efferent nuclei of cranial nerves VII, IX and X and the special visceral efferent nuclei of cranial nerves VII, IX and X, located in an intermediate position between the medial and lateral nuclei (Figs. 13.12 and 13.13). The alar plates contain four groups of nuclei. Listed in order of their medial to lateral positions they are: a general visceral afferent group and a special visceral afferent group of neurons of cranial nerves VII, IX and X, a general somatic afferent group of neurons of cranial nerve V and a special somatic afferent group of neurons of cranial nerve VIII. In addition, cells of the alar plate migrate to a position ventral to the basal plate. These cells form a series of nuclei, the olivary nuclear complex, a structure through which synaptic impulses are relayed to the cerebellum. The medulla oblongata serves as a relay centre for neurological signals from the spinal cord to the brain and from the brain to the spinal cord. Vital centres concerned with the regulation of heart rate, respiration and blood pressure are also present in the medulla oblongata.

Metencephalon

The metencephalon develops from the cranial region of the rhombencephalon. In a manner similar to the formation of the myelencephalon, the lateral walls of the metencephalon diverge so that the alar plate lies lateral to the basal plate. During its development, the metencephalon differs from the myelencephalon by forming two specialised structures, the dorsally positioned cerebellum and a ventral enlargement, the pons. The cerebellum functions as a coordination centre for posture and movement, while the pons serves as a pathway for nerve fibres between the cerebral and cerebellar cortices. The basal plate contains a special visceral efferent nucleus and the alar plate contains a general somatic afferent nucleus, both associated with cranial nerve V.

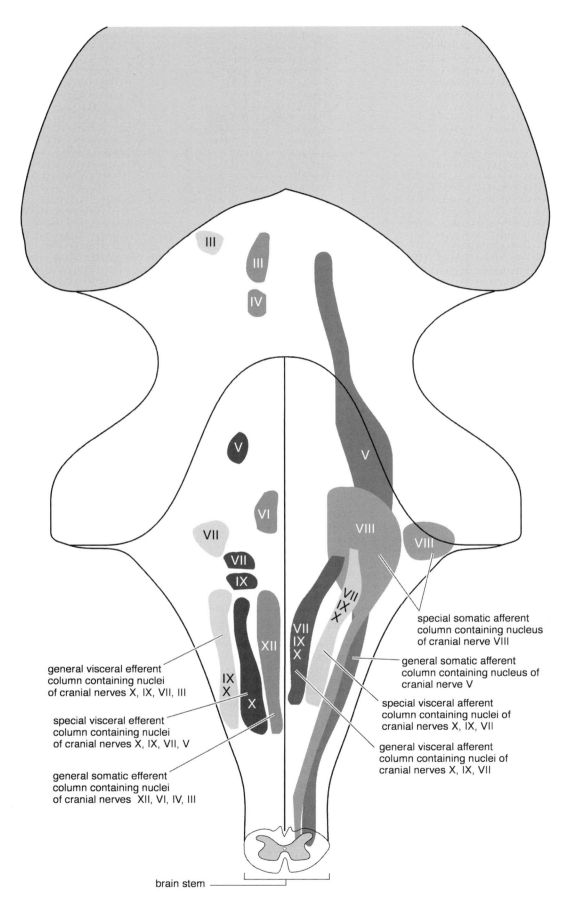

III

III

IV

V

VI

VII

VII

IX

XII

IX
X

X

V

VIII

VIII

VII
IX
X

VII
IX
X

special somatic afferent
column containing nucleus
of cranial nerve VIII

general somatic afferent
column containing nucleus of
cranial nerve V

special visceral afferent
column containing nuclei of
cranial nerves X, IX, VII

general visceral afferent
column containing nuclei of
cranial nerves X, IX, VII

general visceral efferent
column containing nuclei
of cranial nerves X, IX, VII, III

special visceral efferent
column containing nuclei
of cranial nerves X, IX, VII, V

general somatic efferent
column containing nuclei
of cranial nerves XII, VI, IV, III

brain stem

Figure 13.13 Dorsal view of the brain stem, as if it were a translucent structure, showing positions of cranial nerve nuclei and columns within the brain stem. Nuclei and columns which develop in the basal plates are shown on the left; nuclei and columns which develop in the alar plates are shown on the right.

Figure 13.14 Dorsal view of the floor of the fourth ventricle after removal of the roof plate.

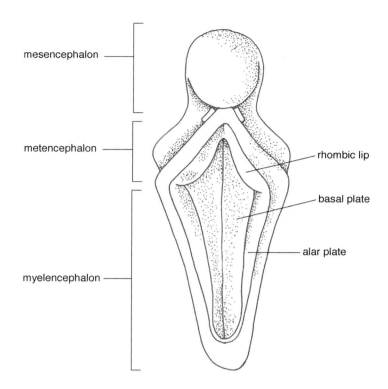

mesencephalon

metencephalon

myelencephalon

rhombic lip

basal plate

alar plate

Cells from the alar plates of the caudal metencephalon and cranial myelencephalon give rise to neurons which migrate ventrally to the pons where they form the pontine nuclei responsible for relaying signals from the cerebral cortex to the cerebellum via the middle cerebellar peduncles.

Cerebellum

The dorso-lateral regions of the alar plates of the rhombencephalon, which fold medially, form the rhombic lips. Viewed from above, the rhombencephalon is a V-shaped structure with the point of the V directed towards the mesencephalon (Fig. 13.14). Thus, the rhombic lips are close together in the region adjacent to the mesencephalon and further apart caudally where they become continuous with the myelencephalon. Towards the end of the embryonic period, the rhombic lips proliferate forming the primordia of the cerebellar hemispheres (Fig. 13.15). As a consequence of continued cellular proliferation, the rhombic lips meet and fuse in the rostral region of the rhombencephalon forming a single structure over the fourth ventricle, the primordium of the cerebellum (Fig. 13.16). In the early foetal period, the developing cerebellum expands dorsally forming a dumbbell-shaped structure. At this stage of proliferation, the developing cerebellum is divided by a transverse fissure into a cephalic and a caudal portion. The larger cephalic portion consists of a narrow medial region, the vermis, connecting the lateral hemispheres. The smaller caudal portion of the developing cerebel-

lum consists of a pair of flocculo-nodular lobes. In an evolutionary sense, these structures are considered to be the most basic components of the cerebellum and are associated with the development of the vestibular apparatus. The cephalic region of the cerebellum develops faster than the caudal flocculo-nodular lobes and later becomes the dominant component of the fully-formed cerebellum. The cerebellar vermis and hemispheres undergo marked growth and expand, occupying a position over the rostral region of the fourth ventricle. This enlargement of the developing cerebellum is characterised by marked folding of its surface, giving rise to closely packed transverse folds referred to as folia (Fig. 13.17).

Initially, the walls of the metencephalon consist of neuroepithelial, mantle and marginal layers. During the early foetal period, cells from the neuroepithelial layer migrate through the mantle and marginal layers to the surface of the cerebellum, forming the external germinal layer. Some cells of the neuroepithelial layer, now referred to as inner germinal layer, give rise to neuroblasts which migrate deep into the cerebellar hemispheres forming four cerebellar nuclei which are responsible for relaying signals to and from the cerebellar cortex. Cells from the inner germinal layer also migrate towards the external germinal layer and give rise to Purkinje cells. Proliferation of the external germinal layer gives rise to neuroblasts which differentiate into the basket, granular and stellate cells of the cerebellar cortex. The granular cells and some basket and stellate cells migrate deep to

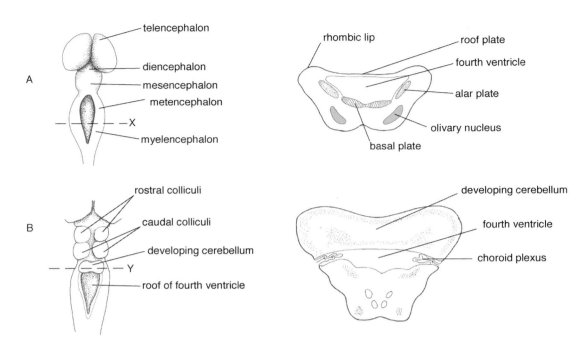

Figure 13.15 Dorsal views and cross-sections at the levels indicated through the myelencephalon, A, and the developing cerebellum and pons, B.

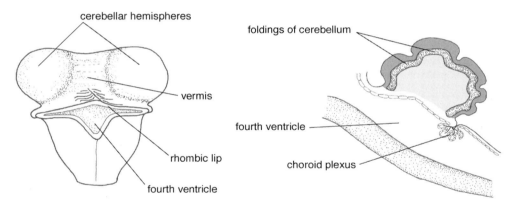

Figure 13.16 Dorsal view and longitudinal section of the developing cerebellum showing the commencement of surface folding.

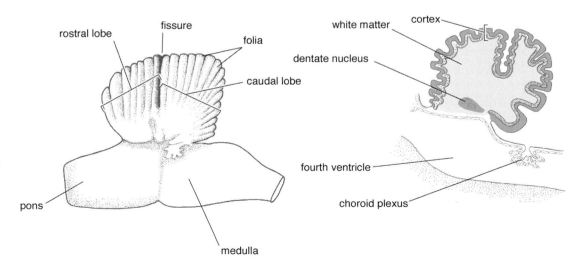

Figure 13.17 Left lateral view and longitudinal section of the developing cerebellum showing marked folding of the surface, the formation of folia.

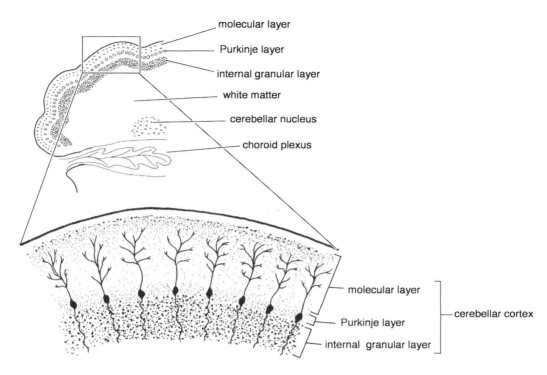

molecular layer
Purkinje layer
internal granular layer
white matter
cerebellar nucleus
choroid plexus

molecular layer
Purkinje layer
internal granular layer
cerebellar cortex

Figure 13.18 Section through the cerebellar cortex. Enlarged view shows the three definitive cellular layers of the cerebellar cortex.

the Purkinje cells, forming an inner granular layer. Thus, in its final form, the cerebellar cortex consists of an outer molecular layer containing basket and stellate cells, a middle Purkinje layer and and an inner granular layer (Fig. 13.18).

The extent to which newborn animals exhibit motor control and co-ordination correlates with the functional capacity of their cerebella at birth. Because the cerebella of newborn foals and calves are fully differentiated and have attained high functional capacity at birth, these animals are able to walk shortly after they are born. In contrast, the inability of pups, kittens and human babies to walk shortly after they are born relates to the incomplete differentiation of the cerebellum in these species at birth.

Mesencephalon

The mesencephalon undergoes fewer developmental changes than other parts of the developing brain. Because of the medial expansion of the alar and basal plates into the roof and floor plates, the neural canal in the mesencephalon is reduced in size, forming the mesencephalic aqueduct. The basal plates give rise to two groups of motor nuclei: a medially positioned general somatic efferent group of cranial nerves III and IV, and a small general visceral efferent group associated with cranial nerve III, in a more dorsal position. The crura

cerebri are formed by enlargement of the marginal layer of each basal plate and these structures serve as pathways for nerve tracts descending from the cerebral cortex to lower centres in the pons and spinal cord (Fig. 13.19).

Neuroblasts from the alar plates migrate into the tectum, the roof of the mesencephalon, and form four aggregations of nuclei, the paired rostral and caudal colliculi, referred to collectively as the corpora quadrigemina, associated with visual and auditory function, respectively. The tegmentum, which arises from the basal plates, is located ventral to the tectum. Although there is uncertainty about the origin of the red nucleus and the substantia nigra, these structures may derive from the alar plates or alternatively they may develop independently *in situ* (Fig. 13.19).

Differentiation of the prosencephalon or fore-brain

The prosencephalon, the most rostral of the three primitive brain vesicles, gives rise to a caudal diencephalon and a rostral telencephalon (Fig. 13.11). From the diencephalon, the optic cups, thalamus, neurohypophysis and epiphysis are formed. The telencephalon gives rise to the cerebral hemispheres and the olfactory bulb. The cavity within the diencephalon is the third ventricle and the paired cavities within the telencephalon are the lateral ventricles.

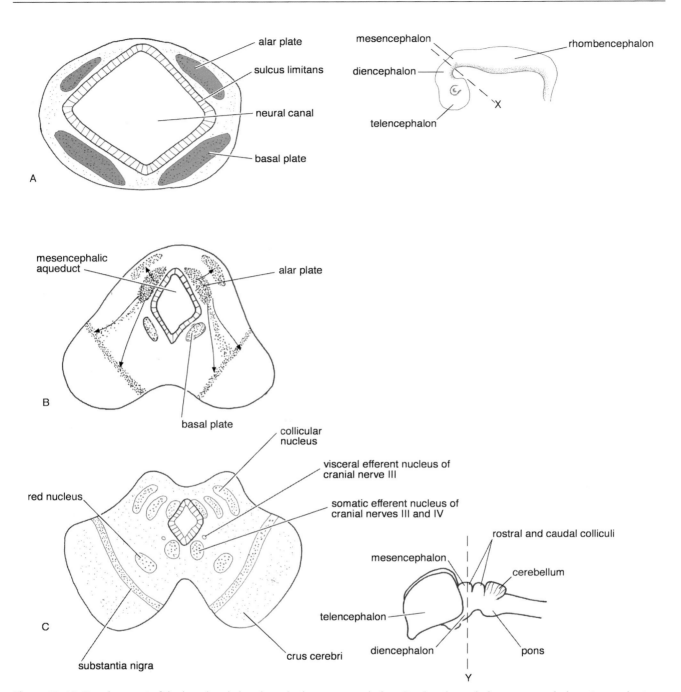

Figure 13.19 Development of the basal and alar plates in the mesencephalon. Section through the mesencephalon at an early stage of development, A, and at a later stage of development, B, showing the alar and basal plates, the wide neural canal and migration of cells from the alar plates (arrows). C, Section through the mesencephalon showing the reduced size of the mesencephalic aqueduct and the development of motor and sensory nuclei from the basal and alar plates. The crura cerebri are also shown. Sections are at the levels indicated.

Diencephalon

As basal plates are absent from the fore-brain, the dien-cephalon is formed from the left and right alar plates and from the roof plate. Three swellings, which occur on the medial aspect of the lateral walls of the diencephalon due to cellular proliferation, form a dorsal epithalamic, a middle thalamic and a ventral hypothalamic mass on each side (Fig. 13.20). Later, the hypothalamic masses fuse forming a single structure. The thalamus and hypothalamus are demarcated by a hypothalamic sulcus. The thalamus develops rapidly on each side and bulges into the cavity of the third ventricle (Figs. 13.21 and 13.22). In some species of animals, including domestic species, these thalamic structures fuse forming an inter-thalamic mass or adhesion, reducing the cavity of the third ventricle to a circular space. The thalamus acts primarily as a centre for relaying sensory impulses,

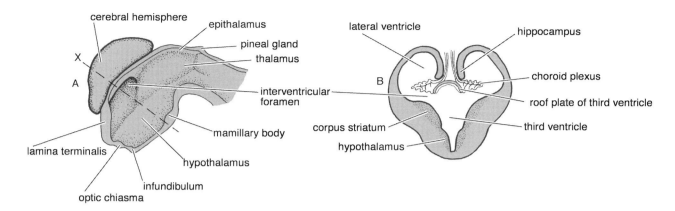

Figure 13.20 Midline longitudinal section through the fore-brain showing the medial wall of the right cerebral hemisphere and the right thalamus and hypothalamus, A. Cross-section through the fore-brain at the level indicated, X, showing the lateral ventricles, the hippocampal lobes, the third ventricle and the choroid plexus, B.

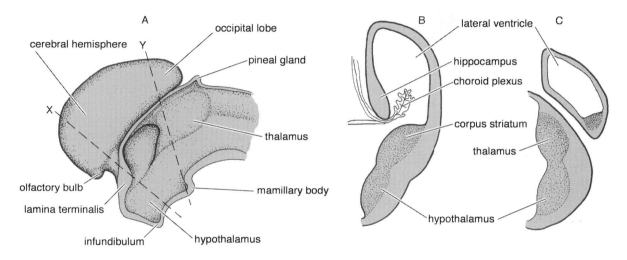

Figure 13.21 A, Midline longitudinal section through the fore-brain at a later stage than that shown in Fig. 13.20A. B, Cross-section through the fore-brain at the level indicated, X. C, Cross-section through the fore-brain at the level indicated, Y.

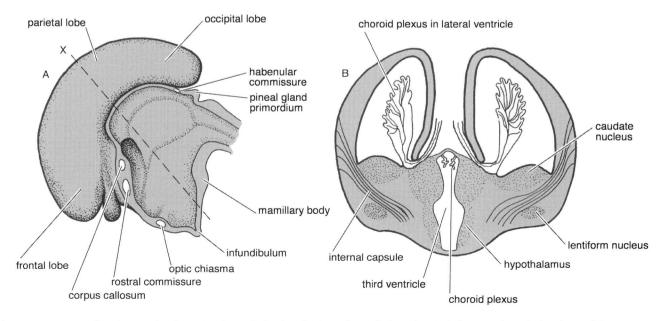

Figure 13.22 A, Midline longitudinal section through the fore-brain in the early foetal period showing the relationships of the developing brain structures. B, Cross-section at the level indicated, X.

along with signals from the cerebellum and basal ganglion, to the cerebral cortex. A number of nuclei which regulate visceral function, sleep, digestion, body temperature and, in humans, emotional behaviour arise in the hypothalamus. The hypothalamus also regulates the endocrine activity of the pituitary gland and influences many autonomic responses. Paired sub-thalamic nuclei, referred to as the mamillary bodies, form distinct protuberances on the mid-ventral surface of the hypothalamus. In addition, a ventral downgrowth from the diencephalon forms the infundibulum of the neurohypophysis, which is discussed in Chapter 20. The most caudal portion of the roof plate of the diencephalon forms a small medial diverticulum which, as a result of cellular proliferation, develops into a cone-shaped structure, the epiphysis cerebri or pineal gland (Fig. 13.21). The cranial region of the roof plate consists of a single layer of ependymal cells covered by vascular mesenchyme. These combined layers invaginate into the third ventricle forming the choroid plexus of the third ventricle. In the early stages of development, two lateral vesicles form in the diencephalon, the primordia of the optic cups. Differentiation of the optic cups is discussed in Chapter 21.

Telencephalon

The telencephalon, the most rostral derivative of the prosencephalon, consists of a central portion, the lamina terminalis, and two lateral diverticula, the walls of which form the future cerebral hemispheres. The cavities of these two diverticula, the lateral ventricles, communicate with the lumen of the diencephalon, the third ventricle, through the interventricular foramina. Initially, the openings between the lateral ventricles and third ventricle are wide. Later, with the expansion and growth of the cerebral hemispheres, the lumen of each interventricular foramen decreases in size. The developing telencephalic vesicles extend initially in a rostral direction. At a later stage, they extend in a dorsal direction, then in a caudal direction and finally in a ventral direction, assuming a C-shaped appearance (Fig. 13.23). In their final form, the cerebral hemispheres are located over the diencephalon, mesencephalon and the rostral area of the hind-brain. The medial walls of the expanding cerebral hemispheres are separated by a longitudinal fissure. Towards the end of the embryonic period, cellular proliferation in the floor of each hemisphere gives rise to prominent swellings which bulge into the lateral ventricles, forming the corpora striata (Fig. 13.21B). A collection of nuclei, the basal nuclei, which contribute to the control of muscle tone and complex body movements, are located in each corpus striatum.

In the ventral medial walls of the cerebral hemispheres, grooves referred to as choroid fissures develop and project into the lateral ventricles. Later, the vascular pia mater covering these grooves invaginates into the lateral ventricles and when covered by a thin layer of ependymal cells forms the choroid plexuses of the lateral ventricles (Fig. 13.21). Dorsal to the choroid fissures, the medial walls of the hemispheres increase in thickness forming the hippocampi. In mammals, each hippocampus forms a specific gyrus which results from an infolding in the hippocampal region into the lateral ventricle, contributing to its medial and ventral walls. The hippocampi, which form part of the limbic system, are closely associated with memory.

The expansion of the hemispheres over the diencephalon and mesencephalon results in fusion of the medial walls of the hemispheres with the lateral walls of the diencephalon. This fusion brings the corpus striatum and thalamus into close contact. The growth and curvature of the hemispheres also affects the shape of the lateral ventricles contained within them, imparting to the ventricles a C-shaped configuration with rostral, caudal and ventral horns. The choroid plexuses which are arranged around the walls follow the contours of the expanding lateral ventricles. With the differentiation of the cerebral cortices from the hemispheres, fibres which arise from the cortices and fibres which relay signals to the cortices pass through the corpus striatum and divide it into a dorso-medial portion, the caudate nucleus, and a ventro-lateral portion, the lentiform nucleus (Fig. 13.22B). The fibre tract dividing the caudate and lentiform nuclei is known as the internal capsule. In association with hemisphere development, both the caudate nucleus and the internal capsule become C-shaped.

Prior to the differentiation of the cerebral hemispheres into cortical structures, their walls have the same three basic layers as those present in the neural tube. Cells which derive from the ependymal layer migrate in a wave-like manner to the surface of the cortex. Three waves of cellular migration occur during the formation of the cerebral cortex, each in turn giving rise to a distinct layer. The first wave of migration gives rise to a layer of cells which, in the final arrangement, constitutes the deepest or third layer of the cerebral cortex. The cells which constitute the second layer of the cortex migrate through the layer already established during the first wave of migration. During the final wave of migration, cells move through the two previously established layers and occupy the most superficial position within the cerebral cortex.

As the hemispheres differentiate during the late foetal period, the surface of each hemisphere becomes folded forming small elongated elevations known as gyri, which contain a superficial layer of grey matter and a central core of white matter. Gyri are separated from

Figure 13.23 Outline of sequential stages in the development of structures in the fore-brain and hind-brain. Arrows indicate direction of growth of the telencephalon.

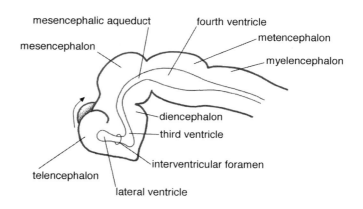

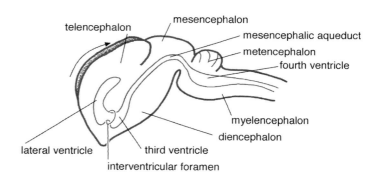

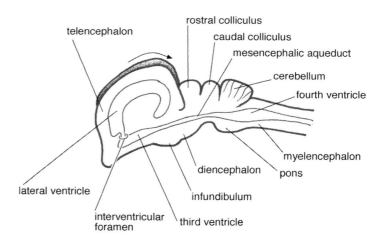

each other by shallow grooves referred to as sulci. As the patterns of gyri and sulci are species-specific, the names applied to these structures in one species are not applicable to gyri and sulci in other species. The cerebral cortex is conventionally subdivided into frontal, parietal, occipital and temporal lobes, according to the bones of the cranium to which these areas of the brain are related.

As the cerebral cortex develops, neuronal fibres synapse with neurons within the same hemisphere, between the left and right hemispheres and also between the hemispheres and other regions of the brain. When they synapse with neurons of the same hemisphere, such fibres are classified as association fibres. Commissural

fibres interconnect corresponding regions of the two hemispheres and projection fibres connect cerebral neurons with neurons in other regions of the brain and spinal cord. The largest and most important of the commissural fibre bundles is the corpus callosum which connects the non-olfactory area of each hemisphere. Initially, fibres of the corpus callosum extend through the lamina terminalis. However, as the hemispheres develop, the corpus callosum expands and eventually extends over the diencephalon. Smaller commissural fibre bundles also develop, including the hippocampal, caudal, and habenular commissures, and the rostral commissure which connects the olfactory bulbs of each hemisphere (Fig. 13.22A).

Table 13.2 Functional roles of brain regions.

Brain region	Functional role
Medulla oblongata	Contains centres for the regulation of involuntary functions, including cardiovascular, respiratory and digestive system activities; relays sensory information to the thalamus
Pons	Contains involuntary somatic and visceral motor centres; has a central role in the regulation of breathing; relays sensory information to the cerebellum and thalamus
Cerebellum	Specialised functions of this structure include processing of sensory information, coordination of movement and maintenance of equilibrium. Sensory input into the cerebellum derives from somatic receptors in the periphery of the body and from receptors for equilibrium and balance located in the inner ear
Mid-brain	Control of eye movement; relays signals for visual and auditory reflexes
Thalamus	Major relay and processing centre for sensory information
Hypothalamus	Contains centres for regulating body temperature, appetite, fluid balance and sexual responses; has a central role in the control of endocrine gland secretion
Cerebrum	Contains centres concerned with learning and memory. In humans the cerebrum is also concerned with intellectual capability and emotional responses. Other functions include voluntary and involuntary regulation of somatic motor activity
Cerebral cortex	Perception, skeletal muscle movement, integration of information; interpretation of sensory information from skin, musculoskeletal system, viscera and taste buds

Outgrowths from the rostral region of the telencephalon, the olfactory bulbs, receive axons of neurons from the olfactory mucosa. These axons, which form the olfactory nerve, synapse with neurons in the olfactory bulb. The axons of the bulb neurons, which comprise the olfactory tract, synapse with neurons in the olfactory centres of the cerebral hemispheres. Functional roles of brain regions are summarised in Table 13.2.

Ventricular system of the brain and cerebrospinal fluid circulation

The cavities of the brain vesicles and the lumen of the neural tube persist and subsequently give rise to the ventricular system of the brain and the central canal of the spinal cord respectively. The ventricles and the central canal, which are lined by ependymal cells, contain cerebrospinal fluid. The lateral expanded cavities of the telencephalic outgrowths are termed the left and right lateral ventricles. The central cavity of the telencephalon and the cavity of the diencephalon form the third ventricle which surrounds the inter-thalamic adhesion of the diencephalon. The central lumen of the mesencephalon remains narrow and forms the mesencephalic aqueduct while the expanded cavity of the hind-brain forms the fourth ventricle. Regions along the floor of each lateral ventricle and the roof of the third and fourth ventricles, which are composed of ependymal cells and vascular pia mater, form the tela choroidea. Projections of the tela choroidea invade the cavity of the ventricles giving rise to villous structures, the choroid plexuses, which form the cerebrospinal fluid. From its site of production, cerebrospinal fluid has a well defined circulatory pathway (Fig. 13.24). Fluid formed in the lateral ventricles passes to the third ventricle by the inter-ventricular foramen and from the third ventricle to the fourth ventricle through the mesencephalic aqueduct. Most of the fluid passes into the sub-arachnoid space from the fourth ventricle through two lateral apertures which develop in the roof of the fourth ventricle in domestic animals. In humans, a third aperture, located in a medial position, also develops. A small amount of fluid enters the central canal of the spinal cord. Thus, the brain and spinal cord are shielded against shock by fluid, both internally and externally. Under normal conditions cerebrospinal fluid, which is produced continually, returns to the venous system at a rate which closely matches the rate of production. As the pressure of cerebrospinal fluid exceeds the venous pressure within the dural venous sinuses, re-absorption of cerebrospinal fluid occurs through the arachnoid villi which project into the venous sinuses. Additional sites at which cerebrospinal fluid returns to the venous system include the veins and lymphatics around the roots of spinal nerves. Cerebrospinal fluid is formed by a combination of filtration of blood plasma and active transport of some plasma constituents, together with secretions of ependymal cells. The concentration of glucose and amino acids in cerebrospinal fluid is lower than that of plasma. Normal cerebrospinal fluid is free of cells. The fact that cerebrospinal fluid and the brain's extra-cellular fluid are in equilibrium helps to maintain a stable environment within the central nervous system. The immediate environment of brain cells is further stabilised by the blood–brain barrier which assists in regulating the composition of the extra-cellular fluid. The capillaries of the brain, unlike capillaries in other organs of the body, act as a selective barrier which excludes macromolecules. These capillaries permit passage of most plasma constituents except proteins. This selective exclusion of macromolecules is attributed to the arrangement of endothelial cells of capillaries which have tight junctions. The perivascular feet of astrocytes, which are

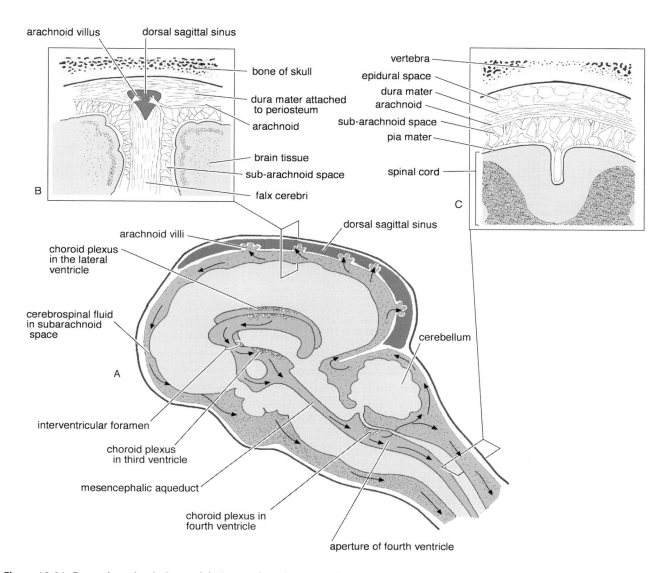

Figure 13.24 Formation, circulation and drainage of cerebrospinal fluid in the cranial region, A. The relationships of the meninges to contiguous structures in the cranial region, B, and in the spinal region, C. Arrows indicate direction of cerebrospinal fluid circulation.

attached to the basal lamina of capillaries of the nervous system, may also contribute to the formation of a selective barrier. The blood–brain barrier allows transportation of substances which dissolve readily in lipids such as oxygen, carbon dioxide and alcohol. Molecules such as glucose and amino acids, which are not lipid soluble, are transferred across the blood–brain barrier by special mechanisms. The highly selective permeability of the brain capillaries helps to protect the brain cells against some toxic substances and against fluctuating levels of hormones, ions and neurotransmitters present in the circulation.

Molecular aspects of brain development

Signals derived from homeobox genes, which are expressed in the notochord, prechordal plate and neural plate, influence the regional specification of the brain into fore-brain, mid-brain and hind-brain.

Genes containing homeodomains specify the fore-brain and mid-brain regions. At the neural plate stage, Lim-1 and orthodenticle homologue 2 (Otx-2), which are expressed in the prechordal plate and neural plate respectively, influence the demarcation of the fore-brain and mid-brain. Following formation of the neural folds and pharyngeal arches, homeobox genes, including *Otx-1*, *Emx-1* and *Emx-2*, which are expressed in overlapping nested patterns, further specify the identity of the mid-brain and fore-brain regions. Upon establishment of these regions, two organising centres, the anterior neural ridge (ANR), which is positioned between the cranial border of the neural plate and the non-neural ectoderm, and the isthmus, positioned between the mid-brain and the hind-brain, influence embryonic brain development. The ANR secretes Fgf-8, which induces expression of brain factor 1 (Bf-1) in early embryogenesis. This factor has a major role in influencing fore-brain regional specification and formation of the cerebral

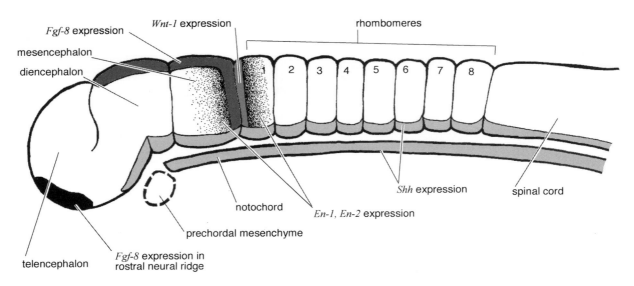

Figure 13.25 Signalling patterns associated with the developing brain and rhombomeres.

hemispheres. Shh secreted by the prechordal plate and notochord influences ventral patterning of the brain, while Bmp-4 and Bmp-7, secreted by the adjacent non-neural ectoderm, control dorsal patterning of the brain. The organising centre in the isthmus also secretes Fgf-8 which induces expression of the homeobox-containing genes, *engrailed 1* and *2* (*En-1* and *En-2*). Subsequently, these genes are expressed in gradients cranially and caudally from the isthmus. *En-1* regulates development of the dorsal mid-brain, and both *En-1* and *En-2* participate in the development of the cerebellum. *Wnt-1*, which participates in the development of the cerebellum, is induced by Fgf-8 (Fig. 13.25).

The hind-brain is composed of segments or rhombomeres the identity of which is specified by a range of homeobox-containing genes. The gastrulation brain homeobox 2 transcription factor, Gbx-2, defines the boundary between the mid-brain and hind-brain. Segmentation genes such as *Krox-20* and *Kreisler* establish the segmentation pattern of the rhombomeres, while homeobox genes of the antennapedia class define the segmental identity of the rhombomeres. Hox gene products are not expressed in rhombomere 1 (r1) as they are antagonised by the Fgf-8 expressed by the isthmic organiser present at the anterior end of r1. The overlapping patterns of expression of Hox paralogues can be detected from rhombomere 2 to rhombomere 8, with Hox genes at the 3′ region of the chromosome expressed in the more cranial regions of the hind-brain. Another family of genes, the ephrins, and their receptors, also influence the differentiation of the rhombomeres. Ephrins are expressed in the even-numbered rhombomeres 2, 4, 6 and 8, and ephrin receptors are expressed in the odd-numbered rhombomeres 3, 5 and 7. This pattern of expression may account for the absence of cell

migration between rhombomeres and also for the maintenance of the distinct groupings of neural crest cells associated with each rhombomere. Accordingly, neural crest cells retain their unique positional association with their respective rhombomeres.

Brain anomalies

Exencephaly

Failure in the closure of the rostral neuropore, resulting in abnormal fore-brain development and interference with fusion of the bones of the cranium, gives rise to the condition referred to as exencephaly. When the cranial defect is small, the meninges can herniate and the anomaly is referred to as cranial meningocoele. A large cranial defect, which allows the meninges and part of the brain to herniate, is referred to as encephalocoele.

Microencephaly

Development of an abnormally small brain is referred to as microencephaly. The hypoplastic brain is often accompanied by a cranial cavity of reduced size. External features of the condition include a flattened and narrow frontal area of the cranium, with cranial bones which are thicker than normal. This condition has been reported in calves, lambs and piglets.

Hydranencephaly

A marked or complete loss of cerebral cortical tissue due to destruction of the germinal epithelium of the telencephalon, leaving only membranous sacs filled with cerebrospinal fluid and enclosed by the meninges, is known as hydranencephaly. Although the cranium usually appears normal, some slight doming of the frontal bones may be evident. The brain stem usually has a normal appearance; occasionally some degree of cerebellar hypoplasia may be observed. This condition may occur sporadically in calves, lambs and piglets. Viral teratogens are often implicated in the development of this condition and occasionally groups of susceptible animals may be affected.

Hydrocephalus

Accumulation of excessive amounts of cerebrospinal fluid in the cranial cavity is referred to as hydrocephalus. Three forms of the condition occur. In internal hydrocephalus the cerebrospinal fluid is within the ventricular system, while in external hydrocephalus the fluid accumulates in the sub-arachnoid space. When excess cerebrospinal fluid is present both in the ventricular system and in the sub-arachnoid space, the condition is referred to as communicating hydrocephalus. The external and communicating forms of hydrocephalus are uncommon in domestic animals. Internal hydrocephalus is usually associated with stenosis or closure of the mesencephalic aqueduct, resulting in accumulation of cerebrospinal fluid in the lateral ventricles. This causes the developing cerebral hemispheres to expand against the developing cranium, the bones of which have not yet fused, causing cranial doming. Pressure from the accumulating cerebrospinal fluid causes atrophy of the brain tissue and results in the formation of thin cranial bones. The degree of cranial malformation varies from slight doming to enlargement which may cause dystocia. Hydrocephalus, which occurs sporadically in most domestic animals, can appear clinically similar to hydranencephaly. However, in hydrocephalus, unlike hydranencephaly, the ependymal lining of the ventricles is not destroyed.

Cyclopia

A single centrally-located orbit which contains a normal eye, a rudimentary eye or two eyes with differing degrees of fusion, is referred to as cyclopia. Eyelids are usually absent and the nose is distorted. When ingested by pregnant ewes during the second week of gestation, teratogens present in the plant *Veratrum californicum* cause this condition in their offspring.

Arnold–Chiari malformation

A condition in which herniation of cerebellar tissue through the foramen magnum into the cranial cervical vertebral canal occurs is known as Arnold–Chiari malformation. This condition, which is often accompanied by spina bifida, meningomyelocoele and hydrocephalus, has been recorded in domestic animals.

Cerebellar hypoplasia

Because many viral pathogens can infect the developing cerebellum, congenital cerebellar hypoplasia is encountered periodically in domestic animals. Viruses replicating in the external germinal layer of the cerebellum lead to hypoplasia of the cerebellar cortex. Agents associated with the induction of cerebellar hypoplasia are discussed in Chapter 24.

Brain stem and spinal cord

On cursory examination, the manner in which the brain stem develops seems to bear little resemblance to the development of the spinal cord. When developmental features of the brain stem are examined more closely, it becomes evident that the primitive brain stem consists of a dorsal sensory alar plate and a ventral motor basal plate on each side, demarcated by a sulcus limitans. In common with the spinal cord, the cranial alar and basal plates give rise to general somatic afferent, general visceral afferent, general visceral efferent and general somatic efferent columns of neural tissue which contribute to the grey matter of the brain stem. Similarities in the basic structure of the brain stem and spinal cord during early development become altered by developmental changes which modify the architecture of the brain stem. These changes include the lateral folding of the walls of the hind-brain so that the alar plates are positioned lateral to the basal plates with enlargement of the central neural canal. Additional special neuronal columns, namely special somatic afferent columns, special visceral afferent and special visceral efferent columns, develop in the alar and basal plates of the brain stem. The special somatic afferent columns are associated with hearing and vestibular function, the special visceral afferent with taste, and the special visceral efferent with innervation of musculature of structures which arise from the pharyngeal arches. The designation of a special visceral efferent category for the innervation of the pharyngeal arch skeletal musculature was formerly based on the view that pharyngeal arch musculature was not myotomally derived but developed from neural crest-derived head mesenchyme. Although recent research has shown that pharyngeal arch musculature is derived from somitomeres, the designation 'special visceral efferent' is so long established in the literature that it has been retained in this text. At an early stage in development, the functional nuclei of grey matter in the brain stem form continuous columns, like those of the spinal cord. As some cranial nerves do not require the range of functional components present in the neuronal columns of the brain stem, segments of individual columns regress and consequently some cranial nerves arise from the surviving discrete nuclei. These nuclei and the cranial nerves to which they give rise retain the functions of the neuronal columns from which the nuclei derived (Fig. 13.13).

Cranial nerves

Twelve pairs of cranial nerves, two pairs which originate outside the brain and ten pairs which originate within the brain, develop in mammals. By convention, roman numerals are used to designate the cranial nerves according to their sites of origin in the brain, with cranial nerve I the most rostral and cranial nerve XII the most caudal. Cranial nerves are also named in accordance with the regions or structures which they innervate or serve. Thus, cranial nerve I is also known as the olfactory nerve (Table 13.3).

Although they have some features in common, spinal nerves and cranial nerves also exhibit some fundamental differences. Because spinal nerves have sensory and motor components, they are referred to as mixed nerves. In contrast, the cranial nerves can be classified according to their functions and their embryological origins into three categories, namely nerves with special sensory functions, nerves which have exclusively motor functions and those which innervate pharyngeal arch derivatives, which are mixed.

The principal features of the twelve cranial nerves are summarised in Table 13.3. The ganglia associated with the cranial nerves are derived either from neural crest cells (cranial nerve V), or from a combination of neural crest cells and placodal-derived cells (cranial nerves VII, VIII, IX and X).

Special sensory nerves

Three cranial nerves, namely olfactory (cranial nerve I), optic (cranial nerve II) and vestibulocochlear (cranial nerve VIII), are included in this category. The olfactory and optic nerves are often regarded as extensions of brain tracts rather than true cranial nerves.

Cranial nerves with exclusively motor functions

The oculomotor, trochlear and abducens nerves, cranial nerves III, IV and VI respectively, innervate the ocular muscles. The hypoglossal nerve, cranial nerve XII, innervates the lingual muscles. Unlike cranial nerves IV, VI and XII which are exclusively somatic, cranial nerve III also carries general visceral efferent fibres which innervate the ciliary muscles. Although these four cranial nerves are usually classified as having exclusively motor function, they may in addition contain fibres associated with proprioception which relay sensory information from muscles and joints. Unlike the cell bodies of other sensory systems which are located in

dorsal ganglia, the cell bodies of these afferent proprioceptive fibres are located within their respective nerve trunks.

Cranial nerves with both sensory and motor function

Four cranial nerves, the trigeminal (cranial nerve V), facial (cranial nerve VII), glossopharyngeal (cranial nerve IX) and vagus (cranial nerve X), innervate pharyngeal arch derivatives. As these nerves carry both sensory and motor fibres they are classified as mixed nerves.

Peripheral nervous system

The peripheral nervous system comprises the components of the nervous system which are located outside the brain and spinal cord. This system consists of cranial and spinal nerves, associated sensory and autonomic ganglia and their non-neuronal supportive cells. The afferent fibres arise from dorsal root ganglia, while the efferent fibres arise from multipolar neurons in the basal plates of the developing spinal cord or brain stem. The spinal, cranial and autonomic ganglia and their associated glial cells arise from the neural crest. Some neurons of the cranial ganglia derive from placodal tissue.

Autonomic nervous system

The autonomic nervous system, also referred to as the general visceral efferent system, is that sub-division of the nervous system which regulates many of the involuntary functions of the body. This system has a central regulatory role in the functioning of smooth muscle, cardiac muscle, exocrine glands and some endocrine glands. The autonomic nervous system can be further sub-divided into a sympathetic system and a parasympathetic system on the basis of anatomical and physiological features (Fig. 13.26). Unlike the somatic efferent system which is a single-neuron system, the visceral efferent system is a two-neuron system.

Sympathetic nervous system

Towards the end of the embryonic period, neural crest cells on either side of the spinal cord migrate to positions lateral to the developing vertebrae where they form aggregations. From these aggregations segmentally arranged paravertebral ganglia of the sympathetic nervous system develop. Initially, these paravertebral ganglia are distributed along the length of the vertebral column from the cervical to the sacral region, level with the body of each vertebra. The eight paravertebral ganglia in the cervical region form three aggregations. The first three cervical paravertebral ganglia fuse forming the cranial cervical ganglion. The middle cervical ganglion

Table 13.3 Origin, functional role, associated ganglia and structures or regions served by the twelve cranial nerves.

Number and name of cranial nerve	Origin	Functional role of components[a]	Associated ganglia	Structures or regions served
I Olfactory	Sensory neurons in olfactory mucosa	S.V.A.	–	Olfactory mucosa
II Optic	Neuroepithelial cells of retina	S.S.A.	–	Retina
III Oculomotor	Mesencephalon	G.S.E.	–	Dorsal, ventral and medial rectus muscles, ventral oblique muscle, levator palpebri superiori muscle
		G.V.E.	Ciliary	Ciliary and sphincter pupillae muscles
IV Trochlear	Mesencephalon	G.S.E.	–	Dorsal oblique ocular muscle
V Trigeminal	Metencephalon	G.S.A.	Trigeminal	Oral mucous membrane, facial skin
		S.V.E.	–	Muscles of mastication, rostral belly of digastricus, tensor tympani, tensor veli palatini and mylohyoideus muscles
VI Abducens	Myelencephalon	G.S.E.	–	Lateral rectus, retractor bulbi muscles
VII Facial	Myelencephalon	S.V.E.	–	Muscles of facial expression, caudal belly of digastricus, stapedius
		S.V.A.	Geniculate	Taste, rostral two-thirds of tongue
		G.V.E.	Mandibular, pterygopalatine	Mandibular and sublingual salivary glands; lacrimal glands
		G.V.A.	Geniculate	Mandibular and sublingual salivary glands; lacrimal glands
		G.S.A.	Geniculate	Skin of auditory meatus
VIII Vestibulocochlear	Myelencephalon	S.S.A.	Vestibular	Semicircular canals, utricle, saccule
			Spiral	Spiral organ of Corti
IX Glossopharyngeal	Myelencephalon	S.V.E.	–	Stylopharyngeus muscle
		S.V.A.	Distal	Taste, caudal one-third of tongue
		G.V.E.	Otic	Parotid salivary gland; zygomatic glands in carnivores
		G.V.A.	Distal	Carotid sinus, pharynx
		G.S.A.	Proximal	External ear
X Vagus	Myelencephalon	S.V.E.	–	Constrictor muscles of pharynx, intrinsic muscles of larynx
		S.V.A.	Distal	Caudal pharyngeal mucosa and mucosa of larynx
		G.V.E.	Terminal	Trachea, bronchi, heart, smooth muscle of digestive tract
		G.V.A.	Distal	Base of tongue, pharynx, larynx, trachea, heart, oesophagus, stomach, intestines, carotid sinus
		G.S.A.	Proximal	External auditory meatus
XI Accessory	Myelencephalon, cervical spinal cord	S.V.E.	–	Trapezius, sternocephalicus and brachiocephalicus muscles
XII Hypoglossal	Myelencephalon	G.S.E.	–	Muscles of tongue

[a]S.V.A., special visceral afferent; S.S.A., special somatic afferent; G.S.E., general somatic efferent; G.V.E., general visceral efferent; G.S.A., general somatic afferent; S.V.E., special visceral efferent.

derives from the fourth, fifth and sixth paravertebral ganglia, and the caudal cervical ganglion is formed by aggregation of the seventh and eighth ganglia. The combination of the caudal cervical ganglion with the first two thoracic ganglia forms the cervico-thoracic or stellate ganglion.

Neural crest cells also migrate to positions close to the branches of the aorta which supply the abdominal viscera and form pre-vertebral ganglia (Fig. 13.26). In addition, cells of neural crest origin give rise to the ganglionic cells of the adrenal medulla. The neurons of the sympathetic nervous system, located within the lateral

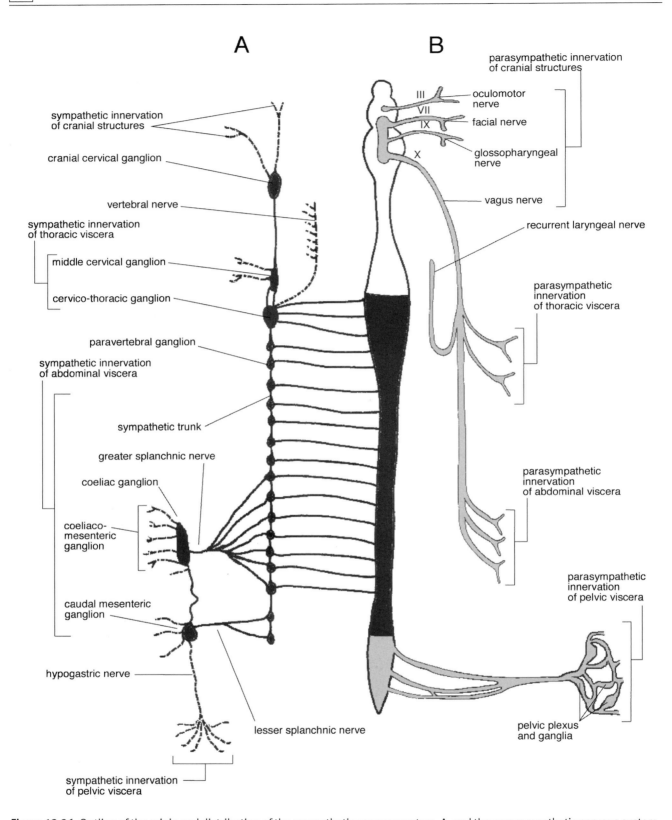

Figure 13.26 Outline of the origin and distribution of the sympathetic nervous system, A, and the parasympathetic nervous system, B. Nerves shown as solid lines represent pre-ganglionic fibres; nerves shown as broken lines represent post-ganglionic fibres. Although nerves of both the sympathetic nervous system and the parasympathetic nervous system arise from both sides of the spinal cord, to ensure clarity, nerves of only one system are shown on each side.

horns of the spinal cord in the thoraco-lumbar region, are referred to as pre-ganglionic neurons. The myelinated axons of the pre-ganglionic neurons grow out from the spinal cord alongside somatic efferent axons in the ventral root and join with the dorsal root forming spinal nerve trunks. After the spinal nerves emerge from the intervertebral foramina, the pre-ganglionic axons emerge from the spinal nerve trunks as the white communicating rami, myelinated axons which extend to the paravertebral ganglia where they form branches. Some branches may synapse with post-ganglionic neurons within the paravertebral ganglion, while other branches may pass cranially or caudally and synapse with neurons within paravertebral ganglia located at positions cranial or caudal to their points of origin. Pre-ganglionic fibres, which carry impulses between the segmental paravertebral ganglia, form the sympathetic chain of the sympathetic nervous system. Some post-ganglionic, non-myelinated fibres of the paravertebral ganglia join the spinal nerve trunks as the grey communicating rami. As the spinal nerves branch, these post-ganglionic, non-myelinated fibres innervate dermal blood vessels, sweat glands and arrector pili muscles. In humans, the white and grey communicating rami can be recognised as distinct structures. In domestic animals, however, the white and grey communicating rami usually form a common trunk containing both myelinated and non-myelinated pre-ganglionic axons. Allowing for some species variations, pre-ganglionic axons of thoracic nerves, which emerge from each side of the spinal cord, may pass through the paravertebral ganglia and leave the sympathetic chains. After they leave the sympathetic chain, they join and form the left and right great splanchnic nerves, the branches of which synapse with pre-vertebral ganglia located around the coeliac and cranial mesenteric arteries. During development, post-ganglionic axons from these ganglia which supply sympathetic innervation to abdominal organs, are distributed in close association with the blood vessels. Pre-ganglionic fibres, which emerge from each side of the spinal cord in the lumbar region, pass through paravertebral ganglia and leave the sympathetic chains. These axons join, forming the left and right lesser splanchnic nerves. Branches of these nerves synapse with a pre-vertebral ganglion associated with the caudal mesenteric artery, referred to as the caudal mesenteric ganglion. Post-ganglionic fibres of the caudal mesenteric ganglion form the left and right hypogastric nerves which supply sympathetic innervation to the caudal abdominal and pelvic viscera (Fig. 13.26). When pre-ganglionic axons enter a ganglion, they branch and each branch synapses with a post-ganglionic neuron in the ganglion. The axon of each post-ganglionic neuron innervates target structures. Accordingly, there may be up to twenty times more post-ganglionic fibres than pre-ganglionic fibres associated with an individual sympathetic ganglion. Thus, the effects of the motor activity of the sympathetic nervous system are widely distributed. Unlike post-ganglionic fibres which are non-myelinated, pre-ganglionic fibres are myelinated. Some pre-ganglionic axons pass through the paravertebral ganglia to the adrenal medulla where they synapse with medullary cells which are homologues of post-ganglionic sympathetic neurons.

Parasympathetic nervous system

Pre-ganglionic neurons of the parasympathetic system are located both in the brain stem, where they form distinct nuclei, and also in the lateral columns of the sacral region of the spinal cord (Fig. 13.26B). The pre-ganglionic parasympathetic axons which emerge from the brain stem as components of the oculomotor, facial, glossopharyngeal and vagus nerves, innervate tissues and structures of the head (Table 13.4). In addition to innervating cranial structures, the vagus nerve innervates viscera in the thoracic and abdominal cavities. The pelvic nerve is formed from the pre-ganglionic axons of the sacral nerves. The ganglia of the parasympathetic system, which develop from neural crest cells, are referred to as terminal or intramural ganglia. These ganglia are located either close to or within the organs which they innervate. Because parasympathetic ganglia are located remote from the neurons in the central nervous system with which they synapse and are usually positioned close to the organs which they innervate, pre-ganglionic myelinated axons are typically longer than post-ganglionic non-myelinated axons. Parasympathetic pre-ganglionic axons may form up to three branches and, accordingly, the ratio of pre-ganglionic to post-ganglionic axons may be approximately 1:3. As a consequence of the reduced branching of parasympathetic pre-ganglionic fibres in comparison with the branching of sympathetic fibres, the effects of parasympathetic stimulation are more localised. The nuclei and distribution of the parasympathetic nerves are presented in Table 13.4.

Enteric nervous system

A system of neurons, nerve fibres and supporting cells, distributed in the submucosal connective tissue and between the layers of the muscularis externa, innervates enteric tissue and some associated structures. This enteric nervous system is composed of reflex pathways which influence gastrointestinal motility and secretion, transport of water and electrolytes across intestinal epithelium, and blood supply to the intestinal mucosa. Neurons of the enteric nervous system derive from neural crest cells originating in the hind-brain region, referred to as vagal neural crest cells, with possible contributions from sacral neural crest cells. Neural crest cells, which migrate into the wall of the developing

Table 13.4 Nuclei of origin, associated ganglia and structures innervated by components of nerves which collectively constitute the parasympathetic division of the autonomic nervous system.

Neural component		Nucleus of origin in brain stem or spinal cord	Ganglion	Structures innervated
Cranial component				
	Oculomotor nerve (cranial nerve III)	Parasympathetic nucleus of cranial nerve III (Edinger–Westphal nucleus)	Ciliary	Ciliary muscles, muscles of iris
	Facial nerve (cranial nerve VII)	Parasympathetic nucleus of cranial nerve VII (rostral salivatory nucleus)	Pterygopalatine Mandibular	Lacrimal and nasal glands Mandibular and sublingual salivary glands
	Glossopharyngeal nerve (cranial nerve IX)	Parasympathetic nucleus of cranial nerve IX (caudal salivatory nucleus)	Otic	Parotid salivary gland and also zygomatic salivary glands in carnivores
	Vagus nerve (cranial nerve X)	Parasympathetic nucleus of cranial nerve X	Terminal ganglia of structures innervated	Trachea, bronchi, heart, smooth muscle of digestive tract
Spinal component				
	Pelvic nerve	Parasympathetic nuclei of sacral nerves in lateral horn of sacral region of spinal cord	Terminal ganglia of structures innervated	Pelvic viscera

gut, form plexuses in the submucosa and between the layers of the muscularis externa. The myenteric plexus, Auerbach's plexus, which is located between the inner circular and outer longitudinal muscle layers, and the submucosal plexus, Meissner's plexus, which is located in the submucosal connective tissue, are interconnected. Enteric neurons are classified as sensory neurons, interneurons and motor neurons. Although the enteric nervous system may function as an independent system, it also receives signals from, and is influenced by, the autonomic nervous system.

Meninges

Along its entire length, the developing neural tube is surrounded by loose mesenchymal tissue. Subsequently, this mesenchymal tissue condenses forming the protective coverings of the central nervous system, the meninges (Fig. 13.24). These coverings develop into an outer ectomenix, considered to be a derivative of the axial mesoderm, and an inner layer, the endomenix, derived from neural crest cells. The ectomenix forms the dura mater, a tough, white, fibrous, tubular, connective tissue sheath composed of collagen and elastic fibres. Along the length of the spinal cord, extensive attachments do not develop between the dura mater and the surrounding developing vertebrae so that in its final form the dura mater has osseous attachments only at its cranial and caudal ends. At its cranial end, the dura mater is attached at the rim of the foramen magnum to the periosteum of the skull. At its caudal end, the dura mater tapers from a tubular structure to a dense cord-

like structure composed of collagen fibres which blend with components of the filum terminale, forming the caudal (coccygeal) ligament, which fuses with the periosteum of a caudal vertebra. The space which develops between the dura mater and the wall of the developing vertebral canal is termed the epidural space. This space contains loose connective tissue, blood vessels and adipose tissue which provide additional support for the spinal cord and for the roots of the spinal nerves which are located within the space.

The dura mater which surrounds the brain differs in its development from the dura mater surrounding the spinal cord in that it is composed of two distinct fibrous layers. The outer layer fuses with the periosteum of the developing bones of the cranium, and the inner layer forms a large fold, the falx cerebri, which projects between the cerebral hemispheres. A smaller transverse fold, the tentorium cerebelli, separates the cerebellum from the cerebral hemispheres. The inner layer of the dura mater which extends over the surface of the pituitary gland is referred to as the diaphragma sellae. Because the outer layer of the dura mater is fused with the periosteum of the cranial bones, no epidural space exists in the vault of the cranium. At the points where the inner layer projects into the major fissures of the brain, venous sinuses are located in the spaces formed between the two layers of the dura mater.

The endomenix gives rise to the leptomeninges, which are composed of an outer arachnoid membrane and an inner pia mater. The arachnoid membrane is a delicate, non-vascular layer beneath the dura mater which consists of an outer layer of flattened fibrocytes and an inner loosely arranged layer of connective tissue. The dura mater and the arachnoid membrane are separated by a thin film of fluid and the space occupied by this fluid is referred to as the sub-dural space. The inner layer of the endomenix, the pia mater, is a thin, highly vascular connective tissue layer which is closely attached to the underlying nervous tissue by reticular and elastic fibres and by the cytoplasmic processes of astrocytes. This delicate vascular layer follows the surface contours of the brain and projects into the sulci. The coalescence of small spaces which form in the mesenchyme between the arachnoid membrane and the pia mater constitute the sub-arachnoid space through which the cerebrospinal fluid circulates. Mesenchyme, which persists between the two membranes, forms trabeculae which attach the arachnoid membrane to the pia mater. Blood vessels in the pia mater supply the central nervous system. As these vessels penetrate into the nervous tissue, they are covered by the pia mater for a short distance. The intervening space between the pia mater and the blood vessels is termed the perivascular space. Intermittently along the lateral surfaces of the spinal cord, the pia mater gives off collagen fibres which cross the sub-arachnoid space and attach to the dura mater. These fibres form the denticulate ligaments which hold the spinal cord in position within the sub-arachnoid space where it is bathed in cerebrospinal fluid.

Further reading

Behan, M. (2004) Organization of the nervous system. In *Duke's Physiology of Domestic Animals*. Ed. W.O. Reece. Comstock Publishing Associates, Cornell University Press, Ithaca, NY, pp. 757–769.

Butler, A.B. and Hodos, W. (2005) Functional organization of the cranial nerves. In *Comparative Vertebrate Neuroanatomy*, 2nd edn. John Wiley and Sons, Hoboken, New Jersey, pp. 173–182.

Carlson, B.M. (2004) Nervous system. In *Human Embryology and Developmental Biology*, 3rd edn. Mosby, Philadelphia, PA, pp. 233–276.

de Lahunta, A. (1983) *Veterinary Neuroanatomy and Clinical Neurology*, 2nd edn. Saunders, Philadelphia, PA.

Jenkins, T.W. (1978) *Functional Mammalian Neuroanatomy*. Lea and Febiger, Philadelphia, PA.

Jubb, K.V.F. and Huxtable, C.R. (1993) The nervous system. In *Pathology of Domestic Animals*. Vol. I, 4th edn. Eds. Jubb, K.V.F, Kennedy, P.C. and Palmer, N. Academic Press, San Diego, pp. 267–292.

King, A.S. (1987) *Physiological and Clinical Anatomy of the Domestic Mammals*. Vol. I. Central Nervous System. Oxford University Press, Oxford.

Kitchell, R.J. (2002) Introduction to the nervous system. In *Miller's Anatomy of the Dog*, 3rd edn. Ed. H.E. Evans. W.B. Saunders, Philadelphia, pp. 758–775.

Noden, D.N. and de Lahunta, A. (1985) Central nervous system and eye. In *Embryology of Domestic Animals, Developmental Mechanisms and Malformations*. Williams and Wilkins, Baltimore, MD, pp. 92–119.

Sadler, T.W. (2004) Central nervous system. In *Langman's Medical Embryology*. 9th edn. Lippincott, Williams and Wilkins, Philadelphia, pp. 433–481.

Sjaastad, O.V., Hove, K. and Sand O. (2003) The nervous system. In *Physiology of Domestic Animals*. Scandinavian Veterinary Press, Oslo, pp. 95–147.

14 Muscular and Skeletal Systems

Differentiation of somites

In mammals, seven paired structures referred to as somitomeres develop cranial to the otic placodes. Somitomeres which develop caudal to the otic placodes give rise to somites. These bilateral segmental structures, which derive from paraxial mesoderm, are located lateral to the developing neural tube and notochord. Somites, transient structures which are formed in a cranio–caudal sequence, are essential for the segmental arrangement of the spinal column and the associated spinal nerves. During the third week of gestation in domestic animals, the outlines of somites first become visible. The number of somite pairs, which is constant for a given species, is usually one pair per vertebra. In domestic animals, differentiation of somites commences around the fourth week of gestation. By the fifth week of gestation, when somite formation is complete, those formed at an earlier stage have already undergone further differentiation. Initially, cells at the periphery of a somite have the appearance of epithelial cells, while those which are centrally located are not arranged in a defined pattern.

With the commencement of differentiation, the epithelial-like cells of the medial and ventral walls of each somite lose their epithelial appearance and differentiate into mesenchymal cells. The differentiating regions of the medial and ventral walls of each somite are referred to as sclerotomes and the mesenchymal cells derived from these regions give rise to connective tissue, including cartilage and bone (Fig. 14.1). The epithelial-like cells of the dorsal and lateral walls of each somite form structures referred to as dermomyotomes. Cells from the dorso-medial and dorso-lateral borders of the dermomyotome form a distinct layer, the myotome, which gives rise to skeletal muscle; cells of the central region of the dermomyotome give rise to the dermatome which contributes to the formation of the dermis of the skin.

Differentiation of the somites is influenced by factors produced by adjacent structures, including the notochord, neural tube, lateral plate mesoderm and surface ectoderm. Signalling molecules from the gene *Sonic hedgehog*, produced by the notochord and the floor plate of the neural tube, induce the medial ventral region of the somite to become the sclerotome. The sclerotome expresses the factors Pax-1 and Pax-9 which induce the cells of the sclerotome to undergo mitosis. The sclerotomal cells lose their intercellular adhesion molecules and undergo transformation into mesenchymal cells which migrate towards the notochord and neural tube (Fig. 14.1).

Muscular system

Skeletal, cardiac and smooth muscle, which develop from mesoderm, comprise the musculature of the body. Skeletal musculature derives from paraxial mesoderm which, in the cranial region, forms somitomeres and, in the regions caudal to the otic placodes, forms somites. Splanchnic mesoderm gives rise to cardiac muscle and also to the smooth musculature of the digestive and respiratory tracts. The smooth muscle of blood vessels and the arrector pili muscles derive from mesenchyme in the regions where these structures develop. The myotome gives rise to the skeletal muscles of the trunk, neck and limbs. In response to two factors secreted by the neural tube, neurotrophin 3 and Mat-1, the dermatome differentiates and gives rise to cells which contribute to the formation of the dermis of the body with the exception of the cranial region. The major contribution to the formation of the dermis, however, is from somatic mesoderm of the body wall.

Skeletal muscle

Under the influence of Wnt proteins produced by cells in the dorsal wall of the neural tube, the dorso-medial cells of the dermomyotome become activated forming the medial myotomal segment of the dermomyotome which expresses the muscle-specific gene product Myf-5. When acted on by Wnt proteins from the body wall and Bmp proteins from the lateral plate mesoderm, the dorso-lateral region of the dermomyotome forms the lateral myotomal segment of the dermomyotome and promotes *MyoD* expression. The transcription factor MyoD influences muscle differentiation. Under the influence of the neurotrophin Nt-3, expressed by cells in the dorsal region of the neural tube, cells of the central region of

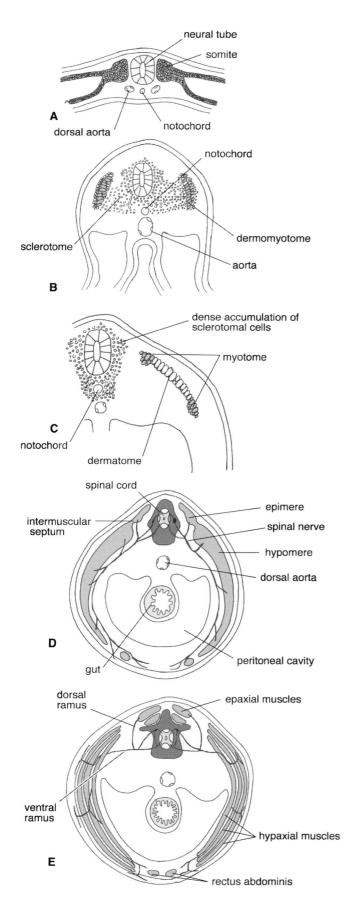

the dermomyotome are induced to differentiate and contribute to the formation of the dermis. Cells of the myotome proliferate and give rise to progenitor muscle cells, myoblasts. The myoblasts derived from the dorso-medial region of the myotome form a structure referred to as the epimere, while a grouping of myoblasts from the dorso-lateral region of the myotome form the hypomere (Fig. 14.1D). The epimere is located dorsal to the transverse process of the developing vertebra, while the hypomere is located ventral to the process. Spinal nerves develop in association with each developing somite, and each nerve gives off a dorsal branch to an epimere and a ventral branch to a hypomere. Because most anatomically defined skeletal muscles of the body derive from more than one myotome, each muscle is innervated by more than one spinal nerve.

As epimeres and hypomeres are somite-derived, the muscle groupings formed are initially arranged segmentally along a cranio-caudal axis. Subsequently, the segmentally arranged epimeric muscles fuse, forming the extensor muscles of the vertebral column, comprising the transverso-spinalis system, the longissimus system and the ileo-costalis system. Collectively, the muscles of these systems are referred to as the epaxial muscles of the body. Epaxial myoblasts are induced to proliferate by the factors Wnt-1 and Wnt-3a which are formed by cells in the dorsal region of the neural tube together with low levels of Shh which arise from cells located in the ventral region of the neural tube.

The segmentally-arranged hypomeric muscle bundles proliferate and extend ventrally into the somatopleure of the body wall, forming the primordial musculature of the body wall which initially remains segmented. Subsequently, with the exception of those in the thoracic region, the hypomeres fuse. In the cervical region, the fused hypomeres give rise to the ventral musculature of the neck. In the thoracic region, the hypomeres, while retaining their segmented arrangement, give rise to three muscle layers, the external and internal intercostal muscles and the transverse thoracic muscles. Ribs develop in the undifferentiated mesenchyme between the segmentally-arranged intercostal muscles. In the abdominal region, individual hypomeres fuse forming a continuous muscular

Figure 14.1 Sections through the abdominal regions of embryos at different stages of development showing structures which derive from somites. A, Location of somites early in gestation. B, Formation of sclerotomes and dermomyotomes from somites. C, Separation of dermatome from myotome and formation of vertebral primordium. D, Division of myotomes into dorsal epimeres and ventral hypomeres. At this stage, innervation of both muscle masses by branches of spinal nerves occurs. E, Section through abdominal region showing the location of epaxial muscles which develop from epimeres and hypaxial muscles which derive from hypomeres.

sheet which subsequently gives rise to three muscle layers, the external and internal oblique abdominal muscles and the transverse abdominal muscles (Fig. 14.1E). The ventral portions of the proliferating hypomeres which separate from the main muscle bands fuse, forming the primordium of the rectus abdominis muscle. Myoblasts from the hypomeres in the lumbo-sacral region give rise to the sub-lumbar muscles, the psoas major and psoas minor muscles and the quadratus lumborum muscles. In the sacro-caudal region, myoblasts give rise to the muscles of the pelvic diaphragm, the coccygeus and the levator ani muscles. Muscles which derive from hypomeres are collectively referred to as hypaxial muscles. Hypaxial myoblasts originating from the dorso-ventral edges of the somites are probably specified by Wnt and Bmp-4 proteins expressed by the lateral plate mesoderm. The musculature of the limbs derives from myoblasts which migrate from hypaxial musculature to the limb buds. The skeletal musculature of the head derives from myoblasts which arise from somitomeres and migrate to the pharyngeal arches. Musculature of the head is discussed in Chapter 19.

Cytodifferentiation of muscle

Smooth muscle

Most of the smooth muscle fibres of the body differentiate from cells which derive from splanchnic mesoderm. The origin of smooth muscle fibres of blood vessels is generally considered to be mesenchyme, while the ciliary and sphincter pupillae muscles of the eye derive from neural crest cells. Although there is some uncertainty about the origin of myoepithelial cells, they probably arise from neural crest-derived mesenchyme.

Cardiac muscle

Cells derived from splanchnic mesoderm surrounding the cardiac tube give rise to cardiac muscle. Unlike skeletal muscle fibres which are formed by the fusion of individual myoblasts, cardiac muscle fibres are formed by the growth and differentiation of single cardiac myoblasts. Growth of cardiac muscle occurs by the formation of new myofilaments. End-to-end adhesion of adjacent cardiac muscle cells occurs at specialised intercellular junctional complexes called intercalated discs. When cardiac muscle cells adhere to each other in a linear fashion, such a structure is referred to as a cardiac muscle fibre. During cardiac development, a group of myoblasts differentiate into special cells which form Purkinje fibres. These cells increase in size, undergo a reduction in the myofibrillar content and acquire an increased concentration of glycogen in their cytoplasm. Purkinje fibres form the intrinsic conducting system of the heart.

Histogenesis of skeletal muscle fibres

Under the influence of the myogenic transcription factors Wnt, Shh, MyoD and Myf-5, cells derived from myotomes are induced to form myoblasts. The myoblasts initially undergo a period of mitosis triggered by fibroblast growth factors and transforming growth factors. As the concentration of these growth factors decreases, myoblasts cease to divide and begin to elongate. The spindle-shaped myoblasts fuse end-to-end and disintegration of their cell membranes at their points of contact results in the formation of long, multinucleated syncytia, termed myotubules. The remaining portions of the cell membranes of adjacent myoblasts, which do not break down, form a continuous external lamina referred to as the sarcolemma. Fusion requires specific molecules, including cadherins, which promote the cell-to-cell adhesion of the developing myoblasts. The final stages in skeletal myotubule differentiation involve the production of specific myofilaments composed of the contractile proteins, actin, myosin, tropomyosin, troponin and other proteins, in a repeating pattern along the length of the myotubule. Myofilaments of actin and myosin become arranged into contractile units referred to as sarcomeres. When arranged in a linear fashion, sarcomeres form myofibrils. Collections of myofibrils grouped together in parallel formation constitute a skeletal muscle fibre. Nuclei are arranged along the periphery of the fibre and mitochondria become orientated parallel to the long axis of the sarcomeres.

A thin layer of connective tissue which surrounds individual skeletal muscle fibres is referred to as the endomysium. Bundles of muscle fibres, referred to as fascicles, are surrounded by a connective tissue layer, the perimysium. The fibrous sheath, composed of dense connective tissue surrounding an entire skeletal muscle, is referred to as the epimysium. Further growth of muscle fibres during foetal and post-natal development results from the fusion of myoblasts which did not initially fuse with the developing myotubules but remained as undifferentiated myoblasts located between the sarcolemma and the basal lamina of the muscle fibres. These undifferentiated cells are referred to as satellite cells. During post-natal life, satellite cells or their progeny can fuse with existing muscle fibres thereby increasing fibre length. Post-mitotic fusion of myoblasts involves adhesion molecules, including N-CAM and V-CAM, cadherins and integrins. Muscle damage is repaired by division and subsequent fusion of satellite cells. Innervation is an essential requirement for normal muscle development. Muscle fibres are first innervated by motor nerve fibres and later by sensory nerve fibres, the latter inducing formation of the specialised stretch receptors of muscle, the intrafusal muscle fibres.

Skeletal system

The skeletal system, which consists primarily of bone and cartilage, provides a supporting framework for other body structures and also protects internal organs. The majority of skeletal structures are composed of bone, while cartilage is associated with bone on articular surfaces and at interosseous connections. Cartilage also functions as a supporting tissue in structures such as the larynx, trachea and external ear.

The cells which give rise to the skeletal system, excluding skeletal structures of the head, derive from paraxial and lateral plate mesoderm. The skeletal structures of the head arise from mesenchymal cells which are of neural crest origin.

Histogenesis of cartilage

The primordial cells of cartilage, chondroblasts, are of mesenchymal origin. The commitment of mesenchymal cells to form cartilage is triggered by Pax 1 and Scleraxis produced by nearby mesodermal cells. These transcription factors activate cartilage-specific genes. At the particular sites where cartilage formation occurs, mesenchymal cells form aggregations and differentiate into chondroblasts. This process of aggregation is promoted by Bmp factors through the up-regulation of N-cadherin. The continued differentiation of the chondroblasts is promoted by Bmp factors, which maintain the expression of Sox transcription factors by chondrocytes. As differentiation continues, mesenchymal cells which give rise to chondroblasts lose their cytoplasmic processes, become rounded and produce the extra-cellular matrix of cartilage which is composed of glycosaminoglycans,

proteoglycans and collagen fibres (Fig. 14.2). Based on the types and distribution of fibres in their matrices, three types of cartilage are recognised: hyaline, elastic and fibrocartilage. Hyaline cartilage contains type II collagen fibres, while elastic cartilage contains type II collagen fibres with elastic fibres scattered throughout the matrix. Fibrocartilage contains dense, coarse, type I collagen fibres arranged in parallel bundles throughout the matrix. This distribution of collagen fibres accounts for the high tensile strength of fibrocartilage.

When they become entrapped in the matrix which they produce, chondroblasts are referred to as chondrocytes. The spaces occupied by cells in cartilage are known as lacunae. The mesenchymal cells surrounding the developing cartilaginous mass give rise to fibroblasts which form a connective tissue sheath, the perichondrium, consisting of an outer fibrous layer and an inner chondrogenic layer. There is a positive reciprocal interaction between chondrocytes and the cells of the perichondrium. Indian Hedgehog secreted from pre-hypertrophic and hypertrophic chondrocytes promotes the maturation of cartilage and perichondrium. In the perichondrium, parathyroid-related peptide, PTHrP, is up-regulated in response to Hedgehog signalling and acts on pre-hypertrophic chondrocytes, inhibiting hypertrophy. By acting as a signal relay between Indian Hedgehog and PTHrP, Tgf-β has a role in regulating hypertrophy of cartilage. As cartilage is avascular, chondrocytes receive their supply of nutrients and oxygen by diffusion from blood vessels in the perichondrium. If the matrix becomes calcified, thereby inhibiting diffusion, the chondrocytes die. A distinguishing feature of cartilage is its ability to grow by two processes. In one of these processes, referred to as interstitial growth, chondrocytes trapped within

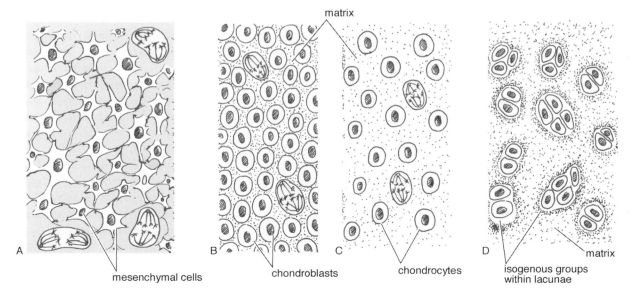

Figure 14.2 Stages in the formation of cartilage from mesenchymal cells.

lacunae retain their ability to divide. An individual chondrocyte can give rise to an isogenous group of up to eight cells. These new cells produce matrix components thereby forming additional cartilage within the existing cartilaginous mass. As individual cells of an isogenous group lay down additional matrix, they become separated from each other and each cell becomes enclosed within its own lacuna. In the second growth process, referred to as appositional growth, chondrogenic cells of the perichondrium give rise to chondroblasts which deposit a new layer of cartilage on the surface of existing cartilage.

Bone formation

Bone is a specialised connective tissue which is composed of cells, an organic matrix and a mineralised inorganic matrix. Three cell types, osteoblasts, osteocytes, and osteoclasts, participate in osteogenesis. The organic matrix, which consists of type I collagen and amorphous ground substance containing proteoglycans, accounts for approximately one-third of the bone mass. The mineralised matrix, which makes up two-thirds of bone mass, is composed of calcium phosphate in the form of hydroxyapatite crystals (Fig. 14.3).

Bone has a remarkable range of physical properties. It is relatively lightweight yet exhibits high tensile strength while retaining a degree of flexibility. It provides the supporting framework of the body, affords protection for vital structures and acts as a storehouse for inorganic minerals. Despite its strength and rigidity, bone is a constantly changing, living tissue which undergoes continual replacement and remodelling. Its structure, shape and composition may be influenced by stress forces and regional immobilisation, and also by metabolic, nutritional and endocrine factors.

Cells of bone

Osteoprogenitor cells

The cells from which osteogenic cells derive, osteoprogenitor cells, differentiate from mesenchymal cells. These progenitor cells, which have pale-staining, oval or elongated nuclei with acidophilic to faintly basophilic cytoplasm, are the stem or reserve cells of bone. When activated, these progenitor cells differentiate into osteoblasts. In both developing and mature bone, osteogenic cells are found on or close to the internal and external surfaces of bone.

Osteoblasts

The cells which are responsible for the synthesis of the bone matrix, osteoblasts, are found on the surface of developing bone and resemble a simple epithelium.

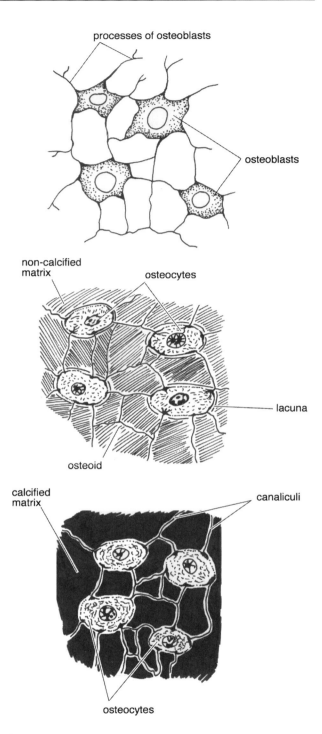

Figure 14.3 Stages in the formation of bone.

During active osteogenesis, osteoblasts are cuboidal or columnar cells with slender cytoplasmic processes which form gap junctions with adjacent osteoblasts. These cells have large round nuclei with prominent nucleoli and numerous mitochondria. Each osteoblast has a prominent Golgi apparatus surrounded by many vesicles. The extensive endoplasmic reticulum is responsible for the basophilia of their cytoplasm. Newly formed organic matrix synthesised by osteoblasts, which has not yet become calcified, is known as osteoid or pre-bone.

When osteoid matrix becomes fully calcified, the resulting tissue is bone. Osteoblasts contribute to the process of calcification through the secretion into the matrix of small vesicles which are rich in alkaline phosphatase. Secretion occurs only during the period when these cells are producing bone matrix. Osteoblasts entrapped in the bone matrix are referred to as osteocytes.

Osteocytes

Approximately 10% of osteoblasts become enclosed in the developing bone matrix. The decline in basophilic staining of osteocytes, due to the reduction in their endoplasmic reticulum content, coincides with the cessation of organic matrix production. As osteocytes become more deeply embedded in mineralised bone matrix, their cytoplasmic content decreases. The cell bodies of osteocytes reside in lacunae within the calcified matrix of bones. Their processes, which are located within channels known as canaliculi, establish contact with processes of other osteocytes, forming gap junctions. This cytoplasmic contact allows for the intercellular transfer of ions and other low molecular weight molecules. Resorption of bone matrix occurs following death of osteocytes. In comparison with cartilage, which grows by both appositional and interstitial growth, bone increases in size only by appositional growth.

Osteoclasts

Large multinucleated cells with acidophilic cytoplasm, which actively resorb mineralised bone and cartilage, are referred to as osteoclasts. Typically, these cells are found in close association with the surface of bone, often in shallow excavations known as Howship's lacunae. In developing bone, it has been estimated that the ratio of osteoclasts to osteocytes is approximately 1:150. Because osteoclasts can be up to 150 μm in diameter, only a small segment of the cell may be observed in a histological section. Up to 50 nuclei, each with a prominent nucleolus, may be present in these large phagocytic cells. Osteoclast cytoplasm contains numerous lysosomes, and the cell membrane interacting with the bone undergoing resorption has multiple cytoplasmic projections and microvilli. This microvillous portion of the cell membrane is referred to as the ruffled border. Reduction in the pH of the environment in the region of the ruffled border due to the active transport of H^+ ions from osteoclasts results in dissolution of the inorganic components of the bone matrix. The organic components of the bone matrix are degraded by the action of proteolytic enzymes secreted by the osteoclasts.

While it was formerly considered that osteoclasts were derived from osteoprogenitor cells, current evidence suggests that they are of the monocyte–macrophage lineage.

Osteoclasts, which have a long life span, are not constantly active. The bone-resorbing activity of osteoclasts is influenced by parathyroid hormone and calcitonin.

Structural and functional aspects of bone

Bone can be considered as a tissue, and individual bones can be considered as organs of the skeletal system. Like other organs, bones are composed of a number of elements including cartilage, connective tissue, haematopoietic tissue, adipose tissue and have a vascular and nerve supply. Long bones support the animal's weight and function as biomechanical levers required for locomotion. If fractured, these mechanical functions of a long bone are lost and can be restored only by osseous cells repairing the fracture. At a macroscopic level, bone as a tissue can be described as either cancellous (spongy) or compact (dense) bone (Fig. 14.4). Cancellous bone is arranged as a network of bone spicules or trabeculae, which enclose cavities, the interosseous spaces. These interosseous spaces contain bone marrow and osteogenic cells. Cancellous bone is found in vertebrae, in the majority of flat bones and in the epiphyses of long bones.

As its name implies, compact bone is a dense tissue with microscopic interosseous spaces. This type of bone, which is found in the shafts of long bones, is arranged in cylindrical lamellae which surround vascular canals forming structures referred to as Haversian systems or osteons. Because Haversian systems may be composed of up to 20 lamellae, their diameters vary widely. In cross-section these structures appear as concentric rings around central vascular channels, and longitudinally they appear as closely spaced lamellae parallel to the vascular channels. A thin cementing line demarcates the peripheral limit of each Haversian system. Volkmann's canals, vascular channels which connect Haversian canals to each other and to the periosteum, are orientated at oblique or right angles to Haversian canals. Interstitial lamellae are located between adjacent Haversian systems.

Osteogenesis

Bone develops by replacement of pre-existing connective tissue. When bone is formed in a sheet of vascular loose connective tissue, the process is referred to as intramembranous ossification. The process whereby bone replaces calcified cartilage is referred to as endochondral ossification. The terms intramembranous and endochondral ossification refer to the local environment in which bone formation takes place and not to the osteogenic process itself. Irrespective of the local environment in which bone formation takes place, the process of osteogenesis always involves the laying down of a fibrous and amorphous matrix by osteoblasts, in which calcium salts are deposited.

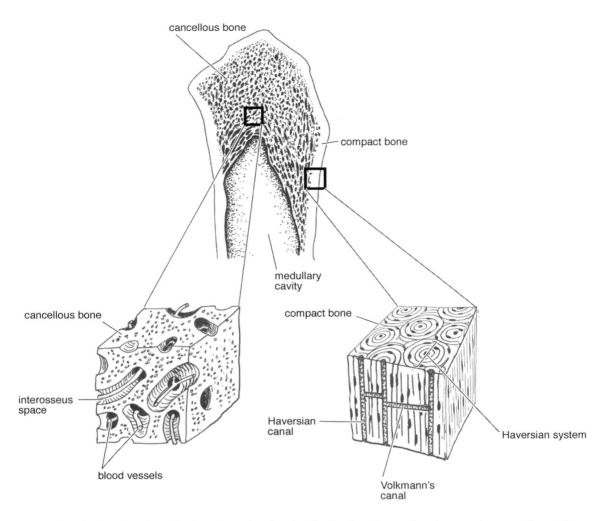

Figure 14.4 Longitudinal section through a long bone showing the distribution of cancellous bone and compact bone. The microscopic appearance of cancellous bone and compact bone is illustrated.

Flat bones of the skull

The flat bones of the skull develop by intramembranous ossification in sheets of well vascularised mesenchyme. Some mesenchymal cells differentiate into osteoblasts which produce an osteoid matrix. Subsequently, this matrix becomes calcified forming bone spicules surrounded by a layer of osteoblasts. When more spicules form in the same location and increase in thickness by the process of appositional growth, they become interconnected forming a trabecular network of cancellous bone, referred to as an ossification centre. Mesenchymal cells, both superficial and deep to the plate-like centre of ossification, give rise to periosteum composed of an inner osteogenic layer and an outer fibrous layer (Fig. 14.5). The osteogenic layer of the periosteum on either side of the centre of ossification forms plates of compact bone. The developing cancellous bone positioned between the two plates of periosteally-derived bone fuses with these two plates of compact bone. Thus, typical flat bones consist of two layers of periosteally-derived compact bone with an intervening layer of can-

cellous bone, referred to as the diploë. The interosseous spaces in cancellous bone contain bone marrow.

Long bones

Formation of long bones begins with the development of a cartilaginous template of the future bone (Fig. 14.6). Mesenchymal cells condense and form a perichondrium along the outer surface of the shaft of the cartilaginous model. Once formed, the cartilaginous template increases in size by both interstitial and appositional growth. Interstitial growth, which occurs at or near the ends of the cartilaginous template, increases its length. Chondrogenic activity of the perichondrium leads to an increase in the width of the cartilaginous template. Enlargement and growth of the chondrocytes, which become arranged in rows parallel to the long axis of the bone, with a thin layer of intercellular matrix between adjacent chondrocytes, is indicative of chondrocyte maturation. The hypertrophied chondrocytes synthesise alkaline phosphatase which promotes calcification of the surrounding matrix. The cells in the hypertrophic zone alter the extracellular

Figure 14.5 Sequential stages in intramembranous ossification leading to the formation of a flat bone (A to D).

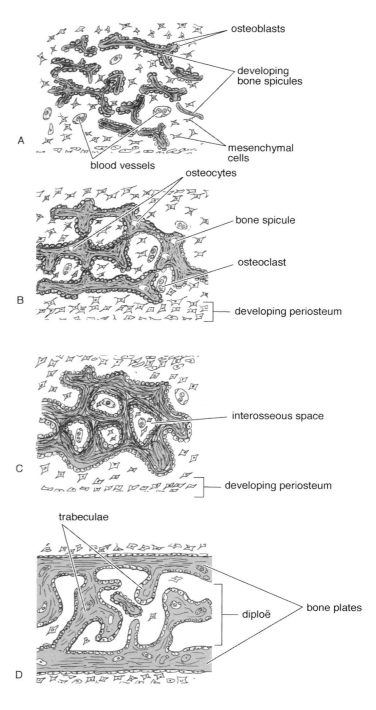

matrix by synthesising collagen X and fibronectin, enabling the matrix to become calcified by the deposition of calcium carbonate. Calcification, which impedes perfusion of oxygen and nutrients through the matrix, results in death of the chondrocytes. Following the death of the hypertrophic chondrocytes, the cells which surround the cartilaginous model differentiate into osteoblasts. These cells express the transcription factor Cbfa-1 which is necessary for both differentiation of the mesenchymal progenitors into osteoblasts and the stimulation of chondrocyte differentiation.

As calcification of the matrix is taking place, there is an increase in the blood supply to the perichondrium around the diaphysis. With the increased vascularisation, the inner mesenchymal cells differentiate into osteoprogenitor cells and the perichondrium becomes converted into the periosteum. Osteoprogenitor cells in the periosteum give rise to osteoblasts which form a collar of bone around the mid-shaft region of the cartilaginous template by intramembranous ossification.

As the calcified cartilage at the centre of the cartilaginous template degenerates, a space, the primitive medullary cavity, forms. Later, this space is invaded by blood vessels, mesenchymal cells, and osteoblasts and osteoclasts from the periosteum, collectively referred to as the periosteal bud. Invasion of the primitive medullary

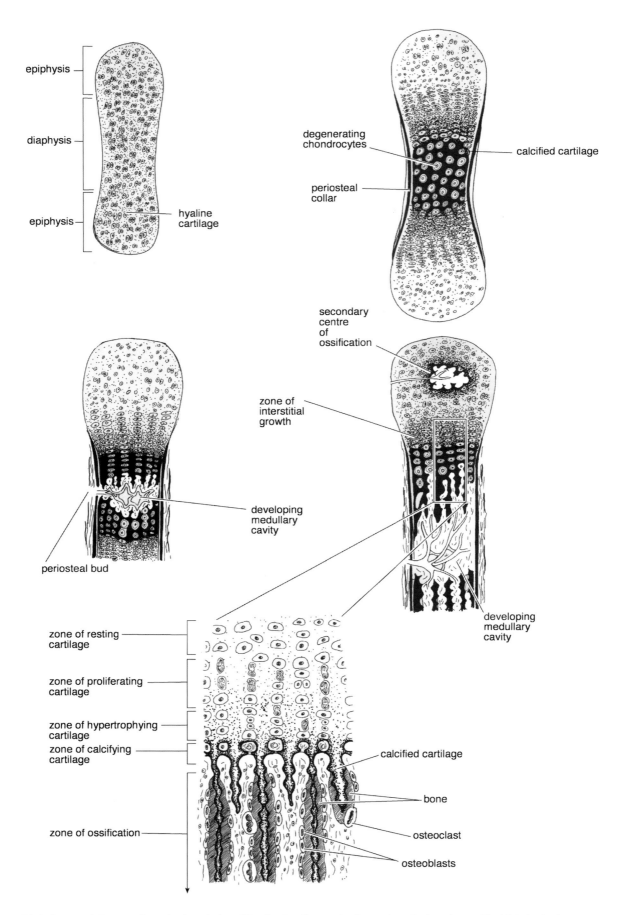

Figure 14.6 Sequential stages in endochondral ossification leading to the formation of a long bone. The histological appearance of a region where calcified cartilage is replaced by bone is illustrated.

cavity by the periosteal bud is indicative of the formation of the primary or diaphyseal centre of ossification of a long bone. Under the inductive influence of Vegf, blood vessels extend into the spaces or tunnels in the calcified cartilage, which result from the removal of the dead chondrocytes by osteoclasts. Osteoblasts, which accompany the blood vessels, line the excavated tunnels and form an osteoid matrix on the non-cellular calcified cartilaginous matrix. The osteoid tissue becomes calcified forming bone spicules with cartilaginous cores, the process of endochondral ossification.

As endochondral ossification proceeds, the primordial long bone has an hourglass-shaped appearance, with a central waisted diaphysis undergoing osteogenesis, and terminal epiphyses composed of hyaline cartilage. Interstitial growth of the hyaline cartilage continues in the regions of the diaphysis adjoining the epiphyses as osteogenesis progresses in the diaphyseal primary centre of ossification. This results in the formation of distinct zones in the cartilage at either end of the diaphysis. In the region where the epiphysis and diaphysis merge, five distinct zones within the cartilage associated with osteogenesis can be recognised in a longitudinal section (Fig. 14.6). The zone of cartilage adjacent to the epiphysis, referred to as the zone of resting or reserve cartilage, exhibits minimal cellular proliferation and matrix production. Next to the zone of resting cartilage, a zone of proliferation exists, characterised by active mitosis among chondrocytes which form parallel rows of closely packed flattened cells aligned parallel to the long axis of the bone. The third zone, the zone of hypertrophy, is characterised by enlargement of chondrocytes which accumulate glycogen, and also by reduction of the matrix between chondrocytes to thin partitions. In the fourth zone, referred to as the zone of calcification, the enlarged chondrocytes begin to degenerate and the matrix becomes calcified. The fifth zone, termed the zone of ossification, is demarcated by the presence of thin layers of bone, deposited on the surface of the calcified cartilage. In this zone, blood vessels and osteogenic cells extend into the spaces left vacant following the death of chondrocytes. As spongy bone undergoes restructuring through osteoclastic and osteoblastic activity, the medullary cavity of the diaphysis enlarges. Despite the long-established and accepted theories on endochondral ossification, data from recent *in vitro* experiments suggest that, following ossification of the intercellular matrix, some hypertrophic chondrocytes may survive and revert to a more undifferentiated cell type capable of giving rise to osteoprogenitor cells.

Secondary centres of ossification

Long bones develop from at least three centres of ossification. The primary centre of ossification is located in the diaphysis, while secondary centres of ossification are located in the epiphyses. The number of secondary centres of ossification in a particular bone is influenced by the shape of the bone and by its function. Irrespective of number, all centres of ossification, other than the primary centre, are referred to as secondary centres of ossification. Although the size and shape of each bone are genetically determined, its final form may be influenced by a range of environmental factors.

The sequence of events which leads to bone formation at the secondary centres of ossification is similar to that described for bone formation at the primary centres of ossification. Chondrocytes mature at the centre of the epiphyseal cartilage. As the central region of the matrix subsequently becomes calcified, the sequential series of osteogenic events corresponds to the steps involved in bone formation at the primary centres of ossification. Bone formation in the epiphyseal regions commences at a central point of ossification and proceeds in a radial manner. There is a progressive reduction in the amount of cartilage in the epiphyses until cartilage remains only as a thin layer on the outer surface of each epiphysis and as plates of cartilage interposed between the epiphyses and the diaphysis. The thin layers of cartilage on the epiphyseal surfaces give rise to articular cartilages, while the cartilaginous plates between the diaphysis and epiphyses are referred to as the epiphyseal plates or growth plates.

Growth in length

The histological organisation of the growth plate is similar to that of the primary centre of ossification. Elongation of the diaphysis results from interstitial growth of the cartilage within the growth plate. Although mitotic activity within the reserve chondrocytic zone continues to add new chondrocytes to this zone and causes elongation of the diaphysis, the growth plate maintains a relatively constant thickness throughout its existence. Because the rate of proliferation of the reserve cartilage is balanced against the rate of osseous replacement, the thickness of the growth plate remains relatively constant. Bones cease to elongate when the rate of cartilage proliferation is exceeded by the rate of osseous replacement, resulting in the eventual replacement of the epiphyseal plate, a process referred to as closure. With these developments, the cancellous bone of the metaphysis becomes continuous with the cancellous bone of the epiphysis.

There is wide variation not only in the times at which growth plate closure occurs in different bones within a given animal, but also in the times at which it occurs in specific bones in different species.

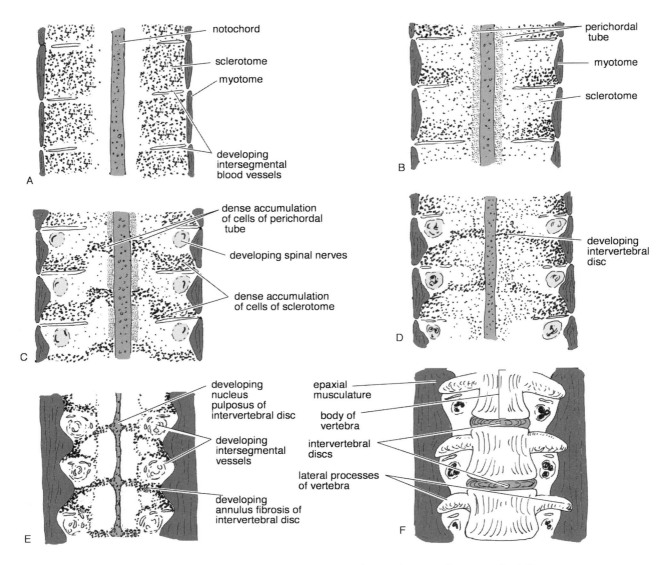

Figure 14.7 Sequential stages in the formation of vertebrae, associated musculature and intervertebral discs.

Growth in diameter

Increase in the diameter of long bones occurs through the deposition of new bone by the periosteum. This appositional growth is achieved by the process of intramembranous ossification. As new bone is added progressively to the outside of the shaft, existing bone lining the medullary cavity is resorbed. These changes ensure that the thickness of the shaft wall increases in a controlled manner until a defined dimension is reached. An associated benefit of this pattern of growth is an increase in the diameter of the marrow cavity. Despite the increase in the size of the marrow cavity, it does not encroach on the extremities of the diaphysis, where cancellous bone persists.

Bone remodelling

As a living tissue, bone can adapt its shape and internal architecture in response to external influences. Changes may result from trauma, disease, use or disuse, or from surgical intervention. Throughout foetal life, bones are constantly undergoing remodelling. These changes are brought about by extensive resorption of bone in some regions and deposition of bone at other sites. During foetal life, osseous tissue is predominantly cancellous bone. Remodelling of cancellous bone takes place through the activity of both osteoclasts and osteoblasts on the endosteal surface of bone spicules. The ongoing remodelling of compact bone involves the development of new Haversian systems from the periosteum and the gradual removal and replacement of existing Haversian systems. Bone remodelling continues throughout the life of an individual.

Vertebral column

The bodies of vertebrae develop from mesenchymal

cells derived from the sclerotomal division of somites, but the actual manner of formation is not fully resolved. Formerly, it was suggested that the bodies of vertebrae developed by the aggregation of cells from the caudal end of one sclerotome with cells from the cranial end of the adjacent sclerotome, a process referred to as re-segmentation. Currently, it is proposed that no re-segmentation occurs and that vertebral bodies arise from chondrogenic centres originating in unsegmented sclerotomally-derived mesoderm which surrounds the notochord throughout its entire length (Fig. 14.7).

Cells, which migrate medially and ventrally from the sclerotomes on either side of the neural tube, form a continuous tube of mesenchymal cells, the perichordal tube, which completely surrounds the notochord. At first, the mesenchymal cells of the perichordal tube are uniformly distributed. Later, there is increased proliferation of cells at regular intervals along the length of the tube which creates an alternating series of dense and less dense accumulations of cells. The cells of the dense accumulations form the annuli fibrosi of the intervertebral discs, while the bodies of the vertebrae develop from the less dense cellular accumulations of the perichordal tube. Mesenchymal cells within the sclerotomes undergo differential proliferation, forming dense caudal accumulations of cells and less dense rostral accumulations. Cells from the dense regions of the sclerotomes on either side of the perichordal tube, which migrate and surround the neural tube, meet dorsally forming primordial vertebral arches. Each arch, in turn, fuses with its corresponding vertebral body. The primordia of the vertebral processes and, in the thoracic region, ribs, also arise from cells in the dense regions of the sclerotomes. The lower cell density of the rostral regions facilitates neural crest cell migration and also permeation by spinal nerves and intersegmental blood vessels. Cells which derive from the less dense regions of the sclerotomes contribute to the formation of intervertebral ligaments.

Myotomes form in close association with the development of their corresponding vertebrae. The muscles which derive from the caudal region of each myotome attach to the caudal region of the vertebra which derives from the corresponding sclerotome. Similarly, the muscles which derive from the rostral region of each myotome attach to the caudal region of the vertebra which derives from the preceding sclerotome. In this manner, muscular derivatives from the caudal region of a given myotome and from the rostral region of the succeeding myotome attach to the caudal region of the same vertebra. Thus, the vertebral musculature overlaps the intervertebral joints contributing to the stabilisation of the vertebral column. Cartilaginous templates replace the mesenchyme of the primordial vertebrae. During the early foetal period, endochondral ossification of these

cartilaginous templates commences. With the exception of the atlas and axis, there are three primary centres of ossification within each cartilaginous vertebra, one for the vertebral body and one for each half of the vertebral arch (Fig. 14.8). Rostral and caudal secondary centres of ossification develop within the body of each vertebra. Prior to complete osseous fusion between the body and arch of each vertebra which does not occur until after birth, proliferation of the cartilage between the centres of ossification facilitates growth of the vertebrae. Each vertebral process has a separate centre of ossification.

Apart from the intervertebral regions, remnants of the notochord become incorporated into the body of each vertebra. The portions of the notochord which persist in each intervertebral region expand, forming the nuclei pulposi of the intervertebral discs. A layer of mesenchymal cells arranged around each nucleus pulposus forms an annulus fibrosus. Accordingly, an intervertebral disc consists of a central gelatinous nucleus pulposus surrounded by a peripheral annulus fibrosus.

Ribs

The ribs develop from mesenchymal costal processes of the thoracic vertebrae. This mesenchymal tissue, which extends between the hypomeres, becomes cartilaginous during the embryonic period and, during the early foetal period, ossifies. Ossification, however, does not extend to the distal end of the primordial cartilaginous rib. The cartilaginous portions of the ribs which do not ossify persist as the costal cartilages. The distal ends of the ribs extend toward the ventral midline. Depending on species, the costal cartilages of a number of ribs articulate with the sternum. The remaining pairs of developing ribs, referred to as asternal ribs, which do not articulate with the sternum, combine, forming the costal arches. In dogs, the costal cartilages of the first nine pairs of ribs articulate with the sternum. Eight pairs of sternal ribs are present in ruminants and horses, and seven pairs in pigs.

Sternum

At an early stage in embryological development, two longitudinal cartilaginous bars develop in the ventral body wall. With the closure of the body wall, these two bars, which are aligned with the long axis of the body, approach each other and fuse (Fig. 14.9). Fusion, which initially occurs in the cranial region of contact, extends caudally, forming the cartilaginous primordium of the sternum. Following fusion, endochondral ossification centres give rise to individual sternebrae within this primordium. The number of ossification centres and the number of sternebrae to which they give rise, although

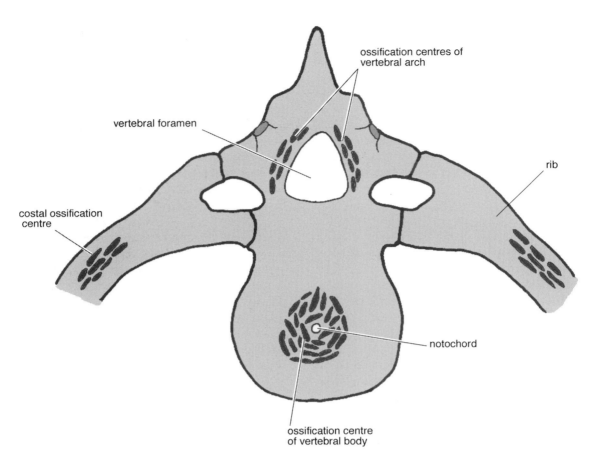

Figure 14.8 Location of centres of ossification which contribute to the formation of the body and arch of a typical vertebra. Costal ossification centres are also shown.

constant for a given species, vary among species. Gradually, the cartilaginous templates of the sternebrae become ossified. The cartilage which persists between the ossified sternebrae contributes to the formation of cartilaginous joints. The first or cranial sternebra is called the manubrium while the most caudal sternebra is the xiphisternum. The sternebrae interposed between the manubrium and the xiphisternum form the body of the sternum. The first pair of costal cartilages articulate with the manubrium and the succeeding costal cartilages form joints which are positioned between adjacent sternebrae.

Joints

Articulations between two or more bones of the body, which are referred to as joints, form early in foetal life. Based on the nature of the attachment between the bones, joints may be classified as fibrous, cartilaginous or synovial (Fig. 14.10).

During the development of a fibrous joint, the mesenchymal cells which form an inter-zonal region between the ends of developing bones differentiate into dense fibrous connective tissue and attach the apposing bones to each other. Minimal movement is possible between the bones in a fibrous joint. Examples of fibrous joints include those formed between the flat bones of the skull and between the radius and ulna. With advancing age, fibrous unions are gradually replaced by bony unions.

In the development of cartilaginous joints, the mesenchymal cells in the interzonal region differentiate into hyaline cartilage or fibrocartilage. Depending on the extent and the flexibility of the uniting cartilage, this form of union allows a limited degree of movement. Examples of cartilaginous joints include the pelvic symphysis, the joints between adjacent sternebrae and the fibrocartilaginous joints between the bodies of vertebrae. With advancing age, cartilaginous joints have a tendency to undergo ossification.

Synovial joints are formed when the mesenchymal cells in the centre of the interzonal region between two developing bones undergo apoptosis leaving a central space referred to as the joint cavity or synovial cavity. The cells at the periphery of the interzonal region give rise to ligaments and to a double-layered joint capsule. The

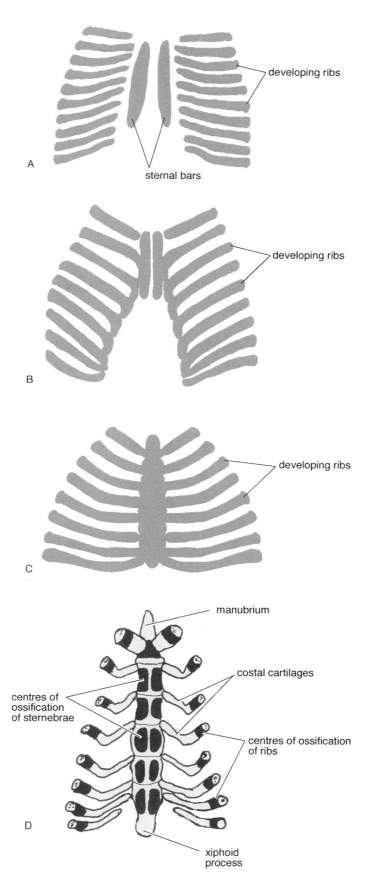

Figure 14.9 Stages in the formation of the porcine sternum, A to D. The dark areas in D represent centres of ossification.

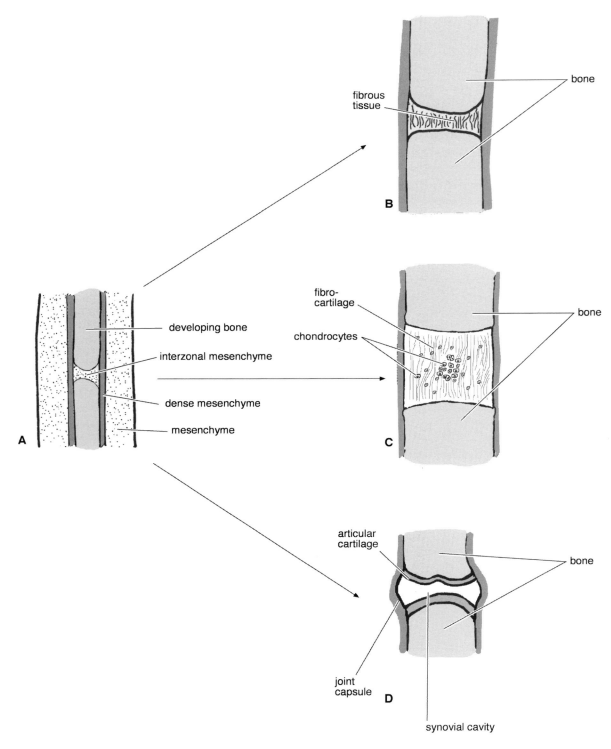

Figure 14.10 Formation of fibrous, B, cartilaginous, C, and synovial, D, joints from a common mesenchymal structural outline, A.

cells of the inner layer of the joint capsule form a secretory epithelial tissue which may develop folds or villi which project into the joint cavity. This inner layer, referred to as the synovial layer, produces synovial fluid for joint lubrication. The outer layer of the joint capsule forms dense fibrous connective tissue. Ligaments, which are composed of white fibrous connective tissue, stabilise the joint. Hyaline cartilage covers the articular surfaces of apposing bones in a synovial joint. The wide variety of movements which can be accomplished by synovial joints include flexion, extension, rotation, adduction and abduction.

Limbs

The forelimbs and hind limbs of terrestrial vertebrates develop at defined positions in the cervico-thoracic and lumbo-sacral regions of the body respectively. In sheep, pigs and cats, limb bud development commences towards the end of the third week of gestation. Limb bud development commences during the fourth week of gestation in humans, cattle and dogs. Although the early developmental processes are similar for the fore-limbs and hind limbs, forelimb development precedes that of hind limb development by up to two days.

Establishment of the limb buds

Under the inductive influence of the signalling molecule Fgf-10, limb bud development begins with the activation of mesodermal cells of the somatopleure, in the region where limb development commences. In this region, referred to as the limb field, proliferation of mesodermal cells gives rise to a mesenchymal outgrowth. This outgrowth, consisting of a core of mesenchymal cells covered by a layer of cuboidal ectodermal cells, constitutes the limb bud. As the limb bud elongates, surface ectodermal cells at its distal border proliferate under the inductive influence of Fgf-10, forming a thickened apical ectodermal ridge (AER).

Limb development is dependent on the interaction between the limb bud mesenchyme and the AER. In the absence of the AER, limb development does not take place. The signalling activity of the AER induces proliferation of the underlying mesenchyme, thereby ensuring sustained growth and differentiation of the limb bud along a proximal–distal axis. The zone of proliferating mesenchyme immediately beneath the AER is termed the progress zone, PZ. This zone in turn induces the AER to synthesise and secrete Fgf-2, Fgf-4 and Fgf-8. These growth factors induce continued proliferation of mesenchymal cells beneath the AER and ensure continued secretion of Fgf-10.

Two models have been proposed to explain the growth and differentiation of the limb bud along its proximal–distal axis (Fig. 14.11). The first model, referred to as the progress zone model, proposes that the patterning and fate of the mesenchymal cells in the PZ are determined by the length of time the mesenchymal cells remain in this zone. Mesodermal cells on the proximal edge of the proliferating progress zone become committed and remain in that region of the limb bud where they give rise to the proximal skeletal elements of the developing limb, the humerus in the forelimb bud and the femur in the hind limb bud. As the progress zone continues to proliferate, succeeding layers of cells at its proximal

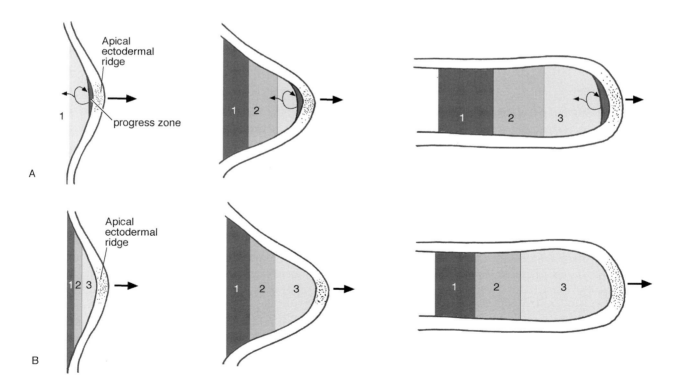

Figure 14.11 Model for the specification of the proximal–distal axis in limb bud development. A. The progress zone model. B. The early specification model. The numbers indicate zones of specification. In the progress zone model, A, it is proposed that cellular proliferation from the apical ectodermal ridge and also from the progress zone contribute to limb formation. The early specification model, B, proposes that cellular proliferation involving subsets of cells within three distinct zones is responsible for the development of the proximal, middle and distal regions of the limb. Straight arrows, direction of limb growth; curved arrows, direction of cell migration.

edge give rise to the middle skeletal elements, the radius and ulna in the forelimb bud and the tibia and fibula in the hind limb bud. The final wave of proliferation gives rise to the distal skeletal elements of the developing limb buds, namely the carpal bones, metacarpal bones and phalanges in the forelimb bud, which constitute the manus, and the tarsal bones, metatarsal bones and phalanges in the hind limb bud, which constitute the pes. An alternative proposal, referred to as the early specification model, attributes limb development to the differentiation of three subsets of cells within the PZ. Cells within one of these subsets give rise to the proximal skeletal elements of the developing limb bud, cells from the second subset give rise to the middle skeletal elements, while cells from the third subset give rise to the distal elements.

Specification of the limb axes

Normal limb development depends on the interaction of signalling centres for each of the three limb axes, proximal–distal, cranial–caudal and dorsal–ventral.

At the sites within the embryo where limb development occurs, retinoic acid appears to be critical for the initiation of limb bud outgrowth. It has been suggested that a gradient of retinoic acid along the cranial–caudal body axis may activate homeotic genes in particular mesenchymal cells destined to form the limb buds. Due to the inductive influences of Hox genes in specifying the regions where the limbs develop, their positions along the cranial–caudal body axis are constant for a given species.

As limb development proceeds, there is variation in Hox gene expression along the proximal–distal limb axis. *Hox-9* and *Hox-10* are expressed in the more proximal regions of the limb, while *Hox-13* expression is confined largely to the regions of manus and pes development (Fig. 14.12). Early in limb bud development, the mesenchymal cells express Fgf-10, and, in addition, express transcription factors which determine whether the limb bud will develop into a forelimb or a hind limb. Two of these transcription factors are members of the T-box family. T-box 5 expression is confined to the forelimb, while T-box 4 is expressed solely in the hind limb. An additional transcription factor, Pitx-1, is a requirement for hind limb development.

Before the limb can be recognised as a distinct anatomical structure, the cranial–caudal limb axis is specified. Experimental evidence suggests that this axis is specified by a small region of mesodermal tissue called the zone of polarising activity, ZPA (Fig. 14.13). The principal signalling molecule in the ZPA is Shh. The *Shh* gene appears to be activated by Fgf arising from the AER. It

has been suggested that the expression of both *Hoxb-8* and *dHand* confers selective competence on the ZPA. Shh initiates and sustains expression of Bmp-4 and Bmp-7 in the interdigital mesoderm which specifies the digits. The signalling molecule Wnt-7, expressed in the dorsal ectoderm, is a major factor in the specification of the dorsal–ventral axis of the developing limb. Wnt-7a induces Lmx-1b in the dorsal mesenchyme of the limb bud, a transcription factor which appears to be essential for differentiation of dorsal limb mesoderm. Ventral limb mesoderm produces En-1 which represses formation of Wnt-7a and consequently formation of Lmx-1b.

The AER is the signalling centre along the proximal–distal axis; the patterning of the cranial–caudal axis is regulated by a cluster of mesenchymal cells at the caudal rim of the limb bud which forms the zone of polarising activity. The dorsal mesoderm of the limb, the AER and the ZPA interact with each other, reinforcing and maintaining each other's inductive influences in early limb bud development. Wnt-7a, produced by the dorsal ectoderm, has a stimulating effect on the ZPA, whereas the Shh from the ZPA stimulates production of fibroblast growth factors by the AER. These growth factors in turn provide positive feedback to the ZPA.

As the developing limb bud elongates, its distal end flattens, forming a paddle-like distal region broader than the cylindrical proximal region. Later, a second constriction divides the proximal region into two segments. In the forelimb, these two segments are the arm and forearm, and in the hind limb the thigh and leg. At defined positions between these segments, the elbow and stifle joints form. The outline of the principal limb regions is evident at this stage of development. As it forms and grows, mesenchymal cells within the limb bud aggregate, forming mesenchymal outlines of the bones in the limb. These mesenchymal models are replaced by cartilaginous templates which subsequently undergo endochondral ossification and form the bones of the limb. Initially, the core of the limb bud consists exclusively of mesenchymal cells derived from lateral plate mesoderm which gives rise to the skeletal elements, connective tissue and blood vessels. Mesenchymal cells of myotomal origin migrate into the limb bud, precursor cells of the limb musculature. Migration of the muscle progenitor cells depends on the tyrosine kinase receptor, c-met, which interacts with its receptor ligand Hgf, produced by mesodermal cells. Mutant murine embryos which lack functional c-met or Hgf receptors have no limb skeletal muscle. Transcription of the *c-met* gene depends on the Pax-3 transcription factor. Another transcription factor, Lbx-1, is also implicated in the migration of muscle progenitor cells from the myotomes. The myogenic determination genes *MyoD* and *Myf-5*

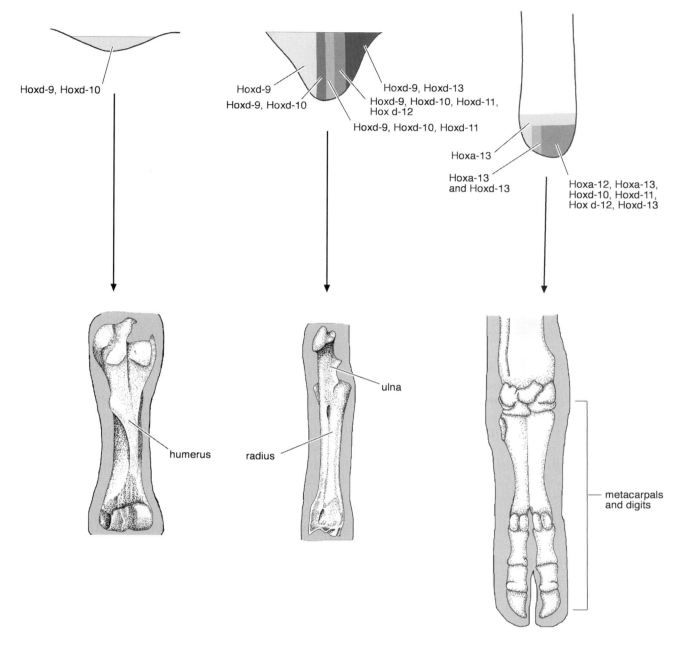

Figure 14.12 The role of Hox gene expression in the specification of structures along the proximal–distal axis during the formation of a mammalian limb bud.

do not become activated until the cells migrating from the somites reach the limb region. Activation of *MyoD* and *Myf-5* may depend on Wnt-7a and Shh produced by the surface ectoderm and the zone of polarising activity respectively. Both before and after activation of these genes, muscle precursor cells undergo extensive proliferation in the limb region. The homeobox factor Msx-1, expressed in migrating muscle progenitor cells, maintains the cells' ability to proliferate and, in addition, is thought to inhibit differentiation during migration. The homeobox *Mox-2* gene is detectable in the lateral dermomyotome and migrating myoblasts. Homozygous mutants for this gene lack specific limb muscles. The

Fgf family of signalling molecules have a major role in the proliferation of myoblasts and their subsequent migration to the limb bud. FgfR-4 and its ligand, Fgf-8, inhibit proliferation of myoblasts which subsequently express muscle-specific genes.

Cells of neural crest origin migrate to the limb bud giving rise to Schwann cells and melanocytes. Schwann cells surround the axons of spinal nerves which innervate the developing musculature. Associated with the development of the limb bud, invading myoblasts form a muscle mass for each developing limb. Later, the muscle mass separates into dorsally-positioned extensor

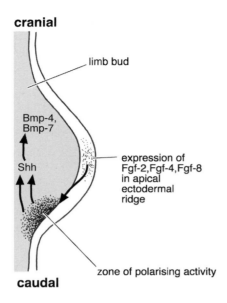

cranial

limb bud

Bmp-4,
Bmp-7

Shh

expression of
Fgf-2,Fgf-4,Fgf-8
in apical
ectodermal
ridge

zone of polarising activity

caudal

Figure 14.13 The major signalling factors in the limb bud associated with specification of digits. Arrows indicate positive influence of signalling molecules.

components and ventrally-positioned flexor components. Subsequently, the muscle masses undergo a series of divisions, giving rise to the individual limb muscles. Contemporaneously, motor axons from the spinal cord extend into the limb bud and innervate the extensor and flexor muscle groups. Later, sensory axons innervate the limb bud. Limb bud vasculature is derived from intersegmental branches of the aorta and also from endogenous vasculogenesis within local mesenchyme. The early vascular pattern consists of a central artery conducting blood into a peripheral marginal sinus which drains into peripheral venous channels. During the late embryonic period, the paddle-like distal region of the limb differentiates into the manus in the forelimb and the pes in the hind limb. The digits are formed by condensations of mesenchymal cells referred to as digital rays. At the tip of each digital ray, a segment of the AER thickens, covering the developing ray; the ectoderm between the thickened regions undergoes apoptosis. The spaces between the rays are initially occupied by loose mesenchyme which gradually undergoes apoptosis, forming notches between the digital rays. Towards the end of the embryonic stage of development, as this process of programmed cell death progresses, individual digits are formed. Bone morphogenic proteins Bmp-2, Bmp-4 and Bmp-7, together with the transcription factors Msx-1 and Msx-2, are considered to be responsible for the induction of digital ray development and the process of programmed cell death which results in digit formation. In the absence of inter-digital cell death, a tissue web connects the digits on each side. The developmental anomaly syndactyly, which is a consequence of failure in the breakdown of the interdigital mesoderm, can result in partial or complete fusion of the digits. In

many aquatic species, such as ducks, webbing between the digits is a normal anatomical feature.

During their development, the limbs undergo a series of rotations. Initially the limbs project laterally from the body and then they bend and are positioned against the body wall. In the forelimb, the first change involves flexion of the elbow and carpal joints so that the weight-bearing surface of the manus faces ventrally. The fore-limbs then undergo partial rotation, which results in the elbow joint pointing caudally and the carpus pointing cranially. Associated with these rotations, the radius and ulna cross over each other and the first digit is positioned medially. Similar changes which occur in the hind limb bring the limb into a position for supporting the body. Flexion of the stifle and tarsus bring the weight-bearing surface of the pes to a ventral position. As the hind limb is brought under the body by the medial rotation of the hip joint, the stifle joint is directed cranially.

In their earliest evolutionary forms, the distal part of the forelimbs and hind limbs consisted of five radiating digits, with digit 1 in a medial position and digit 5 in a lateral position. During evolutionary development, a reduction in the number and size of digits occurred as different species progressed from a plantigrade to a digitigrade form of locomotion. The gradual reduction in the number of digits, which occurred in a sequential order, followed a defined sequence. The sequence of change involved the gradual disappearance of digit 1 followed by digit 5 and then digits 3 and 4. Among ungulates, the equine foot illustrates the ultimate evolutionary reduction in the number of digits. In dogs, digits 2, 3, 4 and 5 are weight-bearing, while the dew-claw, which corresponds to digit 1, is non-weight-bearing. The weight-bearing digits in ruminants and pigs are digits 3 and 4 while digits 2 and 5 are non-weight-bearing. The equine foot has a single weight-bearing digit which corresponds to digit 3.

Additional adaptations observed in the limbs of ungulates include partial or complete fusion of the radius and ulna, tibia and fibula and of the metacarpal and metatarsal bones. These developments are due to the fusion of the respective mesenchymal primordia which form these limb bones.

The human hand can be used as a model for demonstrating the sequential loss of digits during evolution. By placing the hand in the plantigrade position on a flat surface and by gradually raising it to a vertical position, while still maintaining digital contact with the surface, the reduction in the weight-bearing function of individual digits can be simulated. With the hand in a vertical position, only the third digit remains in contact with the surface as a weight-bearing digit.

Skeletal anomalies

Achondroplasia

In the inherited congenital condition referred to as achondroplasia, impaired cell division within growth plates and interference with endochondral ossification, especially in the bones of the appendicular skeleton, results in dwarfism. Changes may also occur in endochondral ossification of the vertebrae and in those bones of the skull which develop by endochondral ossification. Bones which develop by intramembranous ossification are not affected. Achondroplastic animals, which are smaller than normal, have disproportionately short limb extremities, enlarged heads and short flattened faces. This condition, which occurs in humans, cattle and dogs, is due to a mutation in a gene encoding a receptor for Fgf-3. Most affected animals die in the early neonatal period.

Osteogenesis imperfecta

An inherited bone defect in cattle, dogs and cats, characterised by extreme fragility of bones, is referred to as osteogenesis imperfecta. A feature of this condition is that long bones, which are slender with thin cortices, are prone to fracture.

Osteopetrosis

An inherited disease which affects foals, calves and pups, characterised by abnormally dense bones, is referred to as osteopetrosis. In affected animals, obliteration of the marrow cavity within long bones leads to anaemia, and affected long bones are prone to fracture.

Vertebral defects

Defects in sclerotome differentiation can result in anomalous development of the vertebral column. These defects may result in spina bifida occulta, fusion of adjacent vertebrae and hemivertebrae.

If, during development of vertebrae, the left and right vertebral arches fail to fuse, the resulting defect is referred to as spina bifida occulta. As this condition has few clinical manifestations, it is usually diagnosed radiographically.

The condition referred to as block vertebra results from the fusion of two or more adjacent vertebrae.

An anomalous condition, in which only one half of a vertebra develops, is referred to as hemivertebra. The condition, which is usually confined to the thoracolumbar region, results from failure of sclerotome differentiation on one side of the developing vertebral body. If more than one vertebral body is involved, the condition may result in scoliosis, lateral deviation of the vertebral column. Two other congenital defects of the vertebral column, lordosis, abnormal ventral curvature of the vertebral column, and kyphosis, abnormal dorsal curvature, occur in domestic animals.

Congenital stenosis of a vertebral foramen may lead to constriction of the spinal cord resulting in neurological defects. In horses, this condition usually involves the third and fourth cervical vertebrae. The stenosis usually occurs at the entrance or exit of the vertebral foramen. Compression of the spinal cord as a consequence of stenosis affects the ascending spinal tracts involved with general proprioception. Affected horses usually exhibit signs of hind limb ataxia which is characterised by a wobbly gait, hence the term 'wobbler syndrome'. The wobbler syndrome has also been attributed to increased laxity of intervertebral ligaments which predisposes to spinal cord injury. A condition comparable to the wobbler syndrome, with marked stenosis of cervical vertebral foramina, is described in Basset hounds, Doberman pinschers and Great Danes.

A congenital condition, characterised by the marked ventral curvature of the vertebral column in the thoracolumbar region, results in the occipital region of the skull being reflexed backwards until it comes in contact with the sacrum. The condition, referred to as schistosomus reflexus, which is seen most commonly in cattle, includes cleft sternum, dorsal reflection of the ribs and nonunion of the pelvic symphysis. The body wall fails to close, exposing the thoracic and abdominal viscera.

Rib defects

Costal abnormalities, which occur occasionally, are usually associated with malformation of the vertebral column or sternum.

Sternal defects

As a consequence of incomplete fusion of the paired sternal bars during morphogenesis, clefts of the sternum may occur. While the condition may occur independent of other congenital defects, it is more usually associated with ectopic heart or schistosomus reflexus.

Limb defects

Malformations of the limbs may range from absence of a single skeletal element to partial or complete absence of a limb. Although limb malformations may occur alone, they may be associated with developmental anomalies of other systems. The more common forms of limb defects include amelia, absence of an entire limb, meromelia, absence of part of a limb, or ectrodactyly, absence of one or more digits. Additional limb defects include polydactyly, the presence of one or more extra digits, and syndactyly, the partial or complete fusion of digits.

Further reading

Buckingham, M., Bajard, L., Chang, T., Daubas, P., Hadchouel, J., Meilhac, S., Montarras, D., Rocancourt, D. and Relaix, F. (2003) The formation of skeletal muscle: from somite to limb. *Journal of Anatomy* **202**, 59–68.

Christ, B., Huang, R. and Welting, J. (2000) The development of the avian vertebral column. *Anatomia, histologia, embryologia* **202**, 197–194.

Colnot, C. (2005) Cellular and molecular interactions regulating skeletogenesis. *Journal of Cellular Biochemistry* **95**, 688–697.

Dalgleish, A.E. (1985) A study of development of thoracic vertebrae in the mouse assisted by autoradiography. *Acta Anatomica* **122**, 91–98.

Duprez, D. (2002) Signals regulating muscle formation in the limb during embryonic development. *International Journal of Developmental Biology* **46**, 915–925.

Fleming, A., Keynes, R.J. and Tannahill, D. (2001) The role of the notochord in vertebral column formation. *Journal of Anatomy* **199**, 177–180.

Gilbert, S.F. (2003) Development of tetrapod limbs. In *Developmental Biology*, 7th edn. Sinauer Associates, Sunderland, Mass., pp. 523–546.

Haines, L. and Currie, P.D. (2001) Morphogenesis and evolution of vertebrate appendicular muscle. *Journal of Anatomy* **199**, 205–209.

Haldiman, J.T. (1981) Bovine somite development and vertebral anlagen establishment. *Anatomia, histologia, embryologia* **10**, 289–309.

Latshaw, W.K. (1987) Musculoskeletal system. In *Veterinary Developmental Anatomy*. B.C. Decker, Toronto, pp. 127–148.

Laughton, K.W., Fisher, K.R.S., Halina, W.G. and Partlow, G.D. (2005) Schistosomus reflexus syndrome: a heritable defect in ruminants. *Anatomia, Histologia, Embryologia* **34**, 312–318.

Loni, P. (2003) Epithelial mesenchymal interactions, the ECM, and limb development. *Journal of Anatomy* **202**, 43–50.

Marks, S.C. and Popoff, S.N. (1988) Bone cell biology: the regulation of development, structure, and function in the skeleton. *American Journal of Anatomy* **183**, 1–44.

Palmer, N. (1993) Bones and joints. In *Pathology of Domestic Animals*, Vol. l, 4th edn. Eds. K.V.F. Jubb, P.C. Kennedy and N. Palmer. Academic Press, San Diego, pp. 1–181.

Sanz-Esquerro, J.J. and Tickle, C. (2003) Digit development and morphogenesis. *Journal of Anatomy* **202**, 51–58.

Szabo, K.T. (1989) *Congenital Malformations in Laboratory and Farm Animals.* Academic Press, San Diego.

Verbout, A.J. (1985) The development of the vertebral column. *Advances in Anatomy and Cell Biology* **90**, 1–122.

Yoon, B.S. and Lyons, K.M. (2004) Multiple functions of BMPs in chondrogenesis. *Journal of Cellular Biochemistry* **93**, 93–103.

15 Digestive System

Development of the primitive digestive tract commences with the cranial, caudal and lateral foldings of the embryonic disc and the incorporation of the dorsal portion of the primitive yolk sac into the embryo. The endodermally-lined cranial portion of the tract formed within the head fold is termed the foregut, the part formed within the caudal fold is referred to as the hindgut, while the segment of embryonic endoderm between the foregut and hindgut, which is continuous with the yolk sac, is called the midgut. Progressive folding of the embryo constricts the wide connection between the midgut and yolk sac until only a narrow connection remains between these two structures, known as the vitello-intestinal duct. The blind end of the foregut is apposed to an ectodermal depression in the developing head region, the stomodeum, which later forms the oral cavity. A similar ectodermal depression, in contact with the blind end of the hindgut, the proctodeum, later forms the anus. The ecto-endodermal membrane, which separates the stomodeum from the foregut, is called the oro-pharyngeal membrane; the structure between the hindgut and proctodeum is termed the cloacal membrane. Later, with the disappearance of the oro-pharyngeal and cloacal membranes, the oral cavity becomes continuous with the foregut and the hindgut opens to the exterior (Fig. 15.1).

With the folding of the lateral body walls, the embryonic gut, with the exception of the portions which later give rise to the oesophagus and anal canal, is suspended dorsally and anchored ventrally by double folds of mesothelium, the dorsal and ventral mesenteries. From a region caudal to the commencement of the primordial small intestine to a position immediately cranial to the terminal portion of the hindgut, the ventral mesentery atrophies, leaving the gut in this region attached by the dorsal mesentery alone (Fig. 15.2). Absence of a ventral mesentery allows this portion of the gut freedom to elongate and undergo partial rotation. The vascular, lymphatic and neural supply is located in a mesenchymal layer interposed between the folds of the dorsal mesentery. With the exception of the region of the foregut from which the mouth, pharynx and larynx arise, which is closely associated with the development of the head and respiratory system, the remainder of the

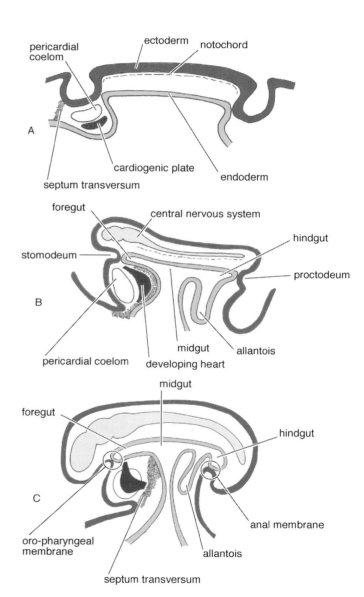

Figure 15.1 Longitudinal sections through an embryo showing sequential stages in cranial and caudal body folding leading to the formation of the foregut, midgut and hindgut.

foregut, together with the midgut and hindgut, constitutes the alimentary tract which extends from the oesophagus to the anus. Two major abdominal organs, the liver and pancreas, arise as outgrowths from the distal region of the foregut.

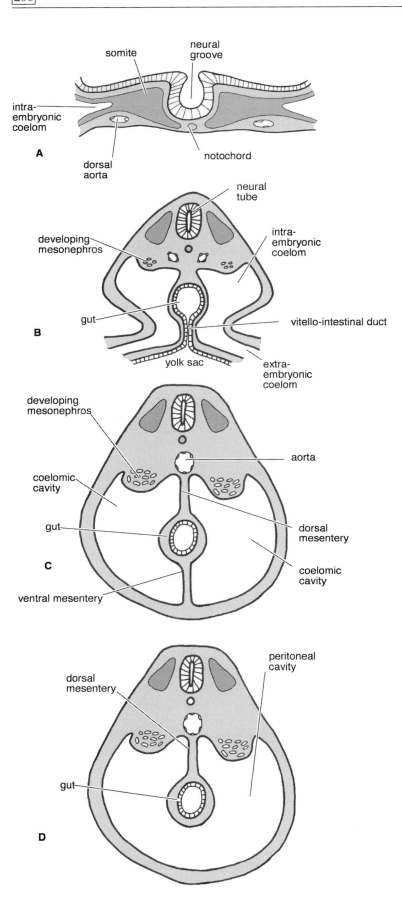

Figure 15.2 Sequential stages in lateral body folding leading to the formation of the abdominal wall, the gut and its associated mesenteries. A, Cross-section through an embryo prior to the formation of lateral body folds. B, Advanced stage of lateral body folding showing formation of the gut and the vitello-intestinal duct. C, Closure of the body wall and positions of the dorsal and ventral mesenteries. D, Atrophy of the ventral mesentery leading to formation of the peritoneal cavity.

If abnormalities occur in the processes controlling the formation of the foregut and hindgut early in development, they are invariably fatal. Accordingly, studies on the molecular mechanisms relating to these processes in transgenic mice provide inconclusive information. The transcription factor GATA-4, which is expressed in the endoderm at an early stage in development, is believed to be important in foregut formation and also in lateral body folding.

Molecular interactions between the endoderm and the mesoderm are prerequisites for normal alimentary tract development. The Sonic Hedgehog transcription factor, which is expressed in the endoderm of the gut, acts on mesoderm during gut development and induces Bmp-4 expression in the splanchnic mesoderm. Expression of Bmp-4, in turn, contributes to formation of the smooth muscle of the alimentary tract.

The primitive alimentary tract is composed of an inner lining of endoderm and an outer layer of splanchnic mesoderm. The epithelium of the digestive tract and the glands which derive from it arise from the endoderm while the splanchnic mesoderm gives rise to the smooth muscle and connective tissue of the tract. Subsequently, these tissues become organised into four basic histological layers: mucosa, submucosa, muscularis externa and serosa or adventitia. As the length of the alimentary tract increases, development of the muscularis externa proceeds in a cranio-caudal direction with the circular layer appearing first, followed by the longitudinal layer.

Wide variations, evident in the structure and function of digestive systems of animals, reflect their evolutionary development. These differences apply particularly to structures associated with the prehension, mastication and digestion of food. Carnivores tend to have short, non-voluminous gastrointestinal tracts; in contrast, herbivores usually have long, voluminous, compartmentalised digestive tracts.

Molecular regulation of alimentary tract development

Molecular controls for the pattern of development of the tissues and organs of the alimentary tract influence development in three directional planes, cranial–caudal, dorsal–ventral, left–right, and also radially.

Cranial–caudal pattern of development

There is evidence that homeobox (Hox) genes play an important role in establishing regional development of the alimentary tract along the cranial–caudal axis of the embryo. Hox genes are expressed in nested overlapping patterns along the cranial–caudal axis (Fig. 15.3). At defined regions of demarcation, sphincters of different size develop under the influence of a combination of homeobox genes together with other genes including Nkx-2.5. Several Hox genes are required for the formation of the pyloric, ileo-caecal and anal sphincters. The formation of sphincters seems to coincide with large shifts in Hox gene expression patterns. Along the cranial–caudal axis, expression of paralogous groups of Hox genes in defined anatomical regions in a craniocaudal direction corresponds to the 3′ to 5′ location of these genes within their respective gene clusters. As an example, Hox-12 and Hox-13 are expressed in the caudal regions of the developing gut and are located on the 5′ end of their respective chromosomes.

Dorsal–ventral pattern of development

In early alimentary tract development there is uniformity along the dorsal–ventral axis and Shh is expressed diffusely and uniformly. Later, in defined regions where active budding occurs, expression of Shh is inhibited. Ventral specification of the foregut, which is required for organogenesis of the thyroid gland and the lung, involves the transcription factor Nkx-2.1.

Positioning of the alimentary tract along the left–right axis of the embryo

Within a given species, the alimentary tract exhibits a consistent arrangement along the left–right axis of the body. Expression of Shh on the left side during early embryonic development results in the unilateral upregulation of other factors such as Nodal, Pitx-2, Nkx-3.2 and Fgf-8 which are expressed exclusively on the left side of the embryo. Despite the fact that the overall controls for left–right orientation are similar, it has been suggested that each organ responds to these signals independently. The precise mechanisms which regulate organ-specific responses are unknown.

Radial development of the alimentary tract

The cytodifferentiation of the endodermal lining along the length of the alimentary tract is strongly influenced by specific mesodermally-derived factors in each defined region. Hence, the characteristics of the epithelium are specific for a given region along the cranial–caudal axis of the alimentary tract. Despite these regional differences, a cross-section through any region of the alimentary tract exhibits radial organisation from serosa to lumen. Early differentiation events which influence the pattern of radial development involve a number of signalling molecules including Shh. As villi and glands develop and the cells in these regions become increasingly differentiated, Shh expression decreases.

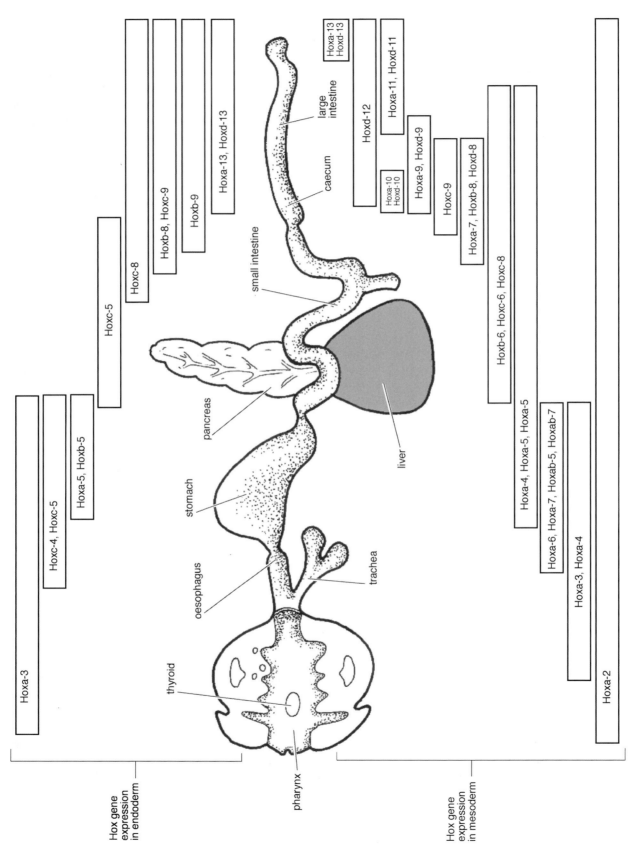

Figure 15.3 Regions of Hox gene expression in endodermally-derived and mesodermally-derived tissues along the cranial-caudal axis of the developing alimentary tract.

Oesophagus

The oesophagus, which at first is a short tube, extends from the tracheal groove to the fusiform dilatation of the foregut, the primordial stomach. In association with the elongation of the cervical region of the embryo, the oesophagus increases in length. Along its length, the endoderm of the oesophagus is surrounded by somatic mesoderm of the head, which develops into striated muscle. Species variation is evident in the extent to which the oesophagus is invested with skeletal muscle. In ruminants, the muscular component consists entirely of striated muscle. With the exception of a short terminal portion where the inner circular muscle layer is composed of smooth muscle, oesophageal muscle in carnivores is striated. In the porcine oesophagus, a short region near the stomach is composed of smooth muscle, while in horses and cats the smooth muscle extends over the caudal third of the oesophagus.

In the early stages of development, oesophageal epithelium is columnar. Later, this epithelium becomes stratified and squamous in all species, with keratinisation evident in herbivores. Oesophageal glands, which develop from the epithelium, are located in the submucosal layer. In domestic animals, these branched, tubulo-alveolar oesophageal mucous glands vary in their distribution along the length of the oesophagus.

Stomach

The stomach, which can be recognised early in embryological development as a fusiform dilatation of the caudal part of the foregut, is attached to the dorsal abdominal wall by the dorsal mesogastrium, and to the ventral wall by the ventral mesogastrium (Fig. 15.4). Because the dorsal region of the stomach grows at a greater rate than the ventral region, this organ changes morphologically resulting in the formation of a greater dorsal curvature and a lesser ventral curvature. Further growth at the cranial aspect of the greater curvature gives rise to the primordium of the fundus of the simple stomach. During its early development, the stomach undergoes two partial rotations. In the first rotation, the organ moves through an angle of 90° to the left about a cranial–caudal axis, which results in the organ assuming a position to the left of the medial plane. Thus, the former left side assumes a ventral position and the former right side a dorsal position. At this stage of development, the stomach is a C-shaped sac, flattened dorsoventrally with greater and lesser curvatures. Subsequent rotation of the stomach through a 45° angle in an anticlockwise direction about a dorsal–ventral axis results in its caudal portion occupying a position to the right of the medial plane. The anatomical region of the stomach into which the oesophagus opens is referred to as the cardia. The portion which lies above the level of the cardia is called the fundus. The large middle portion of the stomach is termed the body and the caudal area is referred to as the pylorus.

Evolutionary development accounts in part for differences not only in the shape and size but also in the epithelial lining and glandular development of the stomach. In carnivores, horses and pigs, the stomach, which is termed simple, consists of a single compartment. The canine stomach consists of four anatomical regions namely cardia, fundus, body and pylorus. In contrast with the structure of the canine stomach, the porcine stomach has a conical diverticulum in the fundic region. The fundus of the equine stomach, which extends markedly above the level of the cardia, is large, and is referred to as the saccus caecus or blind sac. In ruminants, the simple gastric primordium gives rise to a four-chambered structure.

In domestic animals the lining of the gastric primordium, which at first is composed of simple columnar epithelium, later exhibits species-specific regional differences. Simple columnar epithelium persists throughout the stomachs of carnivores, while in horses and pigs stratified squamous epithelium replaces columnar epithelium in defined gastric regions. In those regions of the stomach where simple columnar epithelium persists, gastric glands develop which extend into the lamina propria of the gastric mucosa. This zone is known as the glandular region as distinct from that covered by stratified squamous epithelium, which is referred to as the oesophageal region and is non-glandular. The rumen, reticulum and omasum, compartments of the ruminant stomach, are lined by stratified squamous epithelium and, accordingly, are non-glandular. In contrast, the fourth compartment of the ruminant stomach, the abomasum, which is lined by columnar epithelium, contains gastric glands and is physiologically comparable to the simple stomach. Early in evolutionary development, the primary role of the stomach was for food storage. Later, as a consequence of glandular development and the production of digestive enzymes, the stomach acquired a central role in the digestion of food.

As the stomach undergoes partial rotation, the ventral mesogastrium anchoring the stomach, and the dorsal mesogastrium suspending the stomach, also undergo positional changes (Fig. 15.4D). The dorsal mesogastrium, which lengthens, becomes displaced to the left with the stomach and forms a double fold called the greater omentum. The cavity enclosed by this double fold is termed the omental bursa. This space communicates with the peritoneal cavity through the epiploic foramen. Modifications in the arrangement of the

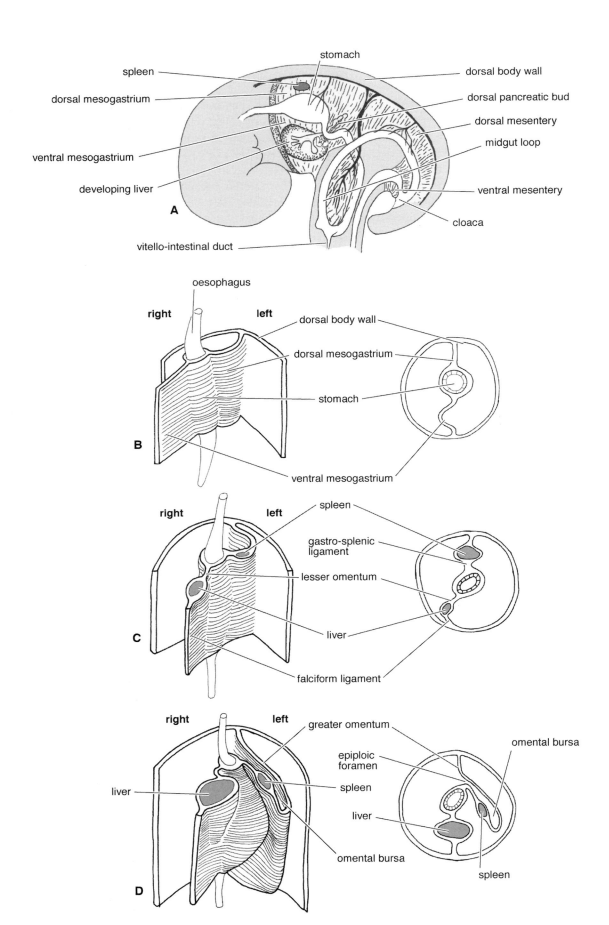

Figure 15.4 Lateral view, A, and ventro-lateral views and cross-sections through the abdominal region at the level of the stomach in a monogastric embryo. B, Developing stomach showing position of the dorsal mesogastrium and the ventral mesogastrium. C, Commencement of gastric rotation to the left and the position of the spleen in the dorsal mesogastrium and the liver in the ventral mesogastrium. D, Elongation of the dorsal mesogastrium and formation of the omental bursa. Growth of the liver in the ventral mesogastrium results in the formation of the lesser omentum dorsal to the liver and the falciform ligament ventrally.

ventral mesogastrium are described with the development of the liver.

Bovine stomach

The gastric primordium of a 30-day-old bovine embryo is a spindle-shaped structure similar to the gastric primordium of monogastric animals at a comparable stage of development. This primordial structure has a greater dorsal and lesser ventral curvature and undergoes rotation to the left in a manner similar to that which occurs in monogastric animals. The fundic region of the gastric primordium extends cranially and to the left of the medial plane. By the 34th day, this cranial expansion, which represents the primordium of the rumen and reticulum, is prominent (Fig. 15.5). An evagination develops along the lesser curvature which forms the embryonic omasum. Caudal to the embryonic omasum, the gastric primordium curves to the right and demarcates the future abomasum. Differential growth of the rumino-reticular primordium results in enlargement both in a cranial direction and to the left of the medial plane. At this stage, the rumino-reticular primordium occupies a position between the developing liver and the left mesonephros. By about the 37th day, a groove called the rumino-reticular groove, which marks the boundary between the rumen and reticulum, is evident on the ventral surface of the rumino-reticular primordium. As the embryonic rumen continues to expand, cranial and caudal grooves partially divide it into two compartments. The primordia of the four compartments of the ruminant stomach are clearly demarcated by the 40th day of development. At this stage of development, the four compartments of the bovine gastric primordium, namely the rumen, reticulum, omasum and abomasum, are lined by columnar epithelium.

The embryonic rumen rotates dorso-caudally through an angle of approximately 150° so that the blind end of the rumen which formerly pointed dorso-cranially occupies a caudal position to the left of the medial plane (Fig. 15.5). As a result of its rotation, the rumen displaces the other gastric compartments and the intestines to the right side of the abdominal cavity, their final position in the adult animal. During the third month of gestation, the four gastric compartments in the bovine foetus, which can be clearly recognised, are miniatures of those in mature animals and the relative sizes of the foetal and adult compartments are comparable. Subsequently, there is progressive enlargement of the abomasum with relatively slower growth of the other compartments. At birth, the capacity of the abomasum is approximately twice the capacity of the other three compartments combined. The lining of the rumen, reticulum and omasum, which was formerly columnar epithelium, is replaced by stratified squamous epithe-

lium. In contrast, the abomasum retains its columnar type of epithelium, in which glands develop, analogous to the glandular region of the stomach of monogastric animals. Changes in the structural arrangement of the mucous membrane of the gastric compartments is first observed in the abomasum where folding occurs at about the 40th day of gestation. At about the 45th day of gestation, leaf-like structures develop along the greater curvature of the omasum. By the 60th day, up to 50 such structures may be present. Reticular folds are evident at three months and ruminal papillae are present by four months. The stages of development, and the final anatomical arrangement of the gastric compartments in ruminants other than cattle, are similar in most respects to the bovine model.

Changes in the compartments of the bovine stomach from birth to maturity

Post-natal development of the gastric compartments in cattle is induced in part by dietary changes. For the first weeks of life, a calf's diet consists mainly of liquids, which bypass the rumen, reticulum and omasum and enter the abomasum by way of the reticular and omasal grooves. The rumen, reticulum and omasum have no role in digestion during this period. With the dietary change from liquids to solids, these compartments become functional and increase in size. Relatively, the capacity of the abomasum changes minimally. Thus, in the newborn calf, the abomasum is about twice the size of the combined rumen and reticulum, while at three months of age the abomasum is only half the size of these combined compartments. At four months of age, the rumen and reticulum are four times larger than the combined omasum and abomasum. From approximately 18 months of age, the rumen accounts for approximately 80% of the total capacity of the four compartments, the reticulum 5%, and the omasum and abomasum can each account for up to 8% of the capacity.

Omental attachments in ruminants

The simple spindle-shaped primordium of the stomach in ruminants is suspended from the dorsal midline of the abdominal cavity by the dorsal mesogastrium, which is attached along its greater curvature. The ventral mesogastrium anchors the lesser curvature to the ventral midline. The development of the simple gastric primordium into a four-chambered organ causes marked changes from this original arrangement, particularly in respect of the attachment of the dorsal mesogastrium. Following developmental modifications of the simple gastric primordium in ruminants, the dorsal mesogastrium forms the greater omentum and the ventral mesogastrium forms the lesser omentum. As the rumen, reticulum and abomasum develop from the wall

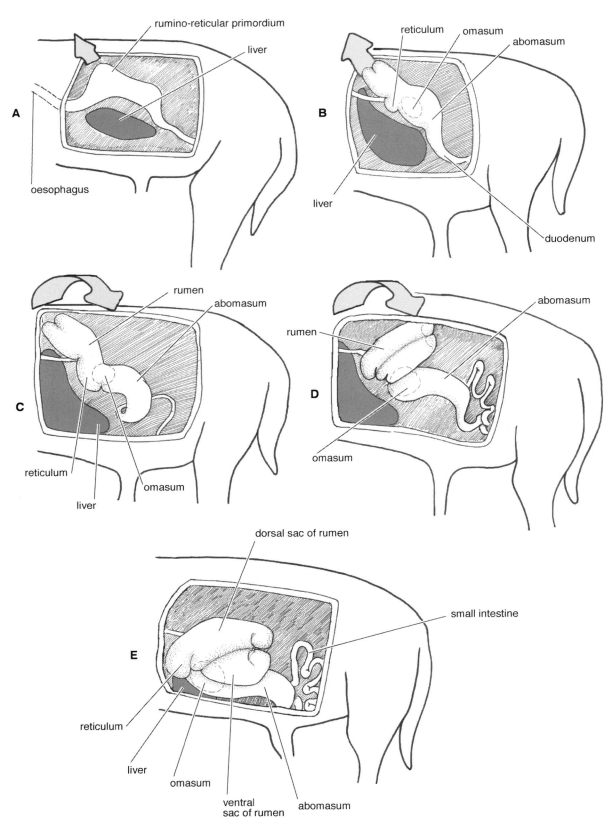

Figure 15.5 Sequential stages in the formation of the four compartments of the ruminant stomach. A, Simple gastric primordium. B, Primordia of the rumen, reticulum, omasum and abomasum and formation of ruminal groove. C and D, Stages in caudal rotation of rumen. E, Final arrangement of the four compartments of the ruminant stomach.

of the greater curvature of the gastric primordium, the greater omentum remains attached to these organs. Since the rumen develops as a cranial extension of the greater curvature, the line of attachment of the greater omentum, which begins at the oesophagus, extends along the right longitudinal groove of the rumen. The line of attachment passes in the caudal groove from right to left and then cranially along the left ruminal groove to the reticulum, and along the greater curvature of the abomasum. The lesser omentum, which extends from the liver to the omasum, has its line of attachment along the lesser curvature of the abomasum.

Avian stomach and related structures

A saccular diverticulum which develops in the ventral wall of the cervical region of the oesophagus in most avian species is referred to as the crop. This diverticulum serves as a short-term reservoir for food, especially grain.

The avian stomach arises from a simple gastric primordium, the cranial part of which becomes the glandular proventriculus, with the caudal muscular region forming the gizzard.

Liver

The liver develops as a hollow ventral diverticulum from the caudal region of the foregut. The diverticulum divides into cranial (hepatic) and caudal (cystic) parts. The hepatic primordium grows cranio-ventrally into the ventral mesogastrium and extends into the septum transversum (Fig. 15.6). The endodermal hepatic diverticulum arises as a result of inductions originating from the hepato-cardiac mesoderm mediated principally by a range of fibroblast growth factors including Fgf-1, Fgf-2 and Fgf-8. In addition, Bmp-2, Bmp-4 and Bmp-7 signals, arising from the septum transversum, specify the development of ventral foregut endoderm into committed precursors of the hepatic epithelium.

The endodermal epithelial cells of the hepatic portion proliferate and form plates of liver cells. As development proceeds, the closely associated mesoderm of the septum transversum continues to support the sustained growth and proliferation of the hepatic endoderm. Hepatic growth factor, which is bound by the receptor c-met, located on the surface of the hepatic endodermal cells, is an example of a specific mesodermally-derived growth factor. Hepatic connective tissue arises from the mesenchymal cells of the septum transversum and splanchnic mesoderm. The hepatic plates disrupt the continuity of the vitelline and umbilical veins, which run through the septum transversum. These vessels, together with additional developing blood vessels, later become the liver sinusoids. The caudal part of the hep-

atic diverticulum forms the gall bladder and cystic duct. That portion of the original diverticulum between the foregut and the area where the hepatic duct and cystic duct join is called the common bile duct. Because the primordium of the gall bladder and cystic duct atrophy during early embryological development in horses, rats and whales, a gall bladder is not formed in these animals. The rapid growth of the liver within the septum transversum causes it to extend caudally beyond the septum so that it gradually protrudes into the abdominal cavity. Mesoderm from the septum, which surrounds the expanding liver, gives rise to the hepatic capsule and associated peritoneal covering. Cranially, the liver remains attached to the tendinous centre of the diaphragm by the coronary ligament, and laterally to the body wall by lateral ligaments. The mesoderm of the septum transversum and ventral mesogastrium between the liver and the lesser curvature of the stomach forms the lesser omentum. That portion of the mesoderm between the liver and the ventral abdominal wall forms the falciform ligament in which the left umbilical vein runs from the umbilicus to the liver (Fig. 15.7). Initially, the liver develops a right and a left lobe. Subsequently, two outgrowths of the right lobe give rise to the caudate and quadrate lobes. In some species, subdivision of the left and right lobes may occur. The final position and orientation of the liver in the abdominal cavity are influenced by the development and rotation of the other abdominal organs. In ruminants, the liver, which is displaced by the developing rumen, lies almost entirely to the right of the medial plane in the abdominal cavity.

The blood-forming role of the embryonic liver, which begins during the second month of gestation, accounts in part for its rapid increase in size during early embryological development. Blood stem cells which migrate from the aorta–gonad–mesonephros region to the liver, initiate haematopoietic activity in this organ.

Pancreas

The pancreas develops as dorsal and ventral endodermal outgrowths of the caudal part of the foregut. The dorsal pancreatic bud, which develops before the ventral bud, occupies a position between the layers of the dorsal mesogastrium. The ventral pancreatic bud, which arises from the hepatic diverticulum near its origin, develops within the ventral mesogastrium (Fig. 15.6). The cells of the pancreatic buds proliferate in an arboreal fashion and give rise to the ducts and associated secretory acini of the pancreas. Some epithelial cells which lose their connections with the duct system develop into the endocrine portion of the pancreas, the pancreatic islets, known as islets of Langerhans. The connective tissue of the pancreas develops from splanchnic mesoderm. As a consequence of gastric and intestinal rotation,

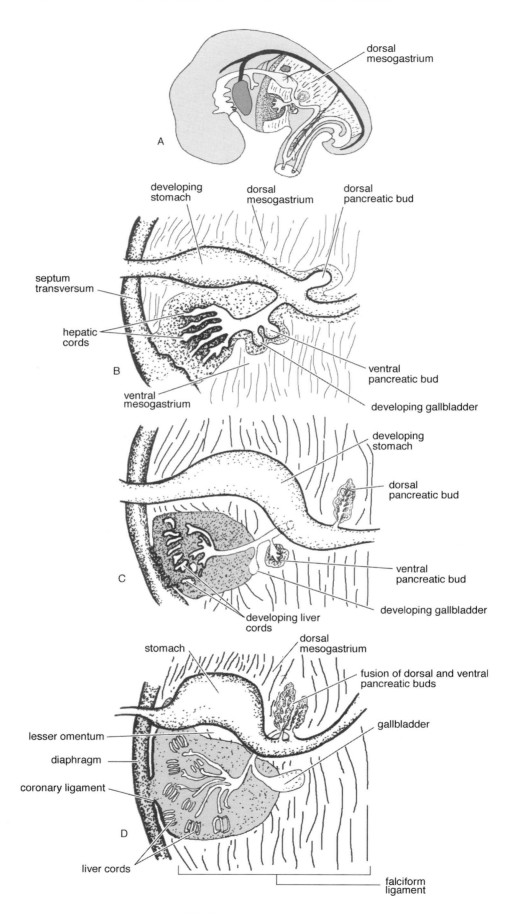

Figure 15.6 Sequential stages in the development of the liver and pancreas.

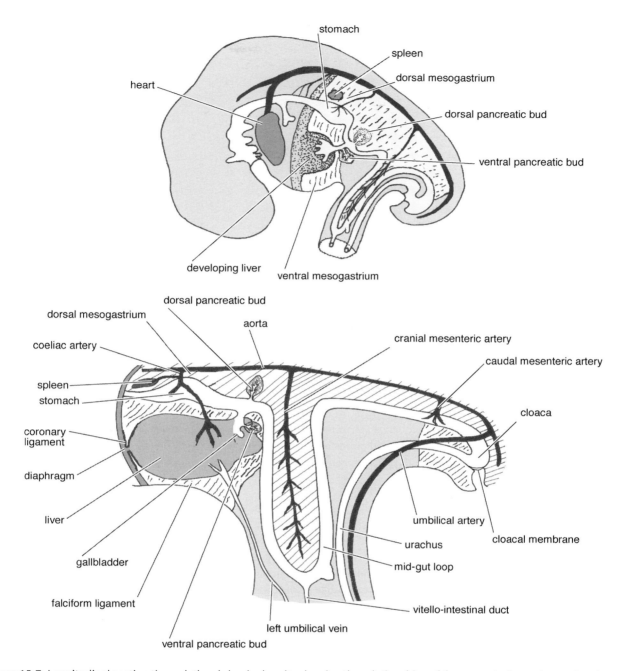

Figure 15.7 Longitudinal section through the abdominal cavity showing the relationships of the mesenteries and associated structures.

the ventral and dorsal pancreatic buds overlap and fuse at their points of contact (Fig. 15.8). This fusion of the pancreatic buds results in a single anatomical structure consisting of a body and left and right lobes. The left lobe develops from the dorsal bud and the right lobe from the ventral bud. The duct of the ventral pancreatic lobe, referred to as the pancreatic duct, joins with the bile duct to form the common bile duct which opens into the duodenum forming an elevation known as the major duodenal papilla. The duct of the dorsal lobe, which enters the duodenum at an elevation of the mucosa known as the minor duodenal papilla, is called the accessory pancreatic duct. Species variation is observed in the arrangement of the terminal portions of the pancreatic ducts. The terminal portions of both ducts may persist or alternatively the terminal portion of either the dorsal duct or the ventral duct may atrophy. In species in which atrophy of the terminal portion of one duct occurs, fusion of the remainder of that duct with the terminal portion of the intact duct permits the secretion of both pancreatic lobes to be conveyed to the duodenum through the intact duct. In humans, horses and dogs, both ducts persist in their entirety; in sheep, goats and cats the terminal portion of the dorsal duct atrophies. The terminal portion of the ventral duct atrophies in cattle and pigs.

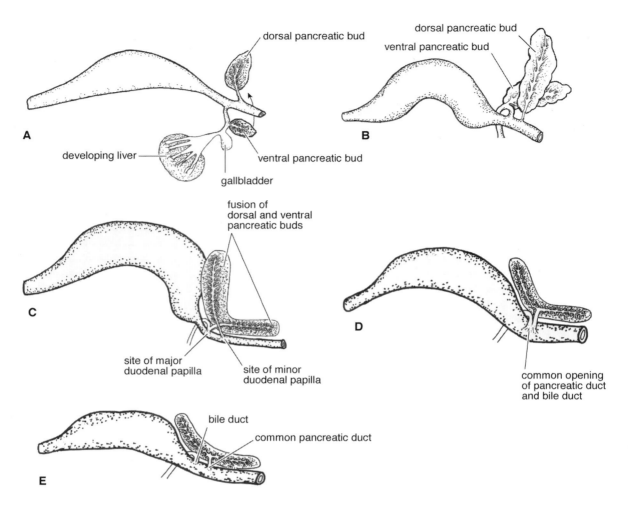

Figure 15.8 Sequential stages in the development of the pancreas, A and B. Final arrangement of the pancreatic duct system in humans, horses and dogs, C, in sheep, goats and cats, D, and in cattle and pigs, E.

Pancreatic development is initiated at the caudal end of the foregut. The dorsal pancreatic bud is induced from the dorsal gut endoderm by activin and fibroblast growth factor signals arising from the notochord. Both of these growth factors repress Shh expression. Subsequently, expression of the pancreatic and duodenal homeobox gene *Pdx-1* is up-regulated in the endoderm of the foregut at regions where both the dorsal and ventral pancreatic buds form. Expression of Shh is restricted to regions of the endoderm which do not express Pdx-1. It has been suggested that Pdx-1 expression is required for normal pancreatic epithelial development but not for pancreatic mesodermal development. The mesodermal pattern of pancreatic development occurs only in the absence of Shh.

Spleen

Although it is a lymphatic organ, development of the spleen is usually considered with the digestive system due to its close embryological association with the

stomach, liver and pancreas. The mammalian spleen develops as an aggregation of mesenchymal cells in the dorsal mesogastrium (Fig. 15.7). As the dorsal mesogastrium and stomach primordium rotate to the left, the spleen primordium is also drawn to the left and becomes apposed to the greater curvature of the stomach to which it is attached by a fold of the dorsal mesogastrium, the gastro-splenic ligament. The mesenchymal cells differentiate and form the splenic capsule and connective tissue; cellular elements of the spleen responsible for haematopoiesis derive from other haematopoietic centres, such as the aorta–gonad–mesonephros. Later, with the establishment of definitive haematopoietic activity in the bone marrow and the development of the lymphoid component of the thymus, B and T lymphocytes populate the spleen and it becomes a functional lymphoid organ. The splenic blood supply derives from a branch of the caudal aorta. By the third month of gestation, the principal structures of the bovine spleen, namely capsule, trabeculae, red pulp, white pulp and blood vessels, can be distinguished.

Development and rotation of the intestines in domestic animals

The intestines are formed from that portion of the foregut which is positioned caudal to the developing stomach and from the entire midgut and hindgut. A short section of the foregut has both a dorsal and ventral mesentery, while the ventral mesentery of the midgut and hindgut atrophies. The midgut, together with its associated mesentery, elongates forming a midgut loop. At the ventral curvature of this loop, the vestige of the vitello-intestinal duct is evident. The descending limb of the midgut loop develops into the distal part of the duodenum, the jejunum and part of the ileum. The ascending limb forms the terminal portion of the ileum, the caecum, the ascending colon, and the proximal portion of the transverse colon. The midgut receives its blood supply from a branch of the dorsal aorta, the cranial mesenteric artery, which is located in the dorsal mesentery. As the loop increases in length, it outgrows its available space in the abdominal cavity and occupies part of the extra-embryonic coelom called the umbilical sac. This herniation of the foetal gut during this period of development, which is a normal occurrence, is referred to as physiological umbilical herniation. These changes occur around the third to fourth week of gestation in cattle, sheep, pigs and dogs. During the time the midgut loop occupies a position in the extra-embryonic coelom, it rotates clockwise, viewed dorso-ventrally, about an axis formed by the cranial mesenteric artery (Fig. 15.9). At first, the rotation is approximately 180° clockwise, so that the descending limb is repositioned caudally and the ascending limb cranially. The descending limb increases in length and forms a series of coiled loops on the right side of the umbilical sac. The ascending limb, which develops a diverticulum, the primitive caecum, grows more slowly than the descending limb, and occupies the left side of the umbilical sac. Due to the lengthening of the midgut, the umbilical sac is unable to accommodate the herniated mass of intestines. Subsequently, the limbs of the midgut loop return to the abdominal cavity where they are accommodated, as proportionately, the liver and kidneys occupy less space in the enlarged cavity than formerly. As the caecal diverticulum impedes the return of the ascending limb, the descending limb is first to return, passing to the left, caudal to the cranial mesenteric artery, and occupying a position medial to the hindgut and its mesentery. As a result, the hindgut, destined to become the descending colon, moves to the left side of the abdominal cavity. The ascending limb of the midgut loop returns to the abdominal cavity passing in front of the cranial mesenteric artery and occupies a position to the right of the midline. The withdrawal of the midgut loop from the umbilical sac results in a further rotation of the intestine

around the cranial mesenteric artery so that the full extent of rotation exceeds 270°.

The development, final position and relationships of the intestines, as described above, relate particularly to carnivores.

Comparative features of the intestines

Although the positions and relationships of the intestine in ruminants, horses and pigs may at first appear different from that of dogs, the position and relationships of the small intestine, caecum, and transverse and descending colon are similar in all domestic species. The length and associated positional changes of the ascending colon are features which distinguish the intestines of domestic animals (Fig. 15.10). As a general rule, carnivores have short intestines and small caeca, whereas herbivores have long intestines and large caeca.

Ruminant intestines

The embryological development and associated rotational changes of the intestines in ruminants follow a pattern similar to that which occurs in carnivores. As the intestines return to the abdominal cavity, the caecal diverticulum increases in size and the ascending colon lengthens forming a loop suspended by a portion of dorsal mesentery referred to as the mesocolon. The loop increases in length, passes to the left side of the mesentery of the small intestine and then coils in a clockwise manner, viewed from the right (Fig. 15.10B). Fusion of the mesocolon with the mesentery of the small intestine can convey the impression that the colon is suspended by the mesentery of the small intestine, when in fact it is suspended by the mesocolon alone. Ingesta passing along the lumen of the coiled colon first travel centripetally for approximately two to three turns and, on reaching the centre of the coil, travel centrifugally. The coils, which are at first conical in arrangement, later assume a circular arrangement in a single plane. In cattle, the changes in the ascending colon occur during the second to the fourth months of gestation. Because the developing rumen displaces the intestines to the right, all of the intestines, with the exception of the rectum, are located to the right of the medial plane in ruminant animals.

Porcine intestines

Porcine intestines initially develop in a manner similar to the development of ruminant intestines. In pigs, however, the coils of the ascending colon remain in a cone-shaped arrangement with the base positioned medially and the apex directed towards the left flank, displacing the caecum to the left of the midline (Fig. 15.10C). The

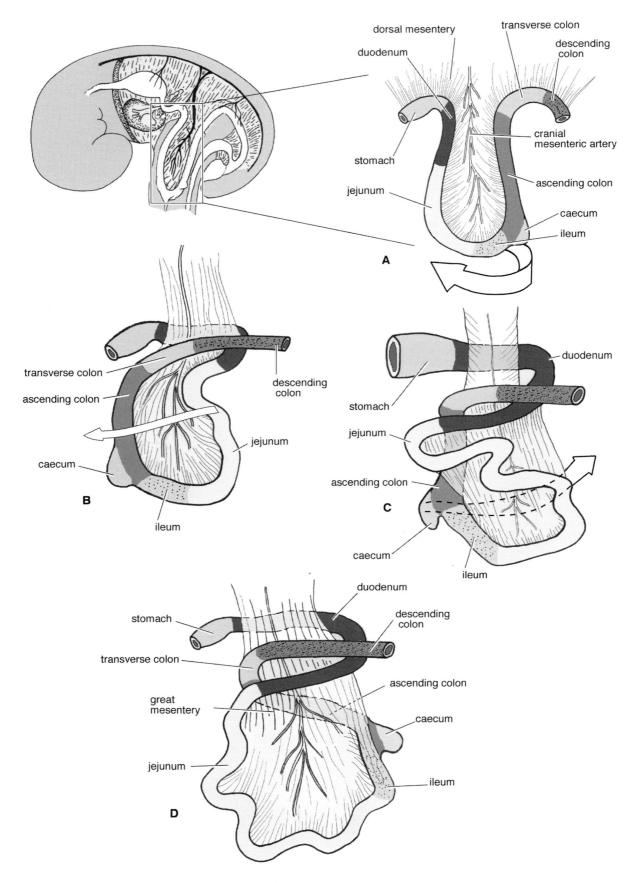

Figure 15.9 Left lateral views showing stages in midgut rotation. A, Descending and ascending limbs of the midgut loop prior to rotation in direction of arrow. B, Change in relative positions of descending and ascending limbs of the midgut loop following initial stage of rotation. C, Further stage in midgut rotation. D, Final arrangement of limbs of the midgut loop in carnivores.

Figure 15.10 Anatomical arrangement of the large intestine of domestic animals showing the comparative features of the caecum and ascending colon. A, Components of the large intestine in carnivores illustrating a simple ascending colon. B, Components of the large intestine of ruminants showing the coiled ascending colon positioned in a single plane. C, Components of porcine large intestine illustrating the cone-shaped arrangement of the coiled ascending colon. D, Components of the equine large intestine illustrating the enlarged caecum and the dorsal and ventral components of the ascending colon.

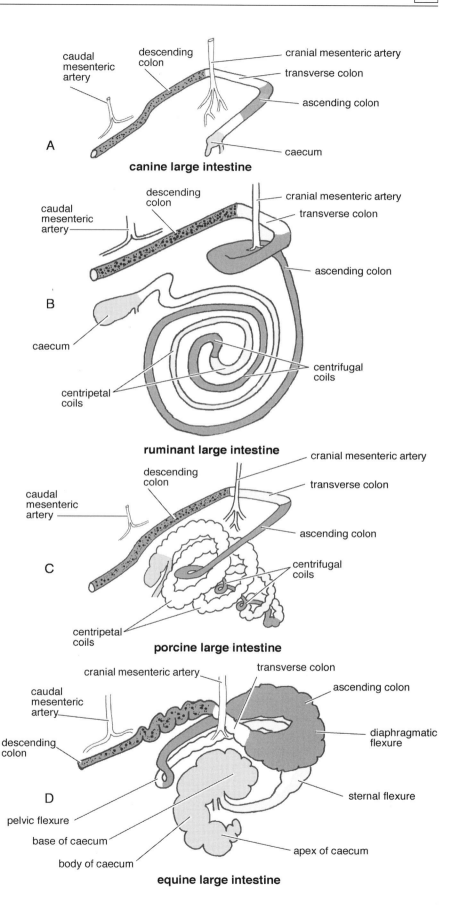

proximal limb of the initial loop gives rise to the centripetal turns, located on the outside of the cone, while the distal limb gives rise to the concealed centrifugal turns. Instead of forming a flat muscular sheet, the outer longitudinal muscle layer becomes arranged into three longitudinal muscle bands or taeniae. The centripetal coil of the ascending colon develops two similar bands or taeniae. These taeniae cause puckering of the caecum and of the centripetal coils of the porcine colon. The major structural changes in the ascending colon of the pig occur during the second month of gestation.

Equine intestines

Unlike ruminants, where microbial fermentation occurs in the pre-intestinal portion of the alimentary tract, the site of cellulose digestion in horses is the large intestine. Accordingly, the caecum and ascending colon are considerably greater in size than other segments of the intestine and have a capacity of up to 100 litres in adult horses. The ascending colon (large colon) elongates, but does not form a coil as in ruminants and pigs. The loop extends cranially on the right side to reach the diaphragm, and then crosses to the left side of the abdominal cavity where it extends caudally to the pelvic inlet. The ascending colon consists of right ventral, left ventral, left dorsal and right dorsal segments (Fig. 15.10D). The flexure between the left and right ventral segments is the sternal flexure; that between the left ventral and left dorsal segments is the pelvic flexure and that between the left dorsal and right dorsal segments is the diaphragmatic flexure. The definitive caecum arises from the foetal caecum with a contribution from the commencement of the ascending colon (Fig. 15.11). The base derives from a dilatation of the wall of the ascending colon opposite the ileo-caecal opening. The foetal caecum elongates cranially to a position between the left and right segments of the ascending colon and gives rise to the body and apex of the definitive caecum. As a result of this differential growth, the base of the caecum has a greater and lesser curvature. Both the ileum and the non-dilated portion of the ascending colon communicate with the caecum on its lesser curvature (Fig. 15.11D). The descending colon elongates and its mesentery lengthens so that its coils mingle with the loops of the small intestine. The longitudinal smooth muscle layers of both the caecum and ventral segments of the ascending colon form four bands. Those on the left dorsal segment form one band and those on the right dorsal segment form three bands; two muscle bands are present in the transverse and descending colon. The characteristic puckering which is a feature of all segments of the equine large intestine is due to the presence of these longitudinal smooth muscle bands. The structural and positional changes relating to the

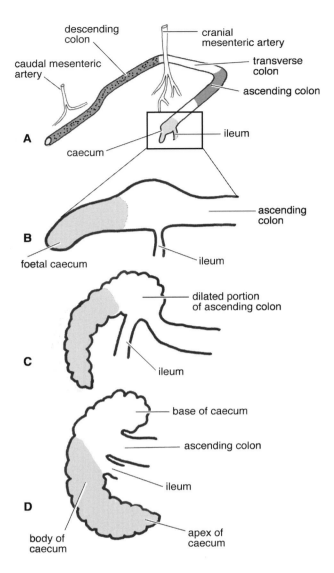

Figure 15.11 Stages in the development of the definitive equine caecum.

ascending colon of the horse occur during the second month of gestation.

Hindgut

The portion of the transverse colon which lies to the left of the medial plane, together with the descending colon, the cloaca and the allantois, arise from the hindgut. The cloaca, the dilated terminal region of the embryonic hindgut, is partitioned by the formation of the urorectal septum into the anorectal canal dorsally and the urogenital sinus ventrally and is separated from the proctodeum by the cloacal membrane (Fig. 15.12). The allantois, which develops as an evagination of the hindgut, extends through the umbilicus and enlarges to

Figure 15.12 Longitudinal sections through the lumbo-sacral region of an embryo showing stages in the division of the cloaca by the urorectal septum into the anorectal canal and the urogenital sinus, A and B.

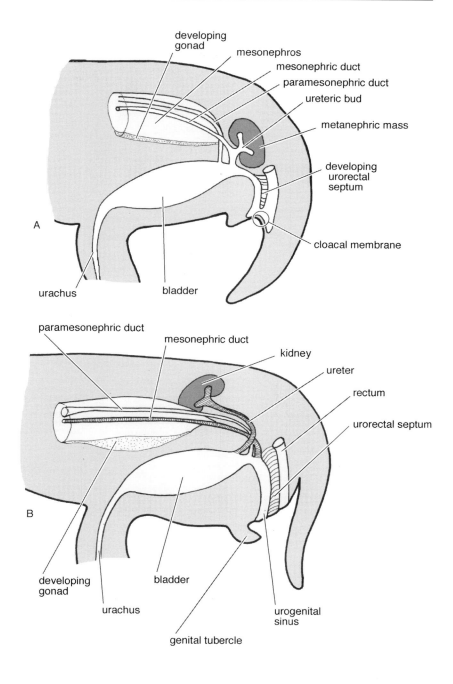

occupy a position in the extra-embryonic coelom. Fusion of the urorectal septum with the cloacal membrane divides the latter into two distinct membranes, the anal membrane dorsally and the urogenital membrane ventrally. An elevation covered by ectoderm surrounding the cloacal membrane, called the cloacal fold, also becomes subdivided into an anal fold dorsally and a urogenital fold ventrally. The urorectal septum gives rise to a fibro-muscular mass referred to as the perineal body. Breakdown of both the anal and the urogenital membranes soon after their formation allows both the alimentary tract and the urogenital tract to communicate with the exterior. In domestic carnivores, two lateral epithelial outgrowths develop at the recto-anal junction and, from these, paranal sinuses and their associated circumanal glands are formed.

Developmental anomalies of the alimentary tract

Stenosis of specific regions of the alimentary tract

An abnormal narrowing or stricture of a portion of the digestive tract is referred to as stenosis. Although this anomaly may occur in any part of the alimentary tract, it is observed more frequently in the small intestine than

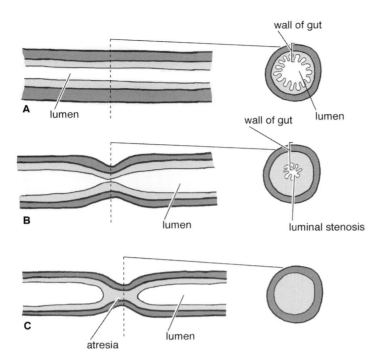

Figure 15.13 Stenosis and atresia of the small intestine. A, Normal intestine. B, Stenosis. C, Atresia. Cross-sections of the normal and abnormal intestines are shown.

elsewhere in the tract. In mice, coincidental mutations in *Hoxa-13* and *Hoxd-13* genes result in anal stenosis.

Atresia

The term 'atresia' describes congenital occlusion of the lumen of the digestive tract. The occlusion itself may occur as a complete membranous partition, as a fibrous or muscular cord between the blind ends of intestine, or there may be a complete absence of a segment of gut. Post-natally, the segment of the intestine proximal to the occlusion is usually dilated. Atresia may occur in the small intestine of cattle, sheep and dogs and in the large intestine of cattle, horses and cats. This condition may result from an inadequate blood supply to a segment of the developing intestine leading to atrophy of the affected portion (Fig. 15.13).

Imperforate anus

Failure of the anal membrane to break down during development gives rise to the condition termed imperforate anus, sometimes described as *atresia ani*. Imperforate anus, which is found in all species, is the most common developmental anomaly of the digestive tract. It is particularly common in cattle and pigs. This condition is often accompanied by atresia of the rectum.

Urorectal fistula

An uncommon anomaly, congenital urorectal fistula results from failure of the urorectal septum to completely separate the anorectal and urogenital sinuses allowing the passage of faecal material into the urogeni-

tal sinus. An acquired urorectal fistula, which may occur during parturition, particularly in mares, is caused by rupture of the perineal body by a foetal limb.

Omphalocoele

If the intestinal loops fail to return to the abdominal cavity from the umbilical sac and protrude through an enlarged umbilical ring, a condition referred to as omphalocoele results.

Congenital umbilical hernia

Incomplete closure of the abdominal wall in the region of the umbilicus results in the anomaly referred to as congenital umbilical hernia. In this condition, loops of intestine protrude through the abdominal wall and occupy a subcutaneous position. The condition occurs more commonly in pigs than in other domestic mammals.

Vitello-intestinal duct anomalies

The vitello-intestinal duct, which connects the midgut loop to the yolk sac, normally atrophies when the yolk sac ceases to function. Persistence of a patent vitello-intestinal duct between the intestine and the umbilicus leads to the development of an umbilical or vitelline fistula. It may also persist as a fibrous cord sometimes with an enclosed cyst. A remnant of the vitello-intestinal duct which occasionally persists as a blind pouch on the border of the intestine, opposite to the line of attachment of the mesentery, is known as Meckel's diverticulum (Fig. 15.14).

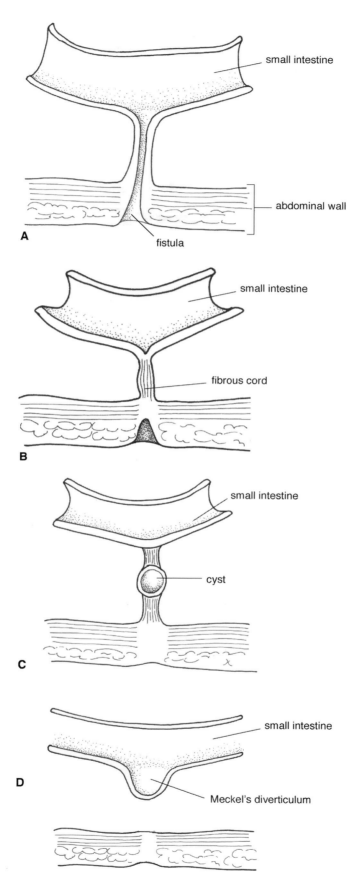

Figure 15.14 Anomalies of the midgut loop and adjacent abdominal wall. A, Umbilical or vitelline fistula. B, Fibrous cord which is the remnant of the vitello-intestinal duct attaching the intestine to the abdominal wall. C, Cyst formation in the fibrous cord remnant of the vitello-intestinal duct. D, Meckel's diverticulum.

'Situs inversus'

A condition in which both the thoracic and the abdominal organs are transferred to the side opposite to that in which they are normally located is referred to as *situs inversus*. In this abnormal position, the organs form mirror images of the normally-located organs. This condition, which is compatible with normal function, is usually detected only when an animal with this anomaly is subjected to diagnostic imaging, surgical procedures or post-mortem examination.

Congenital megaoesophagus

Congenital idiopathic megaoesophagus, oesophageal dilatation, which sometimes occurs in dogs and cats, is usually detected at weaning. The hypomotility and associated dilatation accompanying this condition are attributed to neuromuscular dysfunction.

Megacolon (Hirschsprung's disease)

Dilatation of the colon which occurs cranial to a contracted aganglionic segment of the intestine is referred to as megacolon. This uncommon condition has been described in pigs and dogs. In humans, the condition, which is congenital, is attributed to the developmental failure of enteric ganglia.

Further reading

Asari, M., Wakui, S., Fukaya, K. and Kano, Y. (1985) Formation of the bovine colon. *Japanese Journal of Veterinary Science* **47**, 803–806.

Barker, I.K., van Dreumel, A.A. and Palmer, N. (1993) The alimentary system. In *Pathology of Domestic Animals*, Vol. 2, 4th edn. Eds. K.V.F. Jubb, P.C. Kennedy and N. Palmer. Academic Press, San Diego, pp. 1–139.

Beck, F., Tata, F. and Chavengsaksophak, K. (2000) Homeobox genes and gut development. *BioEssays* **22**, 431–441.

Bryden, M.M., Evans, H.E. and Binns, W. (1972) Embryology of the sheep 2. The alimentary tract and associated glands. *Journal of Morphology* **138**, 187–206.

Carlson, B.M. (2004) Digestive and respiratory systems and body cavities. In *Human Embryology and Developmental Biology*. Mosby, Philadelphia, PA, pp. 353–391.

Dyce, K.M., Sack, W.O. and Wensing, C.J.G. (2002) Digestive apparatus. In *Textbook of Veterinary Anatomy*, 3rd edn. W.H. Saunders, Philadelphia, PA, pp. 100–147.

Kano, Y., Kulfkaya, K., Asari, M. and Eguchi, Y. (1981) Studies on the development of the fetal and neonatal bovine stomach. *Anatomia, histologia, embryologia* **10**, 267–274.

Kapur, R.P., Gershon, M.D., Milla, P.J. and Pachniss, V. (2004) The influence of Hox genes and three intercellular signaling pathways on enteric neuromuscular development. *Neurogastroenterology and Motility* **16** (Suppl.1), 8–13.

Lambert, P.S. (1948) The development of the stomach in the ruminant. *British Veterinary Journal* **104**, 302–310.

McGeady, T.A. and Sack, W.O. (1967) The development of vagal innervation of the bovine stomach. *American Journal of Anatomy* **121**, 121–130.

Noden, D.N. and de Lahunta, A. (1985) Digestive system. In *Embryology of Domestic Animals, Developmental Mechanisms and Malformations*. Williams and Wilkins, Baltimore, MD, pp. 292–311.

Roberts, D.J. (2000) Molecular mechanisms of development of the gastrointestinal tract. *Developmental Dynamics* **219**, 109–120.

Warner, E.D. (1958) The organogenesis and early histogenesis of the bovine stomach. *American Journal of Anatomy* **102**, 33–54.

Zaret, K.S. (2001) Hepatocyte differentiation from endoderm and beyond. *Current Opinion in Genetics and Development* **11**, 568–574.

16 Respiratory System

In mammals, the respiratory system consists of a gaseous conducting portion and a site where exchange of respiratory gases takes place. The conducting portion comprises the nostrils, nasal cavities, paranasal sinuses, pharynx, larynx, trachea, bronchi and bronchioles. The structures involved in gaseous exchange include the respiratory bronchioles, alveolar ducts, alveolar sacs and alveoli. Development of the nostrils, nasal cavities and paranasal sinuses are discussed in association with the development of the head.

The respiratory primordium develops as a ventral groove in the floor of the foregut at the level of the fourth pharyngeal arch. The groove, referred to as the laryngo-tracheal groove, deepens and forms an elongated outgrowth, which extends in a caudal direction and becomes separated from the foregut proper by the formation of two tracheo-oesophageal grooves, one on the left side and one on the right side (Fig. 16.1). When these grooves meet and fuse they form a septum, the tracheo-oesophageal septum. The septum separates the dorsal portion of the foregut, the primordium of the oesophagus, from the ventral portion, the primordium of the laryngo-tracheal tube. That portion of the foregut cranial to the tracheo-oesophageal septum becomes the primordial pharynx.

Formation of the larynx

The larynx, which develops from the cranial region of the laryngo-tracheal tube, communicates with the primordial pharynx. The epithelium of the larynx derives from foregut endoderm, while the cartilages and muscles of the larynx develop from splanchnic mesoderm. The mesoderm of the left and right fourth pharyngeal arches gives rise to two swellings which develop lateral to the laryngo-tracheal groove, the primordia of the arytenoid, thyroid and cricoid cartilages. As these arytenoid swellings develop, they convert the cranial end of the slit-like laryngo-tracheal groove into a T-shaped aperture, the laryngeal glottis. A single swelling which develops from the mesoderm of the left and right third and fourth pharyngeal arches cranial to the developing glottis, referred to as the epiglottic swelling, gives rise to

the epiglottic cartilage. The intrinsic laryngeal muscles, which develop from myoblasts in the fourth and sixth pharyngeal arches, are innervated by branches of cranial nerve X. The crico-thyroid muscles, which derive from the fourth pharyngeal arches, are innervated by the cranial laryngeal branches of cranial nerve X. The other intrinsic laryngeal muscles, which derive from the sixth pharyngeal arches, are innervated by the recurrent laryngeal branches of cranial nerve X.

As the laryngeal cartilages develop, the epithelial lining of the larynx forms a left and a right diverticulum in the lateral walls of the larynx. Cranial vestibular and caudal vocal folds of the larynx, composed of mucosal and muscular tissue, form the boundaries through which the diverticula project laterally. These diverticula, referred to as laryngeal ventricles, are present in humans, horses, dogs and pigs but are not present in ruminants and cats.

Trachea, bronchi and lungs

The laryngo-tracheal tube, which consists of an inner endodermal lining and an outer layer of splanchnic mesoderm, elongates. Bifurcation of the blind end of this tube results in the formation of two bronchial buds, the primordia of the left and right lungs. The portion of the laryngo-tracheal tube from the larynx to the bifurcation gives rise to the trachea. The endodermal lining of the tube gives rise to respiratory epithelium and the mucosal and submucosal glands of the trachea. The connective tissue of the tracheal lamina propria, cartilaginous rings, smooth muscle, blood vessels and lymphatic vessels of the tracheal wall are of mesodermal origin.

Each bronchial bud enlarges, forming a left and a right principal bronchus. These bronchi elongate caudally, between the developing oesophagus dorsally and the developing heart ventrally. Unlike the left bronchus which deviates from the midline in a lateral direction, the right bronchus deviates to a lesser extent, and consequently the right lung is more prone to inhalation pneumonia than the left lung. In domestic animals, with the exception of horses, the right principal bronchus gives off four secondary or lobar bronchi which later give rise

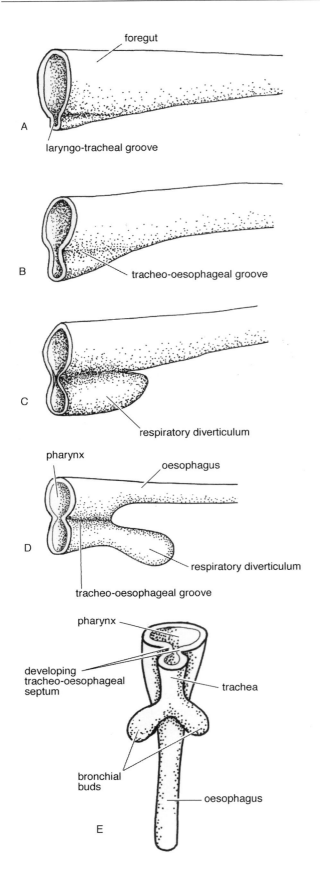

A
foregut
laryngo-tracheal groove

B
tracheo-oesophageal groove

C
respiratory diverticulum

D
pharynx
oesophagus
respiratory diverticulum
tracheo-oesophageal groove

E
pharynx
developing
tracheo-oesophageal
septum
trachea
bronchial
buds
oesophagus

Figure 16.1 Lateral views and a ventral view of sequential stages in the formation of the respiratory diverticulum from the foregut. The development of the laryngo-tracheal groove, tracheo-oesophageal grooves and bronchial buds is also shown.

to the cranial, middle, accessory and caudal lobes of the right lung. A middle lobe is not present in the equine right lung. The right human bronchus gives off three branches and no accessory lobe is present. The left principal bronchus in domestic animals gives off two lobar bronchi which in turn give rise to the cranial and caudal lobes. In ruminants and pigs, the right cranial lobar bronchus, which is given off directly from the trachea, is referred to as the tracheal bronchus. During further development, the lobar bronchi give off tertiary or segmental bronchi which supply large areas within the lobes known as broncho-pulmonary segments. The number of broncho-pulmonary segments within a particular pulmonary lobe in a given species is usually constant. However, the number of broncho-pulmonary segments within a given pulmonary lobe varies from species to species. Stages in lung development, showing the formation of principal and lobar bronchi and their branches, are illustrated in Fig. 16.2.

The segmental bronchi undergo 14 to 18 bifurcations with the diameter of each succeeding branch becoming progressively smaller until a diameter approaching 0.5 mm is reached: tubes of this size are referred to as bronchioles. The final bronchiolar branches, which represent the termination of the exclusively conducting portion of the respiratory system, are referred to as terminal bronchioles. Each terminal bronchiole subdivides into two or more respiratory bronchioles which are structurally similar to terminal bronchioles except that their walls give off numerous saccular alveoli where gaseous exchange takes place. The respiratory bronchioles are transitional zones between the conducting and respiratory regions of the respiratory system. These respiratory bronchioles give off a number of alveolar ducts from which alveolar sacs and alveoli arise. Respiratory bronchioles are present in humans and carnivores. In horses, cattle, sheep and pigs, respiratory bronchioles are either absent or poorly developed and the alveolar ducts arise directly from the terminal bronchioles.

The development of the lungs may be divided into five arbitrary stages based on histological features, namely the embryonic, pseudo-glandular, canalicular, terminal sac and alveolar stages (Fig. 16.3). The embryonic stage extends from the formation of the laryngo-tracheal groove to the formation of segmental bronchi. During this period, the developing lungs, which grow into the common pleuro-pericardial cavity, become surrounded by visceral pleura. In the pseudo-glandular stage, the developing lungs extend into the surrounding mesenchyme in a manner similar to the formation of an exocrine gland. By the end of this period, when up to 14 sequential bifurcations have occurred, all the major conducting branches of the bronchial tree are formed. Subsequently, the histological structure of the bronchial

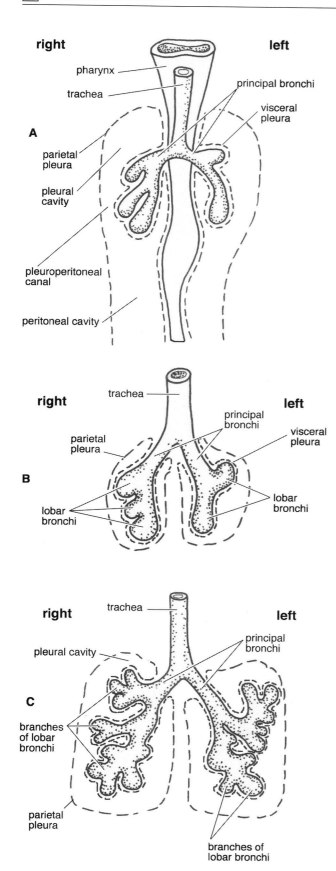

Figure 16.2 Ventral views of sequential stages in lung development showing the formation of the principal bronchi and the origins of lobar bronchi and their branches.

tree undergoes change, a consequence of extensive cellular differentiation. Epithelial cells, cartilage, sub-mucosal glands and smooth muscle are formed, and vascularisation of pulmonary tissue commences. During the canalicular stage, the lumina of the bronchi and bronchioles enlarge and the terminal bronchioles give off a number of respiratory bronchioles. Increased vascularisation is evident with capillaries in direct contact with the epithelium forming a peri-canalicular vascular network. During the penultimate stage of pulmonary development, referred to as the terminal sac stage, large numbers of terminal sacs bud off from the respiratory bronchioles. Initially, the terminal sacs, which correspond to primitive alveoli, are lined by cuboidal epithelial cells. The epithelium lining these primitive alveoli differentiates into two cell types, type I alveolar cells and type II alveolar cells. Type I alveolar cells, which are involved in gaseous exchange post-natally, are squamous epithelial cells, and account for more than 90% of the surface of alveoli, whereas type II alveolar cells are cuboidal cells which secrete surfactant. Surfactant, which forms a phospholipid layer covering the luminal surface of alveoli, reduces surface tension thereby preventing adhesion of alveolar walls during development. This surfactant also facilitates expansion of the alveoli during inspiration and prevents their collapse during expiration. Despite incomplete pulmonary development, and the limited amount of surfactant being produced, human foetuses born towards the end of the terminal sac stage of development may survive with intensive care. During the final stage of pulmonary development, referred to as the alveolar stage, capillaries surrounding the terminal sacs become intimately associated with the alveolar epithelial cells. At the site where gaseous exchange will occur in the neonatal animal, the alveolar epithelial cells are separated from the endothelium of the capillaries solely by the fused basal laminae of the alveoli and the capillaries. Thus, the blood–air barrier is composed of the capillary endothelial cell, the fused basal laminae of both the endothelial cell and the contiguous alveolar epithelial cell, and the alveolar epithelial cell itself. The number of alveolar type II cells increases during this stage of development, resulting in enhanced secretion of surfactant. As the lungs are not fully developed at birth, post-natal alveolar development continues for some time. The duration of the stages of lung development in humans and domestic animals is presented in Table 16.1. Post-natal growth of the lungs is due to the formation of additional respiratory bronchioles and alveoli, either by the formation of additional alveoli or by subdivision of existing alveoli through the formation of septa which increase the surface area for gaseous exchange.

Although lungs are not functional in a respiratory sense during foetal life, they must, however, be sufficiently

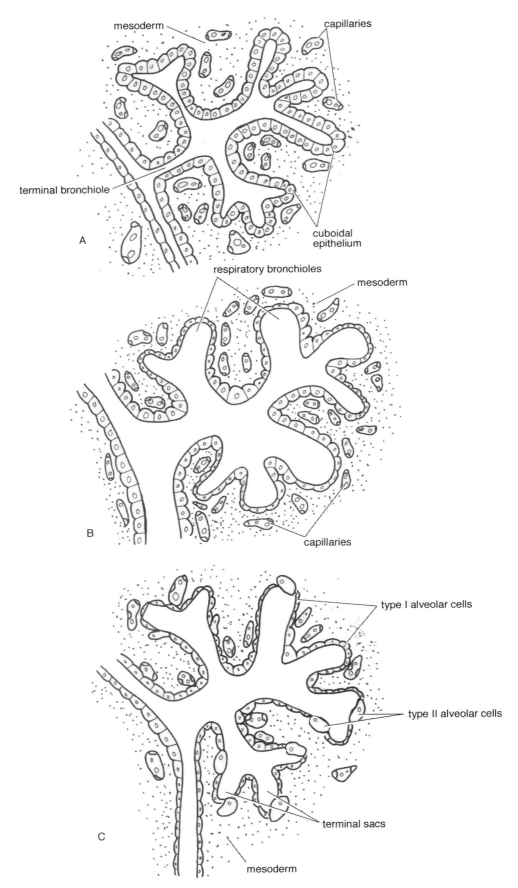

Figure 16.3 Structural changes which occur during stages of pulmonary development. A, Pseudo-glandular stage. B, Canalicular stage. C, Terminal sac stage.

Table 16.1 Duration of the stages of lung development in humans and domestic animals.

Developmental stage	Humans	Horses	Cattle	Sheep	Pigs	Dogs
Embryonic	26 to 42[a]	Up to 50	30 to 50	Up to 40	Up to 55	Up to 32
Pseudo-glandular	42 to 102	50 to 190	50 to 120	40 to 90	55 to 80	32 to 47
Canalicular	102 to 196	190 to 300	120 to 180	95 to 120	80 to 92	47 to 56
Terminal sac	196 to 252	300 to 320	180 to 240	120 to 140	92 to 110	56 to 63
Alveolar	252 to 281	320 to birth	240 to 260	From 140	From 110	Post-natal

[a] Days of gestation.

developed to render them capable of assuming a respiratory role immediately an animal is born. During foetal development, the lungs are filled with fluid. The source of this fluid is primarily from secretions of the pulmonary epithelial cells and mucosal glands. As movements of muscles associated with respiration begin prior to birth, it is possible that a small amount of aspirated amniotic fluid may also be present in the lungs. The presence of fluid is considered to be an important stimulus for expansion of the alveoli as a reduced volume of fluid is associated with pulmonary hypoplasia. Ultrasonic investigation demonstrates that periodic contraction of those muscles associated with respiration occurs throughout the foetal period. These movements are considered essential for post-natal survival as they prepare the respiratory muscles for breathing at birth and they may also promote pulmonary development.

Sub-division of the lung

Lungs of domestic animals are normally sub-divided into relatively large areas called pulmonary lobes. Formerly, these lobes were assigned names based on fissures in their ventral borders and their relationships to neighbouring structures. The extent and depth of the fissures varies from species to species and the position of fissures is constant within a species. The comparison of lung lobation between species, based on the presence of external fissures, relies on superficial evaluation of gross anatomical features. However, the criteria for naming the pulmonary lobes recommended by the *Nomina Anatomica Veterinaria* (NAV) is based not on superficial anatomical features, but rather on the number and location of branches of the principal bronchi. This recommendation offers a defined scientific method for comparing lung lobation among domestic animals (Fig. 16.4). By employing these criteria, all domestic animals with the exception of horses, have four lobes in the left lung, namely cranial, middle, accessory and caudal lobes. Because the right principal bronchus in horses does not have a middle lobar branch, the equine right lung does not have a lobe corresponding to this branch.

Accordingly, the equine right lung is composed of cranial, accessory and caudal lobes. Although the presence of a fissure in the cranial lobe of the left lung of carnivores, ruminants and pigs conveys the superficial impression that this lung is composed of three lobes, based on the NAV classification the left lung is composed of two lobes in all domestic animals.

Based on the area supplied by a bronchus or bronchiole, the following pulmonary functional units are described. A broncho-pulmonary segment is the area supplied by a single segmental bronchus with its accompanying vascular and nerve supply. Adjacent broncho-pulmonary segments are separated by connective tissue septa which are continuous with the pulmonary pleura. Because of this segmental anatomical arrangement, it is feasible to surgically resect a complete broncho-pulmonary segment.

The lung is also described as consisting of units smaller than broncho-pulmonary segments, classified as lobules. However, there is uncertainty as to what constitutes a lobule. A primary pulmonary lobule is defined by the NAV as a respiratory bronchiole with all its associated alveolar ducts, alveolar sacs and alveoli. A secondary pulmonary lobule arises from the branching of a large pulmonary bronchiole and all its branches and accompanying vascular and nerve supply. This secondary pulmonary lobule is demarcated by connective tissue septa which typically outline a pyramidal-shaped lobule with its base towards the pleura and its apex directed towards the hilus of the lung. The inter-lobular connective tissue, which is well developed in cattle and pigs, accounts for the distinct surface lobulation in these species. In carnivores, horses and sheep, the connective tissue framework is less well defined and, accordingly, the surface lobulation is indistinct. The functional unit of lung tissue engaged in respiratory exchange can be defined as a pulmonary acinus which includes all the air spaces distal to one terminal bronchiole including all the respiratory bronchioles, alveolar ducts, sacs and alveoli joining the respiratory bronchioles.

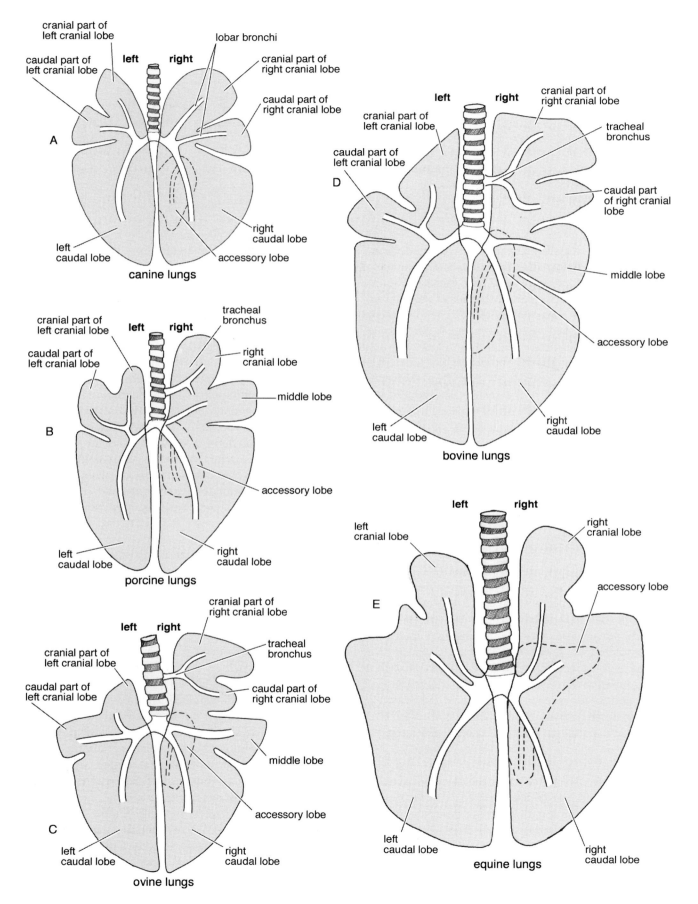

Figure 16.4 Dorsal views of the arrangement of lobar bronchi in the fully formed lungs of domestic animals (A to E). Lung lobation, as illustrated in this diagram, is based on the presence of a lobar bronchus supplying each lobe.

Molecular aspects of respiratory development

At an early stage of embryogenesis, regional specification determines where formation of future respiratory tract structures will occur. This process is attributed to the expression of different combinations of Hox genes along the cranial–caudal axis of the developing embryo.

An array of growth factors associated with the development of the respiratory system influences the anatomical arrangement and functional properties of its regional components. Epithelial cell proliferation is accelerated in expanding regions of the endodermally-derived buds of the branching respiratory tree. Fgf-10 acts as a signaling centre close to the tip of each bud, causing epithelial proliferation and growth in the direction of Fgf-10 secretion. Another locally produced factor, Nkx-2.1, also contributes to apical cell proliferation (Fig. 16.5).

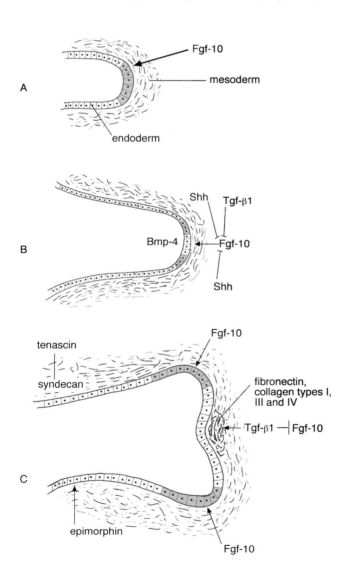

Figure 16.5 Inductive influences of signalling factors on respiratory development. A, Outgrowth; B, growth inhibition; C, branching.

By selective inhibition of cellular proliferation at the apices, secretion of Bmp-4 in discrete regions of the apical epithelial cells initiates branching of the buds. Simultaneously, Shh produced by the epithelium inhibits the formation of Fgf-10, while stimulating growth of the mesenchymal cells on either side of the established apex. As a consequence of the inhibition of Fgf-10 production, growth of the tip is substantially decreased. The mesenchymal cells produce Tgf-β1, which not only further inhibits Fgf-10 production but also promotes the synthesis of extra-cellular matrix molecules, including fibronectin and collagen, distal to the apical epithelium. These molecules stabilise the previously proliferating tip, which does not undergo further branching.

Because Shh and Tgf-β1 are present at low concentrations lateral to the tissue corresponding to the former growing apex and do not effectively inhibit Fgf-10 in this region, two new Fgf-10 signaling centres develop on either side of the previous centre. In these regions, there is increased cellular proliferation resulting in the formation of new buds. As these buds mature, the cycle of inhibition of Fgf-10 commences at this new location, resulting in the formation of new branches.

An epithelial cell-associated proteoglycan called syndecan has an important role in maintaining the established epithelial structures along the developing ducts of the respiratory tree. Syndecan interacts with an extra-cellular matrix protein, tenascin, which is present along developed ducts but absent from regions where branching is taking place.

Expression of *Hoxb-5* can be detected in developing terminal bronchioles but not in regions associated with gaseous exchange, such as alveoli. The protein epimorphin is important in the establishment of epithelial cell polarity and final structural organisation of respiratory ducts.

Anomalies of the respiratory system

Congenital anomalies of the respiratory system are rare. Epiglottic hypoplasia has been recorded in horses and pigs; partial or complete agenesis of the trachea is very rare. Associated with anomalous development of the foregut and upper alimentary tract, ectopic lung tissue may be found in either the thoracic or abdominal cavities or occasionally subcutaneously.

Pulmonary hypoplasia is usually associated with congenital diaphragmatic hernia, with the herniated abdominal organs in the thoracic cavity interfering with pulmonary growth.

Respiratory distress syndrome is a condition manifested in infants born prematurely. These children develop rapid laboured breathing problems at birth. The lungs are underinflated and the alveoli are partially filled with a proteinaceous fluid that forms a membrane over the respiratory surface. The condition is due to insufficient production of surfactant by type II alveolar cells in the developing lungs.

Congenital cysts may develop in the lung or other regions of the respiratory tract. The cysts are formed by dilation of the terminal or larger bronchi. If the cysts are numerous, they can cause respiratory distress and lead to chronic pulmonary infections.

Further reading

Boyden, E.H. and Thompsett, D.H. (1961) The post-natal growth of the lungs in the dog. *Acta Anatomica* **47**, 185–215.

Carlson, B.M. (2004) Respiratory System. In *Human Embryology* and *Developmental Biology*. 3rd edn. Mosby, Philadelphia, PA, pp. 374–379.

Chung, P.-T. and McMahon, P. (2003) Branching morphogenesis of the lung: new molecular insight into an old problem. *Trends in Cell Biology* **13**, 86–91.

Clements, L.P. (1938) Embryonic development of the respiratory portion of the pig's lungs. *Anatomical Record* **70**, 575.

Copland, I. and Post, M. (2004) Lung development and fetal lung growth. *Paediatric Respiratory Reviews* **5**(Suppl. A), S259–S264.

De Zabala, L.E. and Weinman, D.E. (1984) Prenatal development of bovine lung. *Anatomia, histologia, embryologia* **13**, 1–14.

Fukada, Y., Ferrans, V.J. and Crystal, R.G. (1983) The development of alveolar septa in the fetal sheep: an ultrastructural and immunohistochemical study. *American Journal of Anatomy* **167**, 405–439.

Guttentag, S.H. and Ballard, P.L. (1999) Fetal lung development. In *Encyclopedia of Reproduction*. Eds. E. Knobil and J.D. O'Neill. Academic Press, San Diego, pp. 318–326.

Nomina Anatomica Veterinaria (1994) 4th edn. Published by the International Committees on Veterinary Gross Anatomical Nomenclature, Veterinary Histological Nomenclature and Veterinary Embryological Nomenclature. Zürich, pp. 1–198.

Pattle, R.E., Rossdale, P.D., Schock, C. and Creasey, J.M. (1975) The development of the lung and its surfactant in the foal and other species. *Journal of Reproduction and Fertility Supplement* **23**, 651–657.

Shannon, J.M. and Hyatt, B.A. (2004) Epithelial–mesenchymal interactions in the developing lung. *Annual Review of Physiology* **66**, 625–645.

Warburton, D., Schwartz, M., Tefft, D., Flores-Delgado, G., Anderson, K.D. and Cardoso, W.V. (2000) Molecular basis of lung morphogenesis *Mechanisms of Development* **92**, 55–81.

17 Urinary System

With the exception of the epithelial lining of the bladder and urethra, which are of endodermal origin, the urinary system of vertebrates develops from intermediate mesoderm. The urinary system has a number of important functions which include elimination of metabolic waste products by filtration and excretion, and regulation of electrolytes in the body; renal re-absorption of water and low molecular weight molecules is an essential aspect of homeostasis. In addition, the kidney, through the production of the enzyme renin, has a role in the regulation of blood pressure. An important endocrine function of the kidney is the production of erythropoietin in the renal cortex, which has a regulatory role in red cell production by the bone marrow.

Kidney

The primordial kidney essentially consists of tubular units, nephrons, which function by selective filtration, re-absorption and finally excretion of waste products. As species evolved from lower forms to higher forms their functional kidney units likewise evolved from primitive structures to highly complex, efficient filtration units. The changes which occurred on an evolutionary scale are paralleled to some extent by a corresponding increase in the complexity of functional kidney units evident in higher vertebrates during embryological development.

Developing vertebrate nephric tubules exhibit increased complexity as those which form in the cervical region are sequentially replaced in the thoraco-lumbar and sacral regions by more functionally-competent structures. These structures are referred to as the pronephros, mesonephros and metanephros respectively. As the more caudal structures develop and become functional, the pronephric and mesonephric tubules atrophy and the metanephros persists as the definitive functioning kidney. While these three structures are no longer considered as distinct successive functional kidneys, but rather as three successive morphological manifestations of a single excretory organ, the holonephros, the terms pronephros, mesonephros and metanephros have been retained solely for descriptive purposes.

The evolutionary development of the kidney is illustrated by the increasing refinement of renal structure and function evident in vertebrate animals. Lower vertebrates have relatively primitive kidneys in comparison with higher vertebrates. In fish and amphibians, the pronephros, which is replaced by the mesonephros, becomes the functional kidney. In reptiles, birds and mammals, an additional structure, the metanephros, succeeds the two previous structures, which atrophy.

Pronephros

During the early developmental period when somites are present, cells of the intermediate mesoderm in the cervical region separate into an outer parietal layer and an inner visceral layer forming a cavity, the nephrocoele, between the two layers. At the level of each somite, cords of cells referred to as nephrotomes, which grow out from the dorsal (parietal) wall of the intermediate mesoderm, later form pronephric tubules (Fig. 17.1). The distal end of each tubule proliferates and extends initially in a lateral direction and then caudally, before fusing with the corresponding proliferating cells of the tubule developing immediately caudal to it. The primordium of the excretory pronephric duct arises from fusion of the distal end of each tubule. The pronephric duct grows towards the cloaca and becomes canalised. As more caudal pronephric tubules develop, they open into the primordial pronephric duct.

The lumen of each pronephric tubule becomes continuous with the nephrocoele which opens into the coelomic cavity through an aperture termed a nephrostome. Branches from the dorsal aorta form tufts of capillaries, glomeruli, which may invaginate either into the coelomic epithelium, or alternatively into the wall of each pronephric tubule. Glomeruli which invaginate into the coelomic epithelium are referred to as external glomeruli; those which invaginate into the tubular wall are termed internal glomeruli (Fig. 17.1). The term 'Bowman's capsule' is used to describe the invaginated epithelium surrounding each glomerulus. Formation of external glomeruli, a feature of lower vertebrates, results in a filtration arrangement which is less efficient

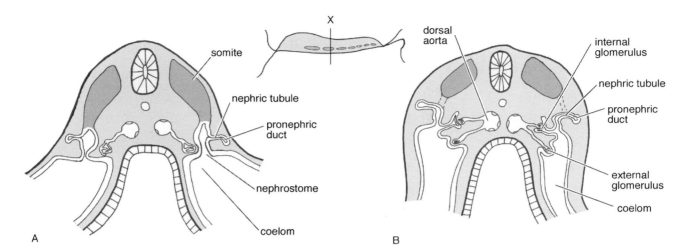

Figure 17.1 Cross-section through an early embryo, A, and an embryo at a later stage of development, B, showing formation of a pronephric duct and an internal and external glomerulus.

than internal glomerular filtration as the filtrate has to be propelled from the coelomic cavity to the pronephric tubule by the ciliary action of cells surrounding the nephrostome. With the formation of internal glomeruli, a feature of higher vertebrates, the connection between the pronephric tubules and the coelomic cavity is lost. Water and some electrolytes are re-absorbed from the pronephric tubules and waste products are conveyed to the cloaca. In placental mammals, these waste products are transported from the foetus to the placenta for excretion by the dam.

Mesonephros

Towards the end of the post-somite stage of development, a column of tissue referred to as the urogenital ridge develops by proliferation of the intermediate mesoderm in the thoraco-lumbar region and projects into the coelomic (peritoneal) cavity. Later, this structure divides into a medial genital ridge and a lateral urinary ridge. Lateral to the urinary ridge, the pronephric ducts, which extend caudally towards the cloaca, induce the mesonephric tissue to form S-shaped tubules within the urinary ridge (Fig. 17.2). Invagination of the medial end of each mesonephric tubule by a glomerular tuft induces the formation of Bowman's capsule by the mesonephric tubule epithelium. The combination of Bowman's capsule and the glomerular tuft forms a filtration unit known as a renal corpuscle. The lateral end of each mesonephric tubule enters separately into the pre-existing pronephric duct, which at this stage is referred to as the mesonephric duct (Fig. 17.3). With the development of the mesonephric system, the pronephric tubules and the cranial portion of the pronephric duct atrophy (Figs. 17.4 and 17.5).

The development of a peritubular capillary network around the mesonephric tubules assists in the re-absorption of water and electrolytes. In contrast to the structure of the pronephros where only one tubule develops at the level of each somite, in the mesonephros multiple tubules may develop at the level of each somite.

The developing left mesonephros and right mesonephros project into the abdominal cavity as distinct anatomical structures in the developing embryo and are especially prominent in porcine embryos up to 35 days of gestation (Fig. 17.4). These structures are less prominent in horses, ruminants, dogs and cats than in pigs; in rodents and humans they are poorly developed. The mesonephros regresses in horses around the 65th day of gestation, in cattle at approximately 58 days, in pigs at around 50 days and in dogs at approximately 36 days. A unique feature of the mesonephric tubules of ruminant embryos is the presence of giant glomeruli associated with the more cranial tubules. The significance of these giant glomeruli is unclear. It has been suggested that they may be related to the large allantoic cavity and the associated high volume of allantoic fluid in ruminants.

Metanephros

The metanephros is formed from two primordial structures: the ureteric bud, which is an outgrowth of the mesonephric duct, and the metanephric blastema located in the sacral region, which forms from the caudal end of the nephric ridge (Figs. 17.4 and 17.5). The ureteric bud extends cranially towards the metanephric blastema and dilates at its cranial end where it becomes almost completely surrounded by metanephric tissue. The dilated portion of the ureteric bud gives rise to the pelvis and the collecting ducts of the definitive kidney. The formation of the collecting ducts induces the metanephric tissue to give rise to metanephric tubules (Fig. 17.6). The manner in which the dilated end of the ureteric bud differentiates

Figure 17.2 Cross-sections through embryos showing successive stages in the formation of a mesonephric tubule and paramesonephric duct.

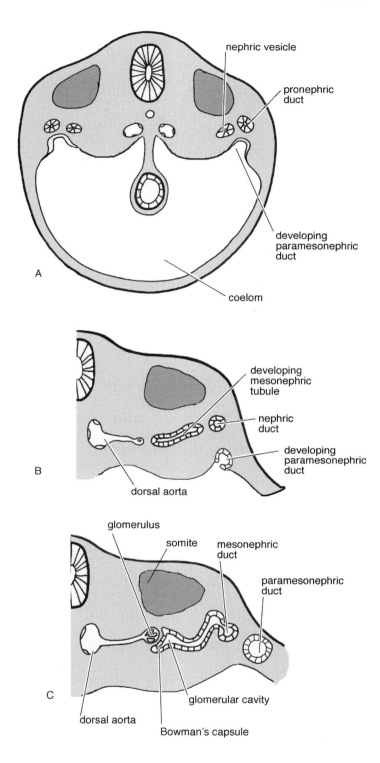

influences the final anatomical arrangement of the fully developed kidney in mammals. Accordingly, the anatomical form of mammalian kidneys ranges from unilobar to distinct multilobar structures, with intermediate gradations of partial and complete lobar fusion.

Molecular basis of metanephros development

During early metanephros development, the ureteric buds and the mesenchyme from which the mesonephric tissue arises promote reciprocal differentiation. *Wilm's tumour suppressor gene 1* (*WT1*), expressed in the mesenchyme, up-regulates the production of glial cell-derived neurotrophic factor, Gdnf, and hepatocyte growth factor, Hgf, which promote development of the ureteric buds. Receptors for these factors, Ret for Gdnf and Met for Hgf, are present on the epithelial cells of the ureteric buds. Associated with ureteric bud branching, repeated tubule induction generates approximately 12,000 nephrons in the mouse kidney and up to 1,000,000 in the

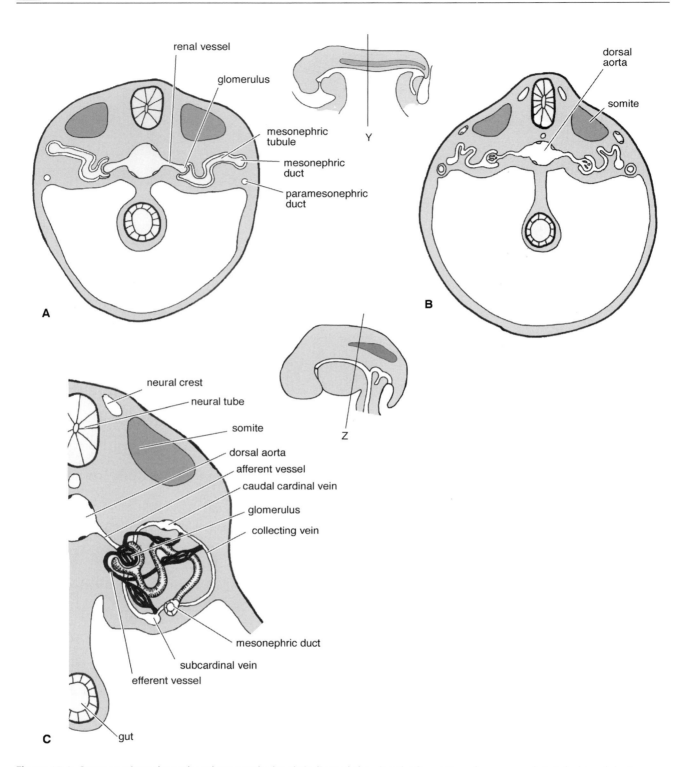

Figure 17.3 Cross-sections through embryos at the levels indicated showing the formation of a mesonephric tubule and duct.

human kidney. Although Gdnf is the primary inducer of ureteric bud branching, other mesenchymal soluble factors such as pleiotrophin and fibroblast growth factors also promote branching and elongation of the ureteric buds. Through negative feedback, the locally-acting inhibitory growth factors Tgf-β and bone morphogenic proteins regulate tubular growth and branching and also maintain tubular lumen size. Matrix metalloproteinases are activated at the leading edges of the branches while proteinase inhibitors protect established tubules from degradation. Extra-cellular matrix molecules such as proteoglycans, and cell adhesion molecules such as integrins, promote branching at the ureteric bud tips and specify the points at which branching occurs.

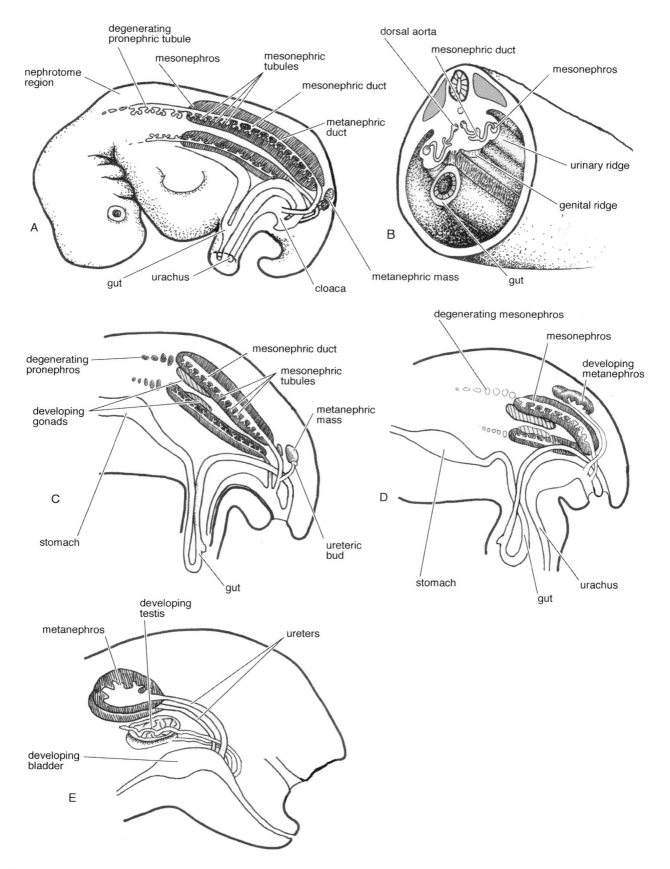

Figure 17.4 Stages in the formation of the pronephros, mesonephros and metanephros and their relationships to other developing structures.

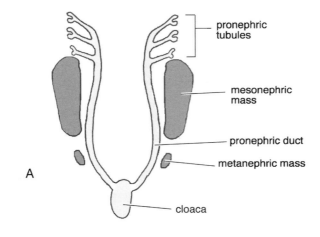

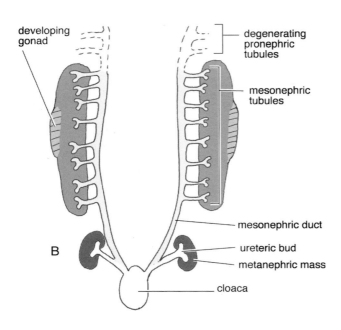

Figure 17.5 Dorsal views of the developing pronephros, mesonephros and metanephros.

Two factors, Fgf-2 and Bmp-4, secreted from the ureteric bud cells, induce mesenchymal differentiation leading to the formation of metanephric tubules. These factors stimulate proliferation and block apoptosis of the metanephrogenic mesenchyme, while maintaining the production of Wt-1. It has been proposed that Wt-1 has a role in enabling the metanephric mesenchyme to respond to signals from the epithelial ureteric buds. Pax-2 and Wnt-4 regulate the differentiation of mesenchyme into epithelium. During this process of differentiation as the extra-cellular matrix proteins undergo modification, fibronectin, type I collagen and type III collagen are replaced by laminin and type IV collagen which are characteristic components of epithelial basal laminae. The cell adhesion molecules, syndecan and E-cadherin, are essential for the differentiation of mesenchyme into epithelium.

Unilobar kidneys

In developing kidneys of rodents and rabbits, the renal pelvis gives off a number of branches which project into the metanephric tissue and become the collecting ducts. Under the inductive influence of the collecting ducts, metanephric tissue forms primitive tubules which later become S-shaped. One end of each tubule joins to the collecting duct and the other, when invaginated by a glomerulus, becomes the cup-shaped Bowman's capsule. The metanephric tubule continues to elongate, forming a U-shaped bend, the loop of Henle, which extends towards the renal pelvis. The portion of the tubule adjacent to Bowman's capsule becomes coiled and is referred to as the proximal convoluted tubule, while the more distant portion of the tubule, which also coils, is referred to as the distal convoluted tubule. Collectively, the renal corpuscle, the loop of Henle and the proximal and distal convoluted tubules constitute a nephron (Fig. 17.6). With the development of the nephron and collecting duct system, the kidney can be descriptively divided into an outer cortical and inner medullary region. The compact cortex consists mainly of renal corpuscles along with proximal and distal convoluted tubules, while the medulla consists principally of the loops of Henle and collecting ducts. The conical arrangement of the loops of Henle and collecting ducts is referred to as a medullary pyramid. The base of the pyramid is capped by the cortex, while the apex forms a papilla which projects into the cup-like pelvis. The medullary pyramid, with its associated cortical covering, constitutes a renal lobe composed of subunits referred to as lobules. A renal lobule consists of a collecting duct and the associated nephrons which drain into it. Because the kidneys of rodents and rabbits consist of a single pyramidal structure, they are referred to as unilobar kidneys.

Each tubule in the pronephros and mesonephros has its own direct blood supply from the aorta. In contrast, the vascular supply to each nephron in the metanephros derives from a branch of the renal artery.

During its differentiation the position of the metanephros changes from the pelvic region to the lumbar region, where it occupies a position dorsal to the degenerating mesonephros and the developing gonad (Figs. 17.4 and 17.5). This change in position may be accounted for in part by migration and also by differential growth of the skeletal and muscular structures in the pelvic and lumbar regions. With the exception of pigs, the right kidney in all domestic animals migrates more cranially than the left kidney. In its final position, the right kidney is in direct contact with the caudate lobe of the liver.

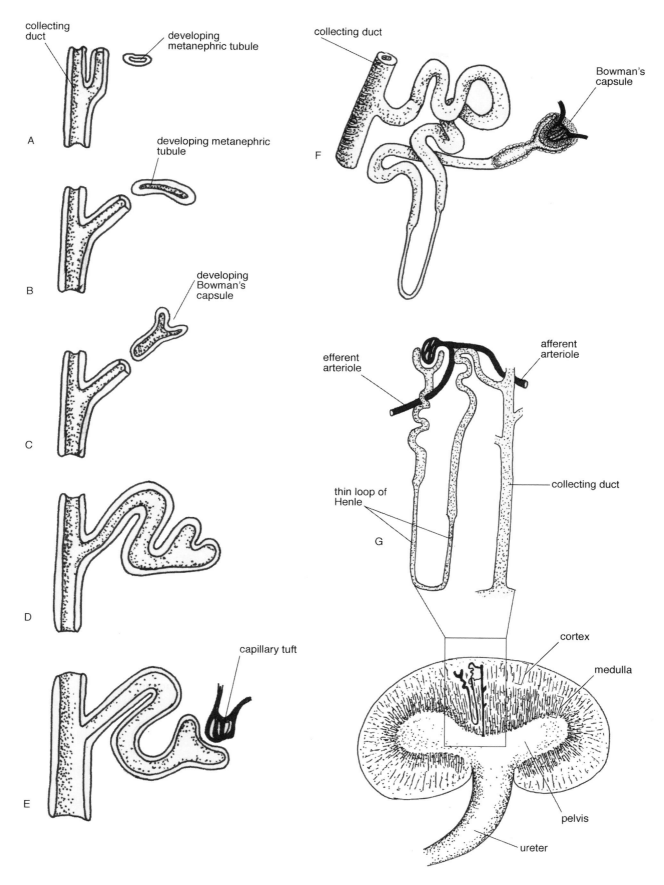

Figure 17.6 Stages in the formation of a nephron, its relationship to a collecting duct and its final arrangement in the functioning unilobar kidney.

Multilobar kidneys

Kidneys of aquatic mammals

In aquatic mammals including seals, otters and whales, the terminal end of the ureteric bud gives rise to a number of branches each capped by metanephric tissue forming a kidney lobe, termed a renculus. Each individual lobe is formed in a manner similar to that described for a unilobar kidney. The multilobar kidney in these species resembles a bunch of grapes, with individual lobes draining separately into a branch of the ureter (Fig. 17.7).

Kidneys of domestic animals

In cattle, the ureteric bud, from which the ureter derives, forms two major branches which subdivide into 12 to 25 minor branches. The dilated ends of the minor branches become invaginated forming funnel-shaped calyces. When capped by metanephric tissue, either singly or in pairs, the resulting structure constitutes a kidney lobe. Collecting ducts which radiate from the calyces into the metanephric tissue induce the formation of metanephric tubules. Bovine kidneys and the kidneys of aquatic mammals have some features in common and some distinguishing features. Superficially, kidneys from these species have a multilobar appearance. However, in bovine kidneys, what superficially appear to be individual lobes in some instances arise from fusion of the cortices of adjacent lobes. Irrespective of whether or not cortical fusion has occurred, each lobe still retains a distinct pyramidal arrangement. The bovine kidney, therefore, is often referred to as a multipyramidal kidney. The fused cortical tissue forms columns which histologically demarcate the boundaries of individual lobes. Unlike the kidneys of other domestic animals, the bovine kidney does not have a pelvis (Fig. 17.7).

The dilated end of the porcine ureteric bud gives rise to the renal pelvis. Two major divisions of the renal pelvis, major calyces, form up to ten funnel-shaped divisions referred to as minor calyces. When minor calyces are capped by metanephric tissue they constitute the renal lobes. Because of fusion of the cortical tissue of adjacent lobes throughout the porcine kidney, its smooth surface imparts the superficial appearance of a unilobar kidney. Despite this superficial appearance, the multilobar structure of the porcine kidney is evident histologically both from its multipyramidal appearance and the separate drainage provided for each lobe by minor calyces.

In domestic carnivores, complete fusion of the cortical areas of adjacent lobes imparts the superficial appearance of a unilobar kidney. Fusion of the apices of medullary pyramids leads to the formation of a ridge-like common papilla, the renal crest, a prominent feature of canine kidneys. This fusion of the pyramidal apices conveys the impression that kidneys of carnivores are unilobar. However, the multilobar structure of kidneys of carnivores is confirmed by the presence of cortical columns and the position of the interlobar arteries which delineate individual lobes. A feature of the kidneys of domestic carnivores is the presence of deep out-pouchings of the lateral walls of the renal pelvis, referred to as lateral recesses.

The kidneys of sheep and goats develop in a manner comparable to those of domestic carnivores with many similar morphological features. Equine kidneys, which consist of 40 to 60 lobes and develop in a manner similar to those of domestic carnivores, have a smooth cortical surface with a common draining area, the renal crest. Extensions of the poles of the renal pelvis form two structures, termed the terminal recesses, into which some collecting ducts drain.

Bladder

During development of the hindgut, the urorectal septum divides the cloaca into the rectum dorsally and the primitive urogenital sinus ventrally. At the point of entry of the mesonephric duct, the primitive urogenital sinus divides into the cranial vesico-urethral canal, the primordium of the bladder, and a caudal urogenital sinus proper (Fig. 17.8). In the male embryo the caudal urogenital sinus gives rise to the penile urethra, and in the female embryo to the urethra and vestibule. As the terminal portions of the mesonephric and ureteric ducts are gradually incorporated into the wall of the developing bladder, each duct system develops its own separate opening into the bladder primordium. Subsequently, in the male embryo, the mesonephric ducts converge before entering the prostatic urethra. As the mesonephric ducts and ureters are of mesodermal origin, a triangular area of the dorsal wall of the bladder, the trigone, is lined by epithelium of mesodermal origin, while the epithelial lining of the remainder of the bladder derives from endoderm. Non-epithelial components of the bladder derive from splanchnic mesoderm.

Developmental anomalies of the urinary system

Renal agenesis

Unilateral or bilateral renal agenesis is associated with developmental failure of one or both ureteric buds. As a consequence of this failure, induction of the metanephric mass, which is required for the formation of renal tubules, does not occur. Survival is not threatened by

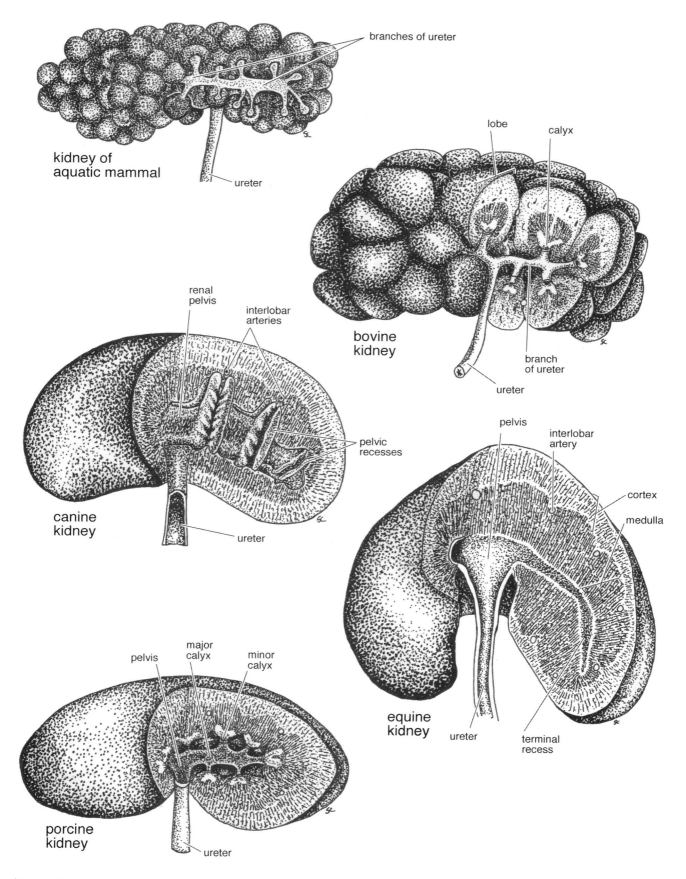

Figure 17.7 Comparative features of the multilobar kidneys of mammals. In aquatic mammals, no fusion occurs between adjacent renal lobes; the degree of fusion between adjacent renal lobes in domestic animals accounts for the gross anatomical appearance of their kidneys.

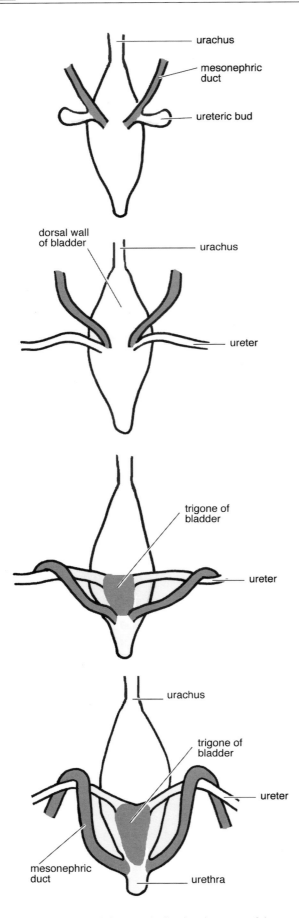

Figure 17.8 Sequential stages in the development of the bladder, ureters and associated structures.

unilateral renal agenesis, whereas bilateral renal agenesis is incompatible with life.

Ectopic kidney

When the metanephros gives rise to a kidney which remains in the sacral region, such a kidney is referred to as an ectopic or pelvic kidney. The frequency of this condition in humans, which may be unilateral or bilateral, is approximately 1 in 400, with a higher incidence in male than in female babies.

Horseshoe kidney

Because of its shape the term 'horseshoe kidney' is used to describe an abnormal renal structure formed by the fusion of the caudal poles of bilateral pelvic kidneys. This anomaly has been reported in humans and in domestic animals.

Congenital cystic kidney

An anomaly which may result either from the failure of developing nephrons to join with their collecting ducts or from the formation of cysts in rudimentary nephrons is referred to as a congenital cystic kidney. Cyst formation arises from the accumulation of urine within nephrons which are isolated from their collecting duct system.

An inherited disease in Persian cats referred to as feline polycystic kidney disease, which has an autosomal dominant pattern of inheritance, is reported to occur at high frequency in the Persian cat population worldwide.

Further reading

Bard, J.B.L. (2002) Growth and death in the developing mammalian kidney: signals, receptors, and conversions. *BioEssay* **24**, 72–82.

Canfield, P.J. (1981) Electron microscopic examination of the developing bovine glomerular filtration barrier. *Anatomia, histologia, embryologia* **10**, 46–51.

Davies, J. (1951) Nephric development in the sheep with reference to the problem of the ruminant pronephros. *Journal of Anatomy* **85**, 6–11.

Davies, J. and Davies, D.V. (1950) The development of the mesonephros of the sheep. *Proceedings of the Zoological Society, London* **120**, 73–93.

Davies, J.A. (2002) Morphogenesis of the metanephric kidney. *Scientific World Journal* **2**, 1937–1950.

Frasier, E.A. (1919) The pronephros and early development of the mesonephros in the cat. *Journal of Anatomy* **54**, 228–304.

Frasier, E.A. (1950) The development of the vertebrate excretory system. *Biological Reviews* **25**, 159–187.

Shah, M., Sampogna, R., Sakurai, H., Bush, K. and Nigam, S. (2004) Branching morphogenesis and kidney disease. *Development* **131**, 1449–1462.

Tiedemann, K. (1976) *The Mesonephros of Cat and Sheep*. Springer-Verlag, Berlin.

Torrey, T.W. (1965) Morphogenesis of the vertebrate kidney. In *Organogenesis*. Eds. R.L. DeHann and H. Upsprung. Holt, Rinehart, and Winston, New York, pp. 559–579.

Woolf, A. (1997) The kidney. In *Embryos, Genes and Birth Defects*. Ed. P. Thorogood. John Wiley and Sons, Chichester, pp. 303–307.

18 Male and Female Reproductive Systems

Although the sex of an embryo is determined chromosomally at fertilisation, an undifferentiated stage of development initially occurs in which the primordia of both male and female genital organs are present. Depending on the genetically determined sex of the individual, the genital organs appropriate for that sex develop while the genital organs for the other sex regress. Sexual identity is not confined solely to the reproductive organs but is evident also in other anatomical features and in physiological and behavioural characteristics.

Primordial germ cells

Primordial germ cells, which eventually populate the undifferentiated gonad, can be detected in the epiblast by specific staining methods at an early stage in embryological development. These cells, which migrate through the primitive streak and then to the yolk sac and allantois, move along the wall of the hindgut to the genital ridge, a structure destined to become the undifferentiated gonad (Fig. 18.1).

In mammals, primordial germ cells arrive at their site of differentiation by active migration, whereas in avian species they reach the genital ridge via the blood stream. It has been suggested that germ cells may be attracted to the genital ridge by chemotaxis. Primordial germ cells can be detected in the genital ridge by day 18 in pigs, by day 21 in dogs, by day 22 in sheep and by day 28 in cattle and humans.

Primordial germ cells divide mitotically during migration to the developing gonads. Soon after entering the primordial gonad, the germ cells become enclosed in specific germ cell compartments, seminiferous cords in the male embryo, and primordial follicles in the female embryo. Both the proliferation and differentiation of primordial germ cells in these particular locations are strongly influenced by locally secreted soluble factors.

Only germ cells which reach the undifferentiated gonad differentiate and survive. Most germ cells outside the gonadal region undergo apoptosis but some which

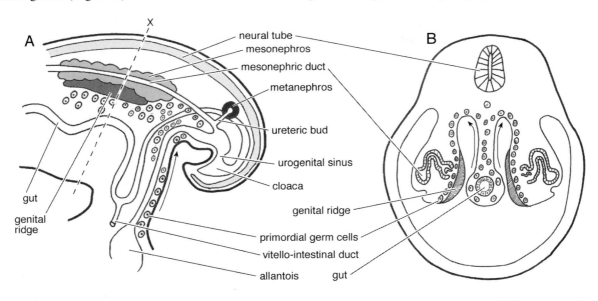

Figure 18.1 A, Route of migration of primordial germ cells from the allantois to the genital ridge, their site of differentiation. B, Transverse section through an embryo at the level indicated showing the migratory pathway of primordial germ cells along the dorsal mesentery to the genital ridge (arrows).

survive outside this region may form germ cell tumours referred to as teratomata. Because these abnormal structures are composed of elements of the three embryonic germ layers, they may contain highly differentiated tissues such as skin, hair, cartilage and teeth.

Undifferentiated stage of gonad formation

Although the origin of the somatic gonadal cells is unresolved, three cellular sources have been proposed: local mesenchymal cells, coelomic epithelium and cells derived from the mesonephric tubules. It is proposed that mesonephric cells from the degenerating mesonephric tubules invade the presumptive gonadal tissue and are the principal cells contributing to the gonadal primordia. Some cells contributing to the gonadal primordia may derive from the coelomic epithelium and also from the underlying mesenchyme. Following proliferation of coelomic epithelium and underlying mesenchyme, gonadal primordia develop as bilateral ridges. These ridges, which develop medial to the mesonephros and project into the coelomic cavity where they become covered by coelomic epithelium, extend from the thoracic to the lumbar region. The outline appearance of the gonadal ridges precedes the arrival of the primordial germ cells in the area. The undifferentiated gonads consist of primordial germ cells and mesodermal cells. The invading mesonephric cells and the mesonephric tubules form a tubular network called the rete system which consists of extra-gonadal cords, connecting cords, and intra-gonadal cords (Fig. 18.2). During development, as a consequence of proliferation in its mid-region, the developing gonadal ridge assumes a globular appearance and remains attached to the mesonephros by a fold of mesothelium. Because of their morphological similarity, it is not possible to distinguish male primordial gonads from female primordial gonads at an early stage of development using histological methods. However, using modern molecular techniques, the sex of an embryo can be reliably confirmed at an early stage of development.

Differentiation and maturation of the testes

In genotypic males, the mesonephric cells at the periphery of the intra-gonadal rete system develop into cords into which primordial germ cells become incorporated. These cords, known as seminiferous cords, become horseshoe-shaped and their extremities join with mesonephric cells at the centre of the developing gonad (Fig. 18.3). The seminiferous cords become convoluted and form the tubuli contorti. During this period of development, the seminiferous cords are solid structures, approximately 40 μm in diameter. On cross-section they are composed of a peripheral layer of 15 to 20 mesonephric cells which are destined to become Sertoli cells.

These mesonephric cells surround a central core of up to four germ cells, the pre-spermatogonia. Later, a layer of mesonephric-derived myoid cells surrounds the cords. Under the influence of the seminiferous cords, mesodermal cells, located between the cords, differentiate into the interstitial cells (Leydig cells) of the testis which produce testosterone. Subsequently, the mesonephric cells at the centre of the developing gonad give rise to the tubules of the rete testis. In cattle and dogs, interstitial cells increase in number until birth and then decrease. In horses, they undergo marked hypertrophy between the 110th and 220th days of gestation and then decrease in number. The highest rate of secretion of testosterone is reached when the interstitial cells are most numerous.

Mesenchymal cells under the coelomic epithelium of the developing testis develop into a fibrous layer known as the tunica albuginea. The mesenchymal cells between adjacent tubuli contorti form connective tissue septa which divide the testis into a number of lobules, while mesenchymal cells surrounding the tubules of the rete testis form a fibrous network called the mediastinum testis. The extent to which the testicular septa and the mediastinum testis become organised varies in individual species. In pigs, dogs and cats, they are well developed but in ruminants they are less well developed. In horses, the testicular septa contain smooth muscle cells, and the rete testis, which is atypical in that it does not occupy an axial position, is confined to the cranial pole of the testis where it extends through the tunica albuginea. Through the secretion of an inhibitory factor, the Sertoli cells, which surround the pre-spermatogonia, prevent further differentiation of the germ cells until, at puberty, the seminiferous cords become canalised and form tubules. Seminiferous tubules form and spermatogenesis begins in sheep at approximately five months of age, in cattle at around six to eight months, in dogs at approximately nine to ten months, in horses at about two years and in humans at 12 to 14 years.

Differentiation and maturation of the ovaries

Although the origin of the sex cords is not known with certainty, in genotypic females it is probable that they derive from the mesothelial cells surrounding the gonads. The sex cords form irregular recognisable structures into which germ cells become incorporated (Fig. 18.4). Following breakdown of the sex cords, germ cells undergo a period of enhanced mitotic activity in the developing ovaries. Irrespective of the duration of oogonial mitosis within a species, in the majority of mammals it ceases before or shortly after birth (Table 18.1). As individual oogonia complete their period of mitotic activity they become surrounded by a layer of squamous somatic cells of mesothelial origin, termed follicular cells. A germ cell enclosed in a basal lamina and surrounded

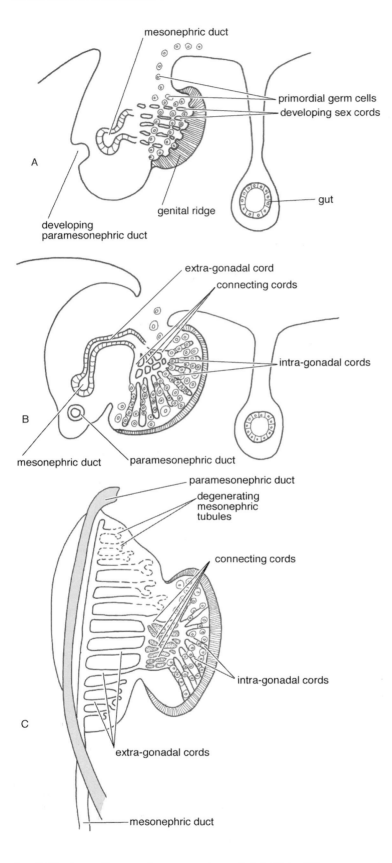

mesonephric duct

primordial germ cells
developing sex cords

gut

genital ridge

A

developing
paramesonephric duct

extra-gonadal cord
connecting cords

intra-gonadal cords

B

mesonephric duct   paramesonephric duct

paramesonephric duct
degenerating
mesonephric
tubules

connecting cords

intra-gonadal cords

C

extra-gonadal cords

mesonephric duct

Figure 18.2 Sequential stages in the development of the undifferentiated gonad. A, Formation of sex cords in the genital ridge. B, Relationship between the mesonephric duct and the developing sex cords. C, Ventral view of the developing gonad shown in B.

by follicular cells constitutes a primordial follicle. The follicular cells induce the enclosed oogonium to enter the prophase of meiosis I. At this stage the germ cells, which are referred to as primary oocytes, undergo a prolonged resting or dictyate stage. Although some maturation of primary oocytes may occur, these germ cells do not progress to the tertiary stage of development until stimulated by gonadotrophic hormones at the

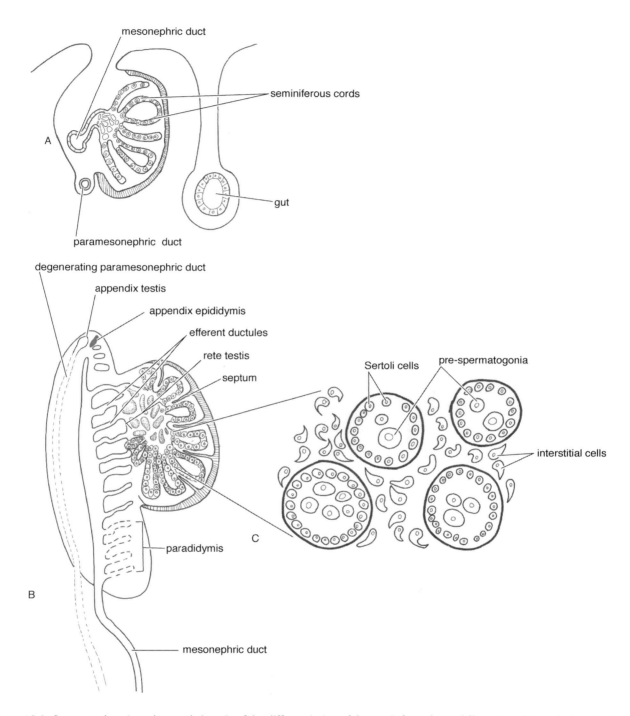

Figure 18.3 Cross-section, A, and ventral view, B, of the differentiation of the testis from the undifferentiated gonad, showing the formation of horseshoe-shaped seminiferous cords. C, Cross-section through seminiferous cords showing Sertoli cells, pre-spermatogonia and interstitial cells.

onset of puberty. Following the advent of puberty, recurring cyclical stages of follicular maturation occur in response to gonadotrophic hormones. As folliculogenesis proceeds, the squamous follicular cells, which become cuboidal, form stratified layers and are referred to as granulosa cells. Female mammals have their full complement of primary oocytes before or shortly after birth. In the ovary, germ cell proliferation and follicular development are confined to the peripheral areas of the

developing gonad. By the end of this developmental period in domestic species, with the exception of horses, the ovary consists of a dense cortical area which contains the follicles, and a less dense central medullary area composed of degenerating intra-gonadal tubules, the rete ovarii. In cattle, sheep and pigs, follicles are randomly distributed in the cortex while in dogs and cats, they occur in clusters. In mammals, a high percentage of oogonia and primary oocytes undergo degenerative

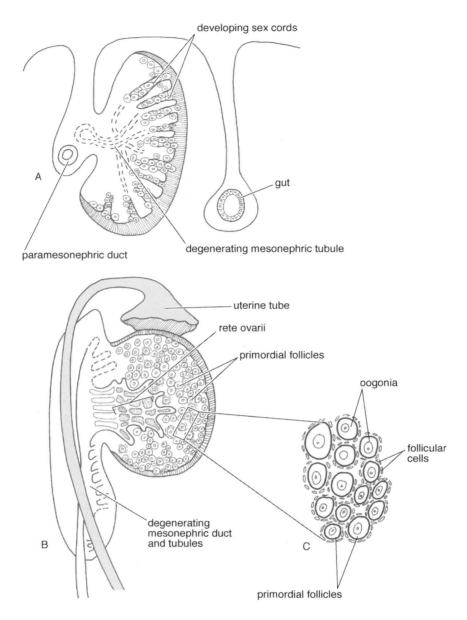

Figure 18.4 Cross-section, A, and ventral view, B, of differentiation of the ovary from the undifferentiated gonad, showing the formation of primordial follicles and the uterine tube. C, Primordial follicles.

Table 18.1 Approximate times of commencement and completion of oogonial mitosis in domestic animals.

| Species | Oogonial mitosis | |
	Commencement	Completion
Cats	32nd day of gestation	37th day after birth
Cattle	50th day of gestation	110th day of gestation
Horses	70th day of gestation	50th day after birth
Pigs	30th day of gestation	35th day after birth
Sheep	35th day of gestation	90th day of gestation

change referred to as atresia, during prenatal and postnatal life. Approximate numbers of germ cells in the ovaries of bovine embryos and foetuses are presented in Table 18.2. Data relating to the approximate numbers of germ cells in canine ovaries from birth to ten years of age are presented in Table 18.3.

Features of equine gonadal development

Development of follicles in the equine ovary is concentrated in the central area corresponding to the medulla in other species, while the non-follicular area is located peripherally. During *in utero* development, the unattached surface of the ovary becomes concave and, because it is from this site that ovulation occurs, the concavity is referred to as the ovulation fossa.

Table 18.2 Estimated germ cell numbers in the ovaries of developing bovine embryos or foetuses at different gestational ages.

Gestational age (days)	Number of germ cells
50	16,000
110	2,700,000
170	107,000
240	68,000

Table 18.3 Approximate numbers of germ cells in canine ovaries from birth to 10 years of age.

Age	Approximate number of germ cells
Newborn	700,000
1 year	350,000
5 years	3,300
10 years	500

The equine foetal gonads exhibit remarkable growth from about the 110th to 220th days of gestation. This enlargement, which occurs in both the developing ovary and testis, is attributed to hyperplasia and hypertrophy of interstitial cells. It has been suggested that gonadal enlargement is due to the action of equine chorionic gonadotrophin produced by endometrial cup cells. However, as the rate of gonadal development is maximal at the time that gonadotrophin activity has declined, this explanation is questionable. An alternative suggestion is that the increased gonadal size is due to the high levels of oestrogens produced by the placenta. However, as gonadal size decreases before maximum oestrogen production is reached, this suggestion seems improbable.

A notable feature of the developing equine testes is the appearance of pigment cells in the interstitial tissue during the ninth month of gestation. Prior to this time, the foetal testes have a yellowish-white appearance but thereafter they gradually acquire a dark appearance. Pigmentation, which persists until after birth, is considered to be associated with degeneration of interstitial cells.

Genital ducts

Irrespective of the genotype of the developing embryo, both male and female genital ducts form during the undifferentiated stages of gonadal formation. Differentiation of the male and female genital duct systems from the undifferentiated duct system is outlined in Figure 18.5. In the male embryo, elements of the mesonephric (Wolffian) duct system which persist are incorporated into the male genital system, while, apart from vestiges, the paramesonephric (Müllerian) ducts largely disappear. In the female embryo, paramesonephric ducts contribute to the formation of the genital duct system, while the mesonephric ducts atrophy except for vestiges. The paramesonephric ducts are located lateral to the mesonephric ducts.

Differentiation of the male duct system in mammals

The mesonephric tubules and mesonephric duct cranial to the developing testes atrophy, except for a small vestige of the mesonephric duct which is called the appendix epididymis. Depending on the species, from 9 to 12 mesonephric tubules, located in the region of the developing testes, lose their glomeruli and become the connecting portion of the rete system which forms the efferent ductules of the testes. Some of the mesonephric tubules at the caudal pole of the developing testes do not join the tubules of the rete testis and gradually lose contact with the mesonephric duct. These vestiges are collectively referred to as the paradidymis. Mesonephric tubules caudal to the developing testes atrophy.

The mesonephric ducts, from the cranial poles of the testes to the urogenital sinus, persist as the male genital ducts. A segment of the mesonephric duct caudal to the point of entry of the efferent ductules elongates and becomes convoluted, forming the epididymis. The remaining caudal segment of the mesonephric duct, which develops a thick muscular wall, becomes the ductus deferens (Fig. 18.5).

With the exception of carnivores, the mesonephric ducts form evaginations near their junctions with the urogenital sinus. These mesodermal evaginations form the seminal vesicles. The primordia of the seminal vesicles are first observed in the bovine foetus around the 55th day of gestation.

The definitive urogenital sinus forms the pelvic and penile urethra. The endodermal epithelium of the pelvic urethra forms outbuddings at its cranial and caudal ends. The cranial outgrowths give rise to the prostate gland in all mammals, and the caudal outgrowths form the bulbo-urethral glands in all domestic mammals, apart from dogs. The cranial vestiges of the paramesonephric ducts give rise to the appendix testis while the caudal vestiges fuse and form the uterus masculinus (prostatic utricle).

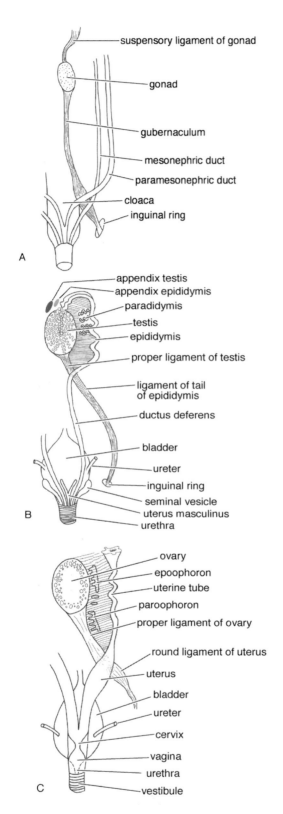

A
- suspensory ligament of gonad
- gonad
- gubernaculum
- mesonephric duct
- paramesonephric duct
- cloaca
- inguinal ring

B
- appendix testis
- appendix epididymis
- paradidymis
- testis
- epididymis
- proper ligament of testis
- ligament of tail of epididymis
- ductus deferens
- bladder
- ureter
- inguinal ring
- seminal vesicle
- uterus masculinus
- urethra

C
- ovary
- epoophoron
- uterine tube
- paroophoron
- proper ligament of ovary
- round ligament of uterus
- uterus
- bladder
- ureter
- cervix
- vagina
- urethra
- vestibule

Figure 18.5 Development of the undifferentiated genital duct systems, A, into the male duct system, B, and the female duct system, C.

Differentiation of the female duct system in mammals

The primordia of the paramesonephric ducts arise from intermediate mesoderm lateral to the cranial ends of the mesonephric ducts. Initially, grooves which form in the coelomic epithelium give rise to paramesonephric ducts which move deeper into the mesenchyme adjacent to the related mesonephric ducts (Fig. 17.2). The cranial portions of the paramesonephric ducts form the uterine tubes while the caudal portions of the ducts give rise to the horns and body of the uterus. At their cranial aspects, the uterine tubes remain open and communicate with the coelomic cavity. Postnatally, this communication persists from the peritoneal cavity to the exterior. In males, a comparable communication between the peritoneal cavity and the exterior does not exist. At first, the portions of the ducts which are closed elongate caudally, lateral to the mesonephric duct (Fig. 18.5). Close to the urogenital sinus, each duct occupies a position ventral to the mesonephric duct and fuses in the midline with its corresponding duct from the opposite side. The closed end of the fused ducts continues to grow caudally and makes contact with the urogenital sinus where it induces cellular proliferation of the endoderm of the urogenital sinus and the formation of the vaginal plate. Differences observed in the final anatomical arrangement of uteri in different species can be attributed to the relative positions of their primordial structures and the extent to which fusion occurs. In rodents, fusion is confined solely to the outer portions of the walls of the ducts while the lumina remain distinct. This results in a separate opening for each uterine lumen into the vagina (uterus duplex). In domestic species, the caudal ends of the ducts fuse. Subsequently, the medial fused walls atrophy resulting in the formation of a single tube, the body of the uterus, which has a single opening into the vagina. Those portions of the ducts cranial to the region of fusion remain distinct and are the primordia of the horns of the uterus and the uterine tubes. Thus, in domestic animals the uterus which consists of two horns and a body is referred to as a bicornuate uterus (Fig. 18.6). In cattle, the primordia of the paramesonephric ducts appear at approximately the 34th day of gestation, and fuse with the urogenital sinus at approximately the 50th day. In primates, including humans, extensive fusion of the paramesonephric ducts occurs with associated atrophy along the medial line of fusion, resulting in the formation of a large uterine body termed a uterus simplex (Fig. 18.6).

The vagina is derived from both the vaginal plate and the fused ends of the paramesonephric ducts. Subsequently, cannulation of these fused structures occurs forming the lumen of the vagina. Initially, the lumen of the vagina is separated from the urogenital sinus by a

Figure 18.6 Final anatomical arrangement of the reproductive tracts in selected mammals. The extent of paramesonephric duct fusion determines the shape of the body of the uterus and the nature of its relationship with the vagina. A, Reproductive tract of rodent, showing a uterus duplex. B, Porcine reproductive tract, showing a bicornuate uterus. C, Primate reproductive tract showing a uterus simplex.

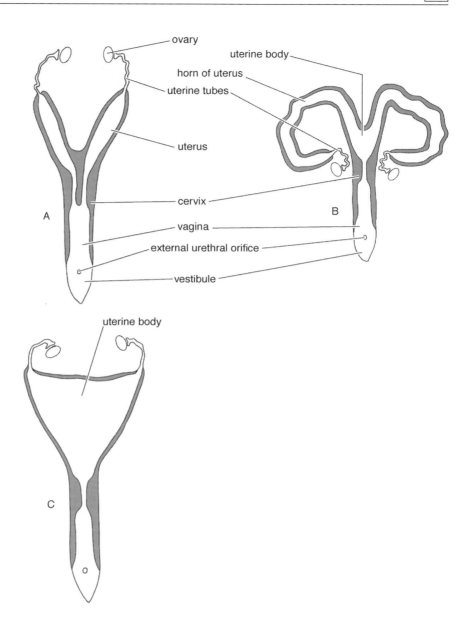

thin membrane, the hymen, which subsequently breaks down. In domestic animals, persistence of hymen remnants is less evident than in primates. The caudal portion of the urogenital sinus forms the vestibule (Fig. 18.7).

Epithelial buds, which arise from the primitive urethra and definitive urogenital sinus, form the urethral and vestibular glands, the female homologues of the prostate and bulbo-urethral glands in the male embryo.

Apart from some remnants of the excretory tubules and a small portion of the mesonephric duct, the female mesonephric system atrophies. The cranial remnants of the mesonephric tubules form the epoophoron (Fig. 18.5). The mesonephric tubules caudal to the developing gonad become the paroophoron and the remainder of the mesonephric duct usually degenerates. Occasionally, a caudal portion of the duct persists as Gartner's duct which may form a cyst in the vaginal wall.

Avian gonads and associated ducts

Two primordial gonads and duct systems develop in avian embryos. In genotypic male embryos, two gonads and two duct systems persist and become functional. In genotypic female embryos, the left gonad and its associated duct continue to develop into functional structures, while the right gonad and associated duct remain rudimentary. The left paramesonephric duct gives rise to the different regions of the female reproductive tract from the ovary to the cloaca.

Formation of the genital fold

The urogenital system, which develops retro-peritoneally, bulges into the peritoneal cavity. With the degeneration of the mesonephros, the gonads and genital ducts become suspended by thin folds of peritoneum. The caudal portions of the genital ducts meet and fuse in

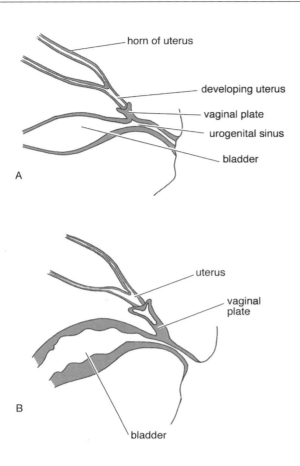

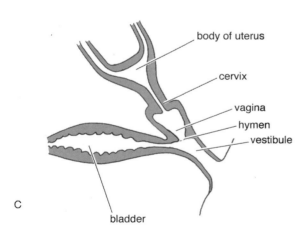

Figure 18.7 Sequential stages in the development of the vagina.

the mid-line. Fusion of their associated peritoneal folds forms the genital fold (Fig. 18.8). In the female, this broad sheet of peritoneum is referred to as the broad ligament of the uterus and is composed of three segments assigned names according to the structures which they support: the mesovarium which suspends the ovaries, the mesosalpinx which suspends the uterine tubes, and the mesometrium which suspends the uterus. In the male, that part of the genital fold which suspends the testes is termed the mesorchium and the portion

which suspends the ductus deferens the mesoductus deferens.

External genitalia

During the undifferentiated phase of sexual development in the embryo, mesenchymal cells from the primitive streak migrate to the region around the cloacal membrane and form two elevated folds, the cloacal folds. These folds fuse ventrally and form the genital tubercle. Later in development, as a consequence of the formation of the urorectal septum, the cloacal membrane is subdivided into an anal and a urogenital membrane. The anal and urogenital membranes subsequently break down allowing communication between the rectum and urogenital sinus and the exterior. Endodermal cells from the urogenital sinus proliferate and grow into the mesoderm of the genital tubercle, forming the urethral plate. The cloacal folds are also divided into the anal folds dorsally and the urogenital folds ventrally. Proliferation of mesoderm lateral to each urogenital fold forms elevations which are termed the genital (labio-scrotal) swellings (Fig. 18.9).

Differentiation of the external genitalia

In the male embryo, the genital tubercle elongates rapidly in a ventro-cranial direction and draws the urogenital folds forwards forming the lateral edges of the urethral plate, the floor of which gives rise to the urethral groove. The urogenital folds fuse converting the urethral groove into a tube, the penile urethra (Fig. 18.10). With closure of the urogenital folds, the penile urethra becomes incorporated into the body of the penis. The urethral plate, however, does not extend to the tip of the penis. An ectodermal bud which invaginates into the tip of the penis fuses with endodermal cells lining the penile urethra. Later, this cord of ectodermal cells becomes canalised and, as a consequence, the penile urethra opens at the tip of the penis (Fig. 18.11). In the feline embryo, the genital tubercle does not extend ventro-cranially and consequently the penis of the cat retains its embryonic orientation with its apex pointing caudally. In rams and male goats, the urethra forms an elongation, the urethral process, which extends beyond the tip of the penis. The corpus cavernosum penis, tunica albuginea, and corpus spongiosum penis derive from genital tubercle mesenchyme. In carnivores, the mesenchymal tissue at the cranial end of the corpus cavernosum penis becomes ossified forming the os penis. The prepuce forms from loose connective tissue and ectoderm surrounding the genital tubercle.

The genital swellings give rise to the scrotal pouches which fuse at their medial aspects forming the scrotum. The line of fusion of the scrotal pouches persists as the

Figure 18.8 Cross-sections through the caudal abdominal regions of female embryos showing sequential stages in the formation of the genital fold.

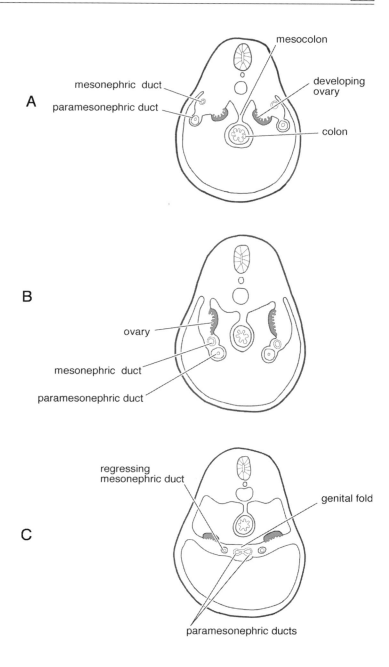

scrotal raphé. The final position of the scrotum differs among domestic species. In horses and ruminants, the genital swellings migrate cranially and the scrotum is located in the inguinal region unlike in cats and pigs where it is positioned beneath the anus. In dogs, the scrotum is located in an intermediate position between the inguinal region and the anus.

In the female embryo, the vestibule arises from the caudal end of the urogenital sinus. The urogenital folds, which do not fuse, develop into the labia of the vulva. The genital tubercle, located on the floor of the vestibule, gives rise to the clitoris which is covered by the labia at the point where these structures meet ventrally (Fig. 18.9).

Factors which influence sexual differentiation in mammals

In amphibians and fish, the sex of the offspring can be definitively determined by a number of environmental factors, including temperature and light. Although gonadal differentiation in mammals is largely determined by the genotype of the zygote, a range of modifying factors can influence gonadal differentiation (Fig. 18.12). In turn, differentiation of the duct system and external genitalia is substantially determined by gonadal hormones. Many abnormalities in sexual development can be attributed to the genotype of the zygote and to the impact of environmental factors which can influence development of the gonads and external genitalia.

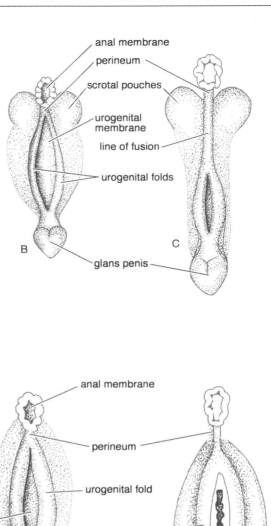

Figure 18.9 Development of the male and female external genitalia. Undifferentiated stage of the external genitalia, A, and sequential stages in the development of the male external genitalia, B and C, and of the female external genitalia, D and E.

Sex determination

In mammals, the genotype of the zygote typically determines the pathway of development of the undifferentiated gonad towards a testis or ovary. The presence of the *sex-determining region Y (Sry)* gene on the short arm of the Y chromosome initiates a series of events which cause the undifferentiated gonad to develop into a testis. Because the female mammalian genotype does not contain a Y chromosome and the associated *Sry* gene, the undifferentiated gonad develops into an ovary. There is evidence that a number of genes play a central role in the differentiation of the testis or ovary (Fig. 18.12). Apart

from the *Sry* gene which determines testicular development, other genes, such as *Sox-9* and *Sf-1*, are considered to be essential for normal spermatogenesis as deletion of these genes results in infertility. *Dax-1* and *Wnt-4* play a central role in ovarian development.

Molecular aspects of gonadogenesis

Using gene knockout studies a number of genes which are essential for the development of the undifferentiated gonad have been identified. Mice lacking functional copies of *Lim*, *Sf-1*, *Wt-1*, *Emx-2* and *Lhx-9* have a complete absence of gonads.

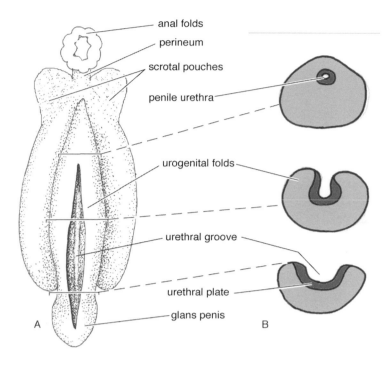

Figure 18.10 Closure of the urethral groove and cross-sections at different levels showing progressive stages in the conversion of the urethral groove into a tube, the penile urethra.

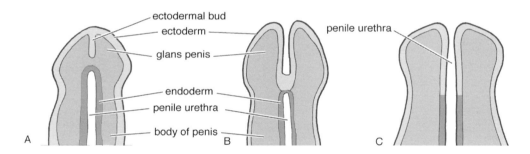

Figure 18.11 Stages in the development of the terminal portion of the penile urethra.

With the development of the undifferentiated gonad into a testicle, a range of soluble factors, encoded by the sex-determining genes including *Sry*, *Sox-9* and *Sf-1*, promote the development of Sertoli cells and Leydig cells. The *Sry* gene initiates a downstream cascade of male sex-determining genes. The *Sox-9* gene is up-regulated under the control of *Wt-1* directly after *Sry* expression. *Sf-1* and *Sox-9* both up-regulate additional genes essential for male sex determination. Subsequently, Sertoli cells secrete paramesonephric inhibitory hormone and Leydig cells secrete testosterone.

Development of the undifferentiated gonad into an ovary is directly influenced by *Dax-1* and *Wnt-4*. *Dax-1* has been shown to inhibit transcriptional activation by *Sf-1* of the male-specific genes through the recruitment of nuclear co-repressor (N-CoR). A member of the nuclear hormone receptor family, *Dax-1*, which is located on the short arm of the X chromosome, acts by down-regulating *Sry*, *Sf-1* and *Sox-9* activity, thereby inhibiting the differentiation of Sertoli cells and Leydig cells. The growth factor Wnt-4 contributes to ovarian differentiation and paramesonephric duct development. Inactivation of *Wnt-4* in early embryonic development causes failure of the formation of the paramesonephric duct derivatives. Studies have shown that duplication of either *Dax-1* or *Wnt-4* has been associated with XY sex reversal, indicating that the inhibitory effect of *Dax-1* on *Sf-1*-dependent genes can override the effects of *Sry* in a dose-dependent manner (Fig. 18.12).

Influence of hormones on development of genital ducts and external genitalia

Development of the male genital duct system and external genitalia is under the influence of the hormones produced by the developing testes. With the formation

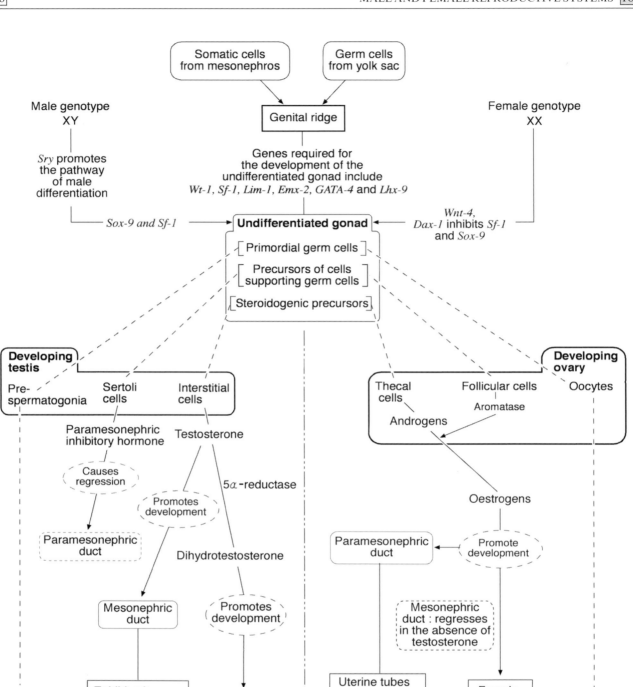

Figure 18.12 Cellular and genetic interactions which specify development of the genital ridge, undifferentiated gonad and either a testis or an ovary. Subsequently, hormones secreted by the testis or ovary promote the development of a male or female duct system and external genitalia.

of the testes, the male duct system and external genitalia develop and the female duct system regresses. The foetal testes secrete two hormones, testosterone and paramesonephric inhibitory hormone (anti-Müllerian hormone). Testosterone, produced by the Leydig cells, induces the differentiation of the paired male duct system, epididymis, ductus deferens and seminal vesicle. When acted on by 5α-reductase, testosterone is converted to

dihydrotestosterone which induces differentiation of the male external genitalia. Paramesonephric inhibitory hormone, secreted by the Sertoli cells, inhibits development of the paramesonephric ducts and induces regression of these structures.

In the female, under the influence of oestrogens, the paramesonephric ducts develop and differentiate into

Table 18.4 Embryonic primordia from which structures in the male and female reproductive systems arise.

Embryonic structure	Derivative in the male reproductive system	Derivative in the female reproductive system
Primordial germ cells	Spermatozoa	Ova
Gonad	Testis	Ovary
Sex cords	Seminiferous tubules, Sertoli cells	Follicular cells
Mesonephric tubules	Efferent ductules	Epoophoron, paroophoron
Mesonephric duct	Epididymis, ductus deferens, seminal vesicles	Gartner's duct
Paramesonephric duct	Appendix of testis, uterus masculinus	Uterine tube, uterus and cranial portion of vagina
Definitive urogenital sinus	Pelvic urethra, prostate gland, bulbo-urethral gland and penile urethra	Vestibule and associated glands
Genital tubercle	Shaft of penis	Clitoris
Urogenital folds	Tissue surrounding the ventral aspect of the penile urethra	Labia of vulva
Genital swellings	Scrotum	None

uterine tubes, uterus and the cranial portion of the vagina. During differentiation, oestrogens act on the external genitalia inducing the formation of the clitoris, caudal portion of the vagina, vestibule and vulva. Although the sites of oestrogen secretion are not definitively established, it is probable that both maternal and foetal tissues secrete this hormone. Embryonic primordia from which structures in the male and female reproductive systems arise are presented in Table 18.4.

Sexual differentiation, associated brain function and subsequent sexual behaviour at puberty

Sex hormones influence the development of regions of the brain associated with sexual behaviour. In female mammals, the hypothalamic nuclei of the brain regulate the rhythmical secretion of gonadotrophic hormones at puberty which ultimately results in the oestrous cycle. In male mammals, testosterone produced by the foetal testis modifies the functioning of the hypothalamus which subsequently inhibits the cyclical pattern of luteinising hormone secretion at puberty, a feature of female reproductive physiology. For testosterone to act

on the hypothalamus, it must first cross the blood–brain barrier. In the brain it is converted by aromatase to oestradiol which abolishes the post-pubertal cyclical pattern of luteinising hormone release. In contrast, although oestradiol is produced by foetal ovaries, it does not cross the blood–brain barrier because it is bound by α-foetoprotein. Accordingly, oestradiol produced by the female foetus does not inhibit the post-pubertal cyclical secretion of gonadotrophic hormones.

Anomalies of sexual development

During the complex series of events involved in the development of the reproductive system, there are numerous opportunities for developmental defects to occur. These anomalies can occur at the chromosomal level, during gonadal differentiation, or at the stage of differentiation of the duct system or of the external genitalia. Manifestations of sexuality can be evaluated at a number of levels: genotypic, gonadal, phenotypic and behavioural. Based on collective conformity to these criteria an animal is considered to be male or female. An animal not conforming to these criteria and which exhibits some of the characteristics of both sexes is described as an intersex animal. Intersexuality in domestic mammals is principally concerned with abnormalities in genotypic, gonadal or phenotypic characteristics. Intersex animals have some of the characteristics of each sex, including physical attributes and reproductive tissue, which may contribute to atypical sexual behaviour. In addition, an intersex animal may be one sex genotypically and the other sex phenotypically.

An individual with cell populations which have derived from two or more separate zygotes is referred to as a chimera. The incorporation of the two cell lines into the developing embryo can occur spontaneously or as a consequence of experimentation. The term 'mosaic' is used to describe an individual with two or more cell populations with different karyotypes which have originated from a single zygote through mutational change.

An individual with gonads of both sexes, either as separate ovaries and testes, or as combined ovo-testes, is termed a hermaphrodite. A pseudohermaphrodite has the gonads of one sex only with duct systems, external genitalia and some of the sexual characteristics of the opposite sex. Such an animal is classified as male or female on the basis of the type of gonad present. Thus, a male pseudohermaphrodite has male gonads but female external genitalia.

What is referred to as true hermaphroditism results from gonadal defects at an early stage of development, so that both testicular and ovarian tissues develop either as separate gonads or as combined ovo-testes. There is evidence that translocation of a fragment of the Y chromosome containing the *Sry* gene to a cryptic site on the X chromosome promotes the development of the testicular tissue. True hermaphroditism has been reported in all species of domestic mammals, especially pigs. This condition has been observed in association with experimentally induced chimerism.

Female pseudohermaphroditism, which is due to androgenic hormones reaching the foetus during the undifferentiated stage of development, is an uncommon condition. Exposure of a female foetus to an external source of androgens may induce differentiation of the mesonephric ducts and development of the urogenital sinus as in a male animal. The paramesonephric ducts develop normally into the female duct system. The sex chromosomal composition of female pseudohermaphrodites is XX.

Male pseudohermaphroditism is one of the most common forms of intersex found in domestic animals. This anomaly of male sexual differentiation can result from a deficiency or decreased secretion of either or both hormones produced by the foetal testes or from insensitivity of target cells to these hormones. In the absence of both testicular hormones, the paramesonephric duct system persists and the animal is born with female external genitalia. Examples of this condition have been described in pigs and dogs. An absence of functional receptors on target cells for dihydrotestosterone, but with secretion of paramesonephric-inhibitory hormone, results in absence of both male and female duct systems and the development of female external genitalia. Male pseudohermaphroditism resulting from a lack of androgen receptors, which has been described in humans, cattle, sheep, pigs, rats and mice, is known as the testicular feminisation syndrome. This X-linked condition renders target organs insensitive to the action of androgens. Individuals with this condition, while phenotypically female, are genotypically and gonadally male with testes retained within the abdomen.

An additional form of male pseudohermaphroditism results from a deficiency of paramesonephric inhibitory hormone but with production of androgenic hormones, giving rise to development of a male duct system and external genitalia along with paramesonephric duct derivatives.

Klinefelter syndrome (XXY) results from non-disjunction of sex chromosomes during meiosis. The presence of the Y chromosome results in male-determining genes inducing the formation of male gonads with production of male hormones and the development of a phenotypic male. The presence of the female chromosomes, however, prevents normal spermatogenesis resulting in hypoplas-

tic testes. This syndrome is recognised in humans, dogs and cats.

Turner syndrome (XO), which is due to non-disjunction, results in a phenotypic female with hypoplastic ovaries, small uterus and under-developed external genitalia. Delayed puberty and small stature are features of Turner syndrome. The condition, which is well recognised in humans, has been observed in horses, pigs, dogs and cats.

Ovarian dysgenesis, involving one or both ovaries, has been reported occasionally in domestic animals. A feature of this condition, which occurs in cattle, sheep and pigs, is that the ovaries, which are smaller than normal, have diminished gametogenic activity. Hypoplasia of both testes and ovaries, which is usually associated with genetic or chromosomal abnormalities, also occurs in domestic animals.

Penile hypoplasia (incomplete growth) is a rare condition which has been observed in dogs and cats. In humans, it has been associated with hypopituitarism and androgen deficiency. Hypospadias is a congenital defect in males due to partial failure of the urogenital folds to close which results in the external urethral orifice being misplaced. The urethral opening may be located on the ventral surface of the penis or in the perineum.

Congenital preputial stenosis, which can vary from narrowing of the preputial orifice to complete occlusion of the orifice resulting in obstruction to urinary outflow, results in the inability to protrude the penis, a condition referred to as phimosis.

Persistent penile frenulum, failure of the normal separation of the glans penis from the preputial epithelium, results in an inability to protrude the penis. The connective tissue attachment usually occurs on the ventral midline of the penis. Normal separation of the glans penis and preputial epithelium is a testosterone-dependent process and occurs ante-natally in some species and post-natally in others.

Freemartinism in cattle

The freemartin syndrome is a form of intersexuality which occurs primarily in cattle. The freemartin is a genotypic female (XX) which is born co-twin to a male calf (XY). Although the basis of freemartinism is disputed, two hypotheses, a hormonal hypothesis and a cellular hypothesis, have been proposed to explain the morphological anomalies in affected animals. In cattle, the vascular tips of adjacent chorio-allantoic membranes fuse in over 90% of pregnancies involving twins with resulting vascular anastomosis between the two embryonic circulations. If anastomosis occurs prior to sexual differentiation, the hormone hypothesis proposes that sex-determining factors from the male co-twin exert a marked influence on the undifferentiated reproductive system of the female twin. In such circumstances, the gonads of the female may have the appearance of normal ovaries or may resemble testes. Development of the paramesonephric duct system is partially inhibited and the mesonephric duct system may undergo varying degrees of differentiation. As a consequence of interference with paramesonephric duct development, the cranial portion of the vagina does not develop. However, the urogenital sinus does develop, giving rise to the caudal vagina closed at its cranial end, an enlarged clitoris and a characteristic tuft of hair at the ventral commissure of the vulva. In affected animals, mammary gland tissue and teats are under-developed.

The cellular hypothesis proposes that XY germ cells from the male co-twin alter the ovarian tissue of the female twin both morphologically and functionally. It is suggested that male germ cells reach the undifferentiated gonad of the female twin where they subsequently promote a degree of differentiation of male gonadal tissue in the female gonad. The extent of alteration of the undifferentiated paramesonephric duct systems reflects the extent to which male gonadal tissue develops and functions in the female gonad.

Although no obvious morphological abnormalities are reported in male animals born as co-twins to freemartins, testosterone production in such animals is lower than in iso-sexual twins and these male animals have reduced fertility.

Transfer of cells between bovine dizygotic twins is not confined to germ cells alone, as haematopoietic stem cells are also exchanged between such twins. As a result of the exchange, each twin has a mixture of red blood cell types and they exhibit mutual immunological tolerance to tissue transplanted from one to the other.

Freemartinism can be confirmed by clinical examination, by demonstration of chromosome chimerism (XX/XY), by blood typing and by the acceptance by one twin of skin grafts from the other.

Freemartinism in species other than cattle

In sheep, dizygotic twinning occurs more frequently than in cattle. The occurrence of vascular anastomosis of the chorio-allantoic blood vessels of ovine twins is reported to range from 1 to 65%. However, cytogenetic tests on heterosexual twins suggest that exchange of cells *in utero* is minimal and the incidence of freemartinism in sheep is approximately 1%. Freemartinism is reported infrequently in pigs and goats.

Segmental aplasia of the paramesonephric ducts

Anomalous embryonic development of the paramesonephric ducts or vaginal plate is reported periodically in cattle and other species. The condition may be characterised by one or more of the following developmental defects: a thickened imperforate hymen, occluded vagina, absence of cervical canal or absence of a segment of the uterine body or of a uterine horn. Although anomalous development of the paramesonephric duct leads to a completely or partially imperforate female tract, the ovaries develop normally and affected animals show normal cyclical behaviour. Normal secretory activity develops. As a consequence of the imperforate state of the affected portion of the tract and normal secretory activity, the lumen of the tract, cranial to the imperforate region, becomes distended with accumulated secretions. Although the condition may occur in all breeds of cattle, formerly it was more commonly described in white shorthorn heifers than in other breeds, with up to 10% of heifers affected. This condition was thought to be due to a sex-linked recessive gene with linkage to the gene encoding for a white coat in the shorthorn breed, a proposal which has been rejected.

Descent of the testes

Migration of the male gonads from their intra-abdominal site of development to an extra-abdominal subcutaneous location, usually in the inguinal region, is referred to as descent of the testes. With the exception of mammals, the testes of vertebrate animals remain within the abdominal cavity. Even among mammals, the process of testicular descent is subject to species variation. In monotremes, such as the duck-billed platypus and spiny anteater, and in some higher mammals, such as armadillos, elephants and aquatic mammals, testicular descent does not occur and the testes remain within the abdominal cavity. In some other species, such as bats, moles, hedgehogs and red deer, the testes, which are retained within the abdominal cavity during the greater part of the year, descend to an extra-abdominal location during the breeding season. In the majority of mammals, however, the testes migrate to an extra-abdominal location, but even in some of these mammals, such as rats, mice and guinea-pigs, the testes may be temporarily withdrawn into the abdominal cavity as a consequence of sensing danger. In those animals in which the testes descend to an extra-abdominal location, a temperature of 2–4 °C below core body temperature is required for normal spermatogenesis.

During testicular development, a mesenchymal column of jelly-like tissue, the gubernaculum, develops and extends from the caudal pole of the mesonephros and testis to the inguinal region (Fig. 18.13). This structure is

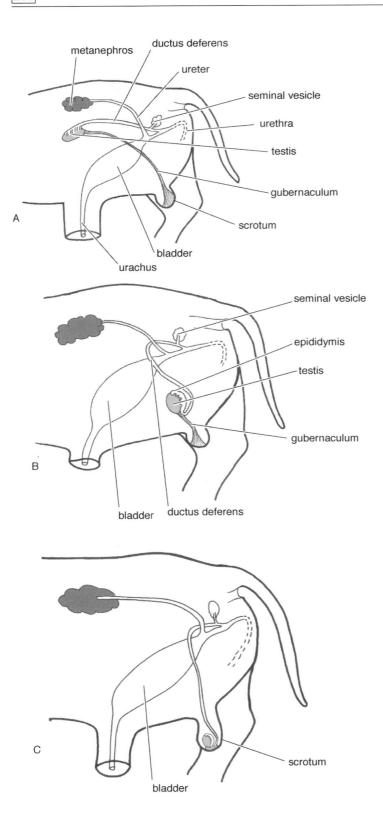

Figure 18.13 Stages in the descent of the bovine testis from a dorsal position in the peritoneal cavity, A, to a ventral position, B, and in its final position in the scrotum, C.

present in both male and female embryos. That portion of the gubernaculum within the abdominal cavity is covered by a fold of peritoneum. The extra-abdominal part of the gubernaculum, which is located in the embryonic abdominal wall, exists prior to the formation of abdominal musculature. This portion gradually extends caudally to the genital swellings and its caudal end acquires

a bulbar shape. As the musculature of the abdominal wall develops around the gubernaculum, openings in the internal abdominal oblique muscle and the external abdominal oblique muscle link the abdominal cavity to the developing scrotal sac. The passageway between these two openings, occupied by the gubernaculum, is referred to as the inguinal canal. A crescentic invagination of peritoneum, referred to as the process vaginalis, which grows into the gubernaculum in dogs at 36 days and in horses and cattle at 48 days, almost completely surrounds it so that a part of the extra-abdominal portion of the gubernaculum, like its intra-abdominal portion, becomes suspended by a fold of peritoneum. Invasion by the process vaginalis divides the gubernaculum into three parts. The proximal part is enclosed by the inner layer of the process vaginalis which forms the visceral layer of the tunica vaginalis. The outer layer of the gubernaculum, which is surrounded by the parietal layer of the tunica, is referred to as the vaginal part. The distal portion, known as the infra-vaginal part, remains attached to the scrotal wall as the scrotal ligament.

The intra-abdominal part of the gubernaculum is attached to both the mesonephric and paramesonephric ducts at a point where the ducts change from a lateral to a medial position. In the male embryo, the part of the mesonephric duct cranial to this attachment becomes the epididymis and the part caudal to it becomes the ductus deferens.

Despite disagreement about the mechanisms involved in testicular descent, it is described as occurring in two stages, intra-abdominal descent and inguino-scrotal descent. Intra-abdominal migration of the testes from the lumbar region to the inguinal ring is considered to be more apparent than real due to the rapid growth of the vertebral column and associated structures relative to the position of the gonads in the lumbar region. In both male and female embryos, the gonads are retained in a fixed position by the gubernaculum. As they remain attached in position and are not drawn cranially by the rapid growth of the vertebral column and associated structures, they appear to have migrated caudally. The metanephros, which initially develops in a position caudal to the gonads, is drawn cranially by this developmental process and occupies a position cranial to the gonads.

Some workers maintain that the entire process of testicular descent is due to contraction of the gubernaculum. However, there are no contractile fibres present in the gubernaculum to account for this proposed mechanism of testicular descent. It has been observed in horses, cattle and pigs that, as the intra-abdominal portion of the gubernaculum decreases in length, the extra-abdominal portion lengthens. Another suggestion is that the change in length of the gubernaculum is due to the increased abdominal pressure on the fluid within the vaginal process. It is claimed that this pressure forces the extra-abdominal part of the gubernaculum caudally, thus drawing the gonad towards the inguinal ring. A further suggestion proposes that the decrease in length of the intra-abdominal gubernaculum is due to the rapid

swelling of the extra-abdominal gubernaculum which pulls it caudally and with it the attached testis. The testes are located at the internal inguinal rings in dogs at 50 days, in cattle at 90 days, in pigs at 70 days, in humans at 150 days and in horses at 240 days of gestation. Testicular migration is influenced by paramesonephric inhibitory hormone which induces enlargement of the gubernaculum (Fig. 18.13).

As the testis approaches the inguinal ring, the tail of the epididymis enters the inguinal canal. Enlargement of the gubernaculum, attributed in part to cell division but primarily to an increase in intercellular fluid, dilates the opening into the inguinal canal, thereby facilitating entry of the testis. It is suggested that abdominal pressure causes tension on the gubernaculum through the process vaginalis and forces the testis through the internal inguinal ring. Once the testis enters the inguinal canal, contraction of the internal inguinal ring, together with contractions of the oblique abdominal muscles, force the testis along the canal and through the external inguinal ring. Passage of the testis through the canal is rapid in cattle and pigs, but slow in horses. As the testis leaves the inguinal canal, the gubernaculum regresses, facilitating descent of the testis into the scrotum. This decrease in gubernacular size is due mainly to a sudden reduction in the intercellular fluid content of the gubernaculum. Inguino-scrotal descent is reported to be androgen-dependent. The approximate times of testicular descent in humans and domestic animals are presented in Table 18.5.

A survey of neonatal foals subjected to post-mortem examination found that testicular descent had occurred in approximately 50% of these animals. Palpation of the scrotum of foals during the first days of life is an unreliable method of determining testicular descent because the gubernacular bulb may be mistaken for a testis. Following descent, the portion of the gubernaculum between the caudal pole of the testis and the epididymis

Table 18.5 Times at which testicular descent occurs in humans and in domestic animals.

Species	Time of testicular descent
Humans	During the 7th month of gestation
Cattle	During the 4th month of gestation
Dogs and cats	3 to 25 days post-natally
Horses	During the 10th to 11th months of gestation
Pigs	During the 3rd month of gestation
Sheep	During the 3rd month of gestation

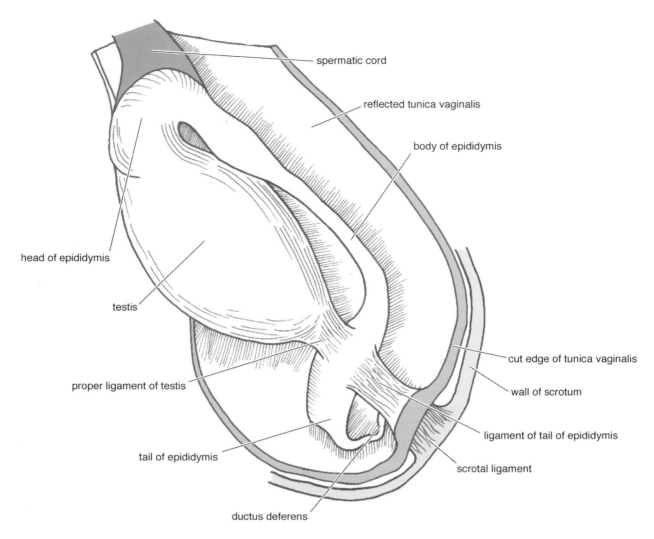

Figure 18.14 The position of the testis in the scrotum and the attachments of the three ligaments which are formed from the gubernaculum. The tunica vaginalis has been reflected.

persists as the proper ligament of the testis. The part of the gubernaculum between the epididymis and the parietal layer of the tunica vaginalis forms the ligament of the tail of the epididymis (Figs. 18.5 and 18.14).

If, following descent through the inguinal canal, a testis migrates to a position other then the scrotum, it is termed an ectopic testis.

Ovarian migration

In females, some intra-abdominal migration of the ovary occurs in particular species. In dogs and cats, the ovaries occupy a position in the sub-lumbar region caudal to the kidneys. The ovaries of mares migrate to a location midway between the kidneys and the pelvic inlet. In cattle and pigs, migration is more pronounced and the ovaries occupy a position at the pelvic inlet. The portion of the gubernaculum between the ovary and

paramesonephric duct forms the proper ligament of the ovary; the remainder of the gubernaculum forms the round ligament of the uterus which occupies a position in the mesometrium. In bitches, the round ligament, which is a prominent structure, enters the internal opening of the inguinal canal and may predispose to inguinal herniation.

Cryptorchidism

Failure of normal testicular descent, cryptorchidism, is a condition which occurs in all mammalian species. It is most frequently encountered in horses and pigs, and in miniature dog breeds. A bilaterally cryptorchid animal is sterile but as the interstitial (Leydig) cells are unaffected by core body temperature, the animal usually has the phenotypic and behavioural characteristics of an entire male. Cryptorchidism has been attributed to abnormal testicular development, failure or abnormal development of the vaginal process, abnormal development of the gubernaculum and hormonal imbalance or deficiency. Whether unilateral or bilateral, cryptorchidism is considered to be an inherited condition. In horses, the mode of inheritance is attributed to a dominant gene, whereas in other species it is probably an autosomal recessive pattern of inheritance. In humans and dogs, there is an increased frequency of neoplastic change in undescended testes, relative to descended testes.

Development of the mammary gland

A definitive characteristic of the class Mammalia, and the one from which this group of animals derives its name, is the presence of mammary glands in the females of all species in the group. These glands have the same basic structure in each of the mammalian subclasses. Mammary glands evolved at a time when increasing parental care of neonatal animals was required to ensure species survival. Milk, the secretion of the mammary glands, is synthesised in specialised epithelial cells, which are organised into small sacs, alveoli. Secretions are released into a duct system, which leads to the surface of the body. Although controversy exists as to the evolutionary origin of mammary glands, existing embryological and comparative anatomical evidence suggests that they evolved from sweat glands.

Monotremes

In the egg-laying monotremes, such as the echidna and the duck-billed platypus, two mammary glands, devoid of teats, are located on the surface of the abdomen. Each gland consists of 100 to 200 separate lobules with lobular duct openings on the skin.

Marsupials

Among marsupials, which are viviparous, a short gestation period of up to four weeks follows implantation. Accordingly, lactation plays an important role in the development and growth of neonatal animals in this group. The mammary glands are usually located close to the pouch or marsupium. From 2 to 25 mammary glands are present in individual marsupial species. The mammary ducts of each gland drain into a single excretory duct which conveys the secretion to a surface teat. The number of teat openings varies with individual species.

Eutheria

Foetal mammals which are sustained by the placenta *in utero* are relatively mature at birth. Although some species, such as guinea-pigs, can survive without milk,

mammary secretions are an important source of nourishment for the newborn of most species. In addition, mammary secretions in the form of colostrum confer passive immunological protection on newborn animals during the first weeks of life.

Development of mammary glands in domestic animals

In higher mammals, the fully functioning mammary gland is a compound tubulo-alveolar structure demarcated by connective tissue into lobes and lobules. In domestic animals, mammary glands arise from two epithelial thickenings on the ventral body wall of the embryo, the mammary lines, which extend from the axillary region to the inguinal region. The number of glands and their location vary with individual species. Among domestic species, dairy cattle occupy a particularly important position as milk-producing animals, a purpose for which they have been selectively bred. Accordingly, the development of the bovine mammary gland will be used to illustrate the sequential stages of differentiation of this secretory organ.

Development of the bovine mammary gland

It is usual to consider mammary gland development in two stages, pre-natal differentiation and post-natal development. In the bovine embryo at approximately 30 days of gestation, the mammary line extends from the forelimb buds to the hindlimb buds. Changes which occur in the epidermis during the development of the mammary line are induced by the underlying mesoderm. That portion of the mammary line caudal to the umbilicus marks the area in which future mammary gland development takes place. Two distinct epidermal thickenings, mammary crests, form on each mammary line and initially appear lenticular in cross-section (Fig. 18.15). With continued epidermal proliferation, the thickenings, which project into the mesenchyme, acquire a semi-lunar appearance and are referred to as mammary buds. The buds are separated from the mesenchyme by well-developed basement membranes. Cellular changes subsequently occur at the centre of the bud. The cells at the periphery become columnar with their long axes pointing towards the centre of the bud, while cells at the central zone are not as densely packed and appear to undergo cornification. During this stage of development, the portions of the mammary line not incorporated into the mammary crests or buds gradually regress. Up to the mammary bud stage, the process of mammary development is similar in male and female embryos. Thereafter, the mammary bud in the female embryo becomes ovoid with its long axis perpendicular to the surface, while in the male embryo it tends to become spherical.

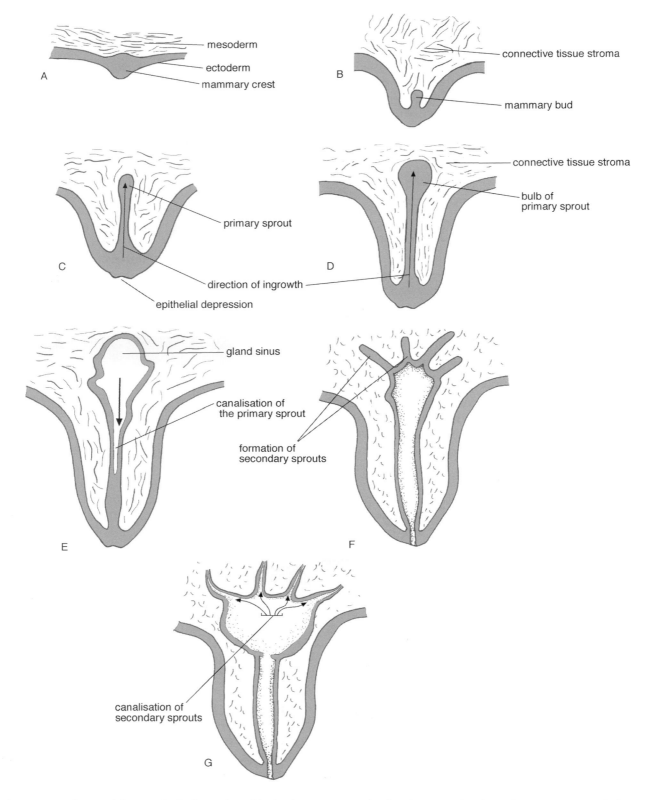

Figure 18.15 Sequential stages in the formation of the bovine mammary gland. A, Cross-section through mammary crest. B, Cross-section through mammary bud as the teat primordium is forming. C and D, Formation of primary sprout. E, Canalisation of primary sprout and formation of gland sinus. F, Formation of secondary sprouts from gland sinus. G, Canalisation of secondary sprouts.

Proliferation of mesenchymal cells surrounding the mammary bud causes outward projection of the tissues forming a conical papilla or primitive teat. The epidermal cells of the bud proliferate and move into the mesenchymal tissue forming a club-shaped structure with the narrower portion pointing towards the tip of the developing teat. This structure is referred to as the primary sprout. The epidermal cells at the apex of the teat become cornified, forming a slight depression at the tip.

At approximately the fourth month of gestation, the primary sprout becomes canalised at its proximal end, forming the gland sinus (gland cistern). As the canalisation continues towards the apex, the teat sinus (teat cistern) and the papillary duct (teat duct) form. The vascular supply, muscle and connective tissue components of the teat wall are of mesenchymal origin. After the fourth month of gestation, eight to 12 secondary sprouts radiate from the gland sinus into the surrounding tissue. When canalised, these secondary sprouts form the lactiferous ducts, which in later development drain the lobes into the gland sinus. Tertiary sprouts arise from the lactiferous ducts which complete the primitive duct system. The rudimentary duct system, which continues to develop until birth, is confined to the body of the gland in the region of the gland sinus.

Differentiation of the body of the bovine mammary gland

The connective tissue support and vascular supply are provided by surrounding mesenchymal cells. Sustained mesenchymal development results in incorporation of the four glands into a distinct anatomical structure referred to as the udder. Spherical masses of mesenchymal cells, which form in the body of the developing gland, differentiate into adipose tissue referred to as fat pads. Adipose tissue formation, which occurs at the base of the developing mammary gland, commences around the 180th day of gestation. The suspensory apparatus of the mammary glands which consists of four sheets of connective tissue, two medial and two lateral, forms from mesenchymal tissue (Fig. 18.16A). The two medial sheets fuse, forming a septum, which divides the udder into left and right sides. The fore and hind mammary glands on either side are not divided by a septum. Hair follicles, which begin to develop around the 120th day of gestation, are confined to the body of the udder and do not cover the teats.

Post-natal development of the bovine mammary gland

Minimal glandular development takes place from birth to puberty. Any increase in size which occurs during this period is attributed to proliferation of connective tissue and fat deposition. With the gradual onset of sexual maturity and release of ovarian hormones, glandular development accelerates. Oestrogens promote development of the duct system while progesterone promotes development of the secretory tissue. Growth hormone and glucocorticoids promote duct development. Under the influence of ovarian and placental hormones, a marked increase in the alveolar tissue of the mammary gland occurs during pregnancy. As alveolar cells replace the adipocytes, the fat depots are replaced by alveolar tissue arranged in a lobular fashion and the amount of alveolar tissue in the gland increases (Fig. 18.16B). Alveolar proliferation, which persists until parturition, may continue into the early stages of lactation. Although bovine mammary glands are capable of secreting milk from the seventh month of pregnancy, it is probable that the high levels of oestrogen and progesterone associated with pregnancy inhibit the action of lactogenic hormones thereby preventing synthesis of milk by the alveolar cells until late in gestation. Due to the removal of this lactogenic inhibition, cows which abort after the seventh month of pregnancy can secrete milk.

Selective breeding of dairy cattle over many decades has resulted in high-yielding animals with greatly enlarged mammary glands. This selective breeding, driven by commercial interests, has given rise to substantial increase in milk yield with enhanced financial return, but has also contributed to a higher incidence of metabolic diseases in such animals and an increased occurrence of mammary infections.

Anomalies in bovine mammary gland development

Polythelia, a condition in which small accessory teats develop as a consequence of additional mammary bud development, sometimes occurs in dairy cattle. These accessory teats, referred to as supernumerary teats, are usually located caudal and dorsal to the normal teats. Although these teats are frequently rudimentary and imperforate, occasionally they are associated with small amounts of glandular tissue which may secrete milk. Congenital absence of one or more mammary glands, amastia, occurs occasionally in domestic animals. Incomplete canalisation of a primary sprout may result in a congenitally imperforate teat. Obstruction of milk flow may occur in the region of the papillary duct or at points between the gland sinus and teat sinus.

Comparative features of mammary gland development in domestic animals

Sheep and goats

The development of mammary glands in sheep and goats is similar to that in cattle. However, in sheep

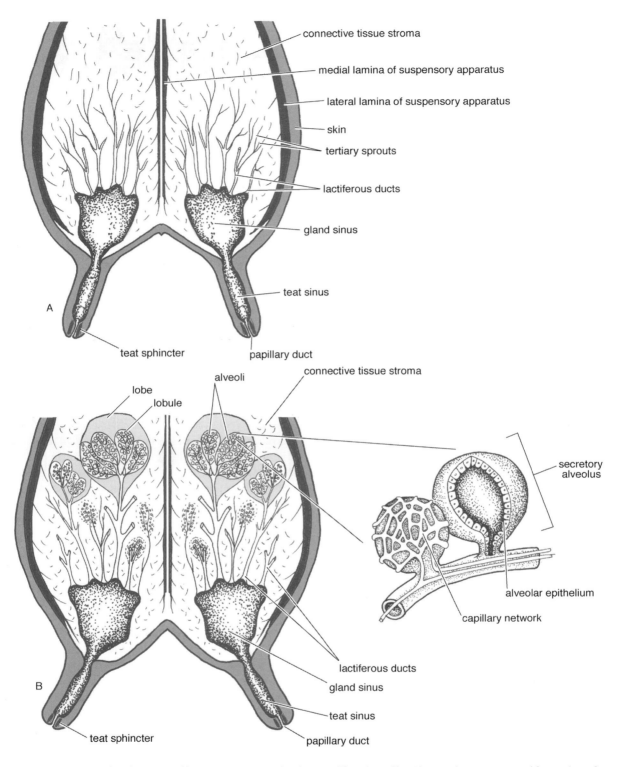

connective tissue stroma

medial lamina of suspensory apparatus

lateral lamina of suspensory apparatus

skin

tertiary sprouts

lactiferous ducts

gland sinus

teat sinus

teat sphincter

papillary duct

alveoli

lobe

lobule

connective tissue stroma

secretory alveolus

alveolar epithelium

capillary network

lactiferous ducts

gland sinus

teat sinus

teat sphincter

papillary duct

Figure 18.16 Post-natal development of bovine mammary gland. A, Proliferation of lactiferous duct system and formation of suspensory apparatus of the mammary gland. B, Formation of alveolar secretory system.

and goats, unlike cattle, only one gland develops on each mammary line and thus the udder is composed of two mammary glands, each with a single papillary duct.

Mares

The udder of the mare consists of two mammary glands located in the inguinal region. The development of the glands in the mare follows a pattern similar to that in ruminants. However, unlike ruminants, two primary sprouts normally develop from each mammary bud in mares. Each sprout, following canalisation, gives rise to a gland and teat sinus and papillary duct. From each primary sprout, a hair follicle and sebaceous gland develop which are associated with the papillary duct.

Sows

The porcine mammary lines extend from the pectoral to the inguinal region. Up to seven mammary buds develop on each line, giving rise to 14 mammary glands. Typically, two glands develop in the thoracic region, three in the abdominal region and two in the inguinal region on each side. Two primary sprouts develop from each bud, giving rise to two to three papillary ducts in each teat, each having its own teat sinus and gland sinus.

Bitches and queens

The mammary lines in bitches and queens extend from the pectoral to the inguinal region. In bitches, two thoracic glands, two abdominal glands and one inguinal gland develop on each side. Queens typically have four mammary glands on each side. In bitches, eight to 14 primary sprouts arise from each mammary bud, each giving rise to a corresponding number of papillary ducts per teat. In queens, in which five to seven primary sprouts arise, a corresponding number of papillary ducts are present in each teat.

Further reading

Baumans, U., Dykstra, G. and Wensing, C.J.G. (1981) Testicular descent in the dog. *Anatomia, histologia, embryologia* **10**, 97–110.

Blackhouse, K.M. and Butler, H. (1960) The gubernaculum testis of the pig. *Journal of Anatomy* **94**, 107–120.

Byskov, A.G. and Hoyer, P.E. (1994) Embryology of mammalian gonads and ducts. In *The Physiology of Reproduction*, 2nd edn. Vol. 2. Eds. E. Knobil and J.D. Neill. Raven Press, New York, pp. 487–540.

Capel, B. (1998) Sex in the 90s: SRY and the switch to the male pathway. *Annual Review of Physiology* **197**, 523.

Edwards, M.J., Smith, M.S.R. and Freeman, B. (2003) Measurement of the linear dynamics of the descent of the bovine fetal testes. *Journal of Anatomy* **203**, 133–142.

Federman, M.D. (2004) Three facets of sexual differentiation. *New England Journal of Medicine* **350**, 323–324.

Graves, J.A. (2001) From brain determination to testes determination: evolution of the mammalian sex-determining gene. *Reproduction Fertility Development* **13**, 665–672.

Hullinger, R.L. and Wensing, C.J.G. (1985) Descent of the testes in the fetal calf. *Acta Anatomica* **121**, 63–68.

Jost, A., Vigier, B. and Prepin, J. (1972) Freemartins in cattle: the first steps of sexual organogenesis. *Journal of Reproduction and Fertility* **29**, 349–379.

Juengel, J.L., Sawyer, H.R., Smith, P.R., Quirke, L.D., Lun, S., Wakefield, S.J. and McNatty, K.P. (2002) Origins of follicular cells and ontogeny of steroidogenesis in ovine foetal ovaries. *Molecular and Cellular Endocrinology* **191**, 1–10.

Kobayashi, A. and Behringer, R. (2003) Developmental genetics of the female reproductive tract in mammals. *Nature Reviews Genetics* **4**, 969–980.

Koopman, P. (1995) The molecular biology of SRY and its role in sex determination in mammals. *Reproduction Fertility Development* **7**, 713–722.

McLaughlin, D.T. and Donahoe, P.K. (2004) Mechanisms of disease, sex determination and differentiation. *New England Journal of Medicine* **350**, 367–378.

Morrish, B.C. and Sinclair, A.H. (2002) Vertebrate sex determination: many ways to an end. *Reproduction* **124**, 447–457.

Pailhoux, B., Mandon-Pepin, B. and Cotinot, P. (2001) Mammalian gonadal differentiation: the pig model. *Reproduction Supplement* **58**, 65–80.

Staack, A., Donjacour, A.A., Brody, J., Cunha, G.R. and Carroll, J. (2003) Mouse urogenital development: a practical approach. *Differentiation* **71**, 402–413.

Turner, C.W. (1952) Development and involutions of the udder of cattle. In *The Mammary Gland. The Anatomy of the Udder of Cattle and Domestic Animals*. Lucas Brothers Publishers, Columbia, MO, pp. 175–219.

Wensing, C.J.G. and Colenbrander, B. (1986) Normal and abnormal testicular descent. In *Oxford Review of Reproductive Biology*, Vol. 8. Clarendon Press, Oxford, pp. 132–164.

19 | Structures in the Head and Neck

From the earliest stages of its formation, the cephalic region of the embryo is associated with the developing nervous, digestive and respiratory systems. One component of the nervous system, the brain, dominates structural development of the head region. Later, elements of the digestive and respiratory tracts contribute to cephalic structural development. A unique feature of the development of the head is that much of the connective tissue and many of the skeletal structures are of neural crest origin. Because of the complexity of cephalic structures, some are dealt with in chapters relating to the special senses and the nervous, cardiovascular, endocrine and respiratory systems. This chapter is concerned with the elements of the digestive and respiratory systems located in the cephalic region and also with the innervation of these particular structures.

Pharyngeal region

A distinguishing feature of the development of the head region of the embryo is the formation of the pharyngeal arches (Fig. 19.1). Development of these structures commences during the fourth week of gestation when

neural crest-derived mesodermal cells migrate into the developing head and neck regions and form discrete aggregations. These aggregations, located between the surface ectoderm and foregut endoderm, give rise to the six pairs of pharyngeal arches. Formation of the mesodermal aggregations results in surface elevations on the lateral aspects of the developing head and neck. The first pair of pharyngeal arches are formed immediately caudal to the oro-pharyngeal membrane.

By the end of the first month of gestation, the first four well-defined pairs of arches, which develop in a cranio-caudal sequence, can be detected on the surface of the developing embryo. The presence of rudimentary fifth and sixth arches is not discernible on the surface. The fifth arch undergoes atrophy, while the sixth arch fuses with the fourth arch, forming a fourth–sixth arch complex. Invaginations of surface ectoderm between adjacent arches are known as pharyngeal grooves or clefts. The endoderm of the lateral wall of the expanding foregut, the primordium of the pharynx, evaginates between the arches forming the pharyngeal pouches. The pouches and clefts establish contact with each other

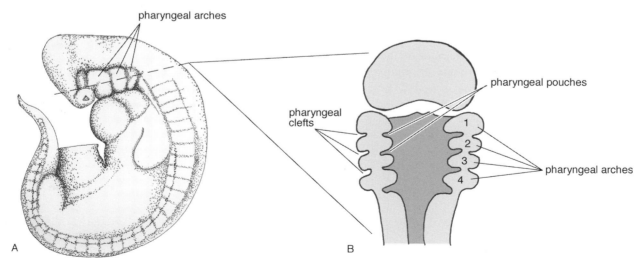

Figure 19.1 Position of pharyngeal arches in a developing mammalian embryo, A, and section through the pharyngeal region showing the pharyngeal arches, pouches and clefts, B.

forming pharyngeal membranes composed of ectoderm and endoderm, the ectodermal component contributed by the clefts and the endodermal component contributed by the pouches. In fish, these membranes break down establishing communication between the oral cavity and the exterior. Because these membranes do not break down in mammals, no communication between the oral cavity and the exterior occurs at these sites. Collectively, the pharyngeal arches, pouches and clefts are referred to as the pharyngeal complex or apparatus.

Associated with each pharyngeal arch are structures which include an aortic arch artery, a muscle component derived from somitomeres and a branch of a cranial nerve which supplies the arch musculature and provides sensory innervation to the epithelia associated with the arch. At this stage of development, the structures in the cranial region of an early mammalian embryo resemble those of a piscine embryo at a comparable stage of development, as each possesses pharyngeal arches, clefts and pouches which have homologous neural and vascular supplies. The term branchial arch is used in fish in preference to pharyngeal arch, which is reserved for terrestrial species. Branchial arches persist as integral structures of fish gills. Towards the end of the embryonic period in mammalian development, the resemblance between the pharyngeal region in fish and mammals is obscured by the remodelling of the various pharyngeal arch derivatives, a necessary step in their evolutionary transition from an aquatic to a terrestrial existence.

Mesoderm of the head is of both paraxial and neural crest origin. The paraxial mesoderm gives rise to whorls of mesodermal cells which form seven paired somitomeres. These somitomeres do not differentiate into classical somites, the origin of sclerotomes and dermomyotomes, but instead form myoblasts which seed the pharyngeal arches and give rise to the musculature of the head. An additional feature of cephalic development is the absence of intermediate and lateral mesoderm.

Derivatives of the pharyngeal apparatus

The pharyngeal apparatus contributes to the formation of the face, nasal cavities, mouth, pharynx, larynx, cervical structures, external and middle ear and elements of the endocrine system.

Pharyngeal arch derivatives

The mesenchyme of the first pair of pharyngeal arches, also referred to as the mandibular arches, gives rise to dorsal maxillary and ventral mandibular prominences. These facial structures grow towards each other and fuse

in the midline enclosing an invagination of ectoderm, the stomodeum. Fusion of the stomodeal ectoderm with the blind end of the foregut gives rise to the oropharyngeal membrane. This membranous structure separates the stomodeum, the primordium of the oral cavity, from the foregut. Later, atrophy of the oropharyngeal membrane establishes an opening between the stomodeum and the pharynx. The mandibular prominences on either side contribute to the formation of the lower jaw while the paired maxillary prominences contribute to the formation of the upper jaw. Initially, a plate of cartilage, referred to as Meckel's cartilage, forms in each mandibular prominence and a cartilaginous core forms in each maxillary prominence. These cartilaginous structures, which initially support the prominences, later atrophy and are replaced by bone formed by intramembranous ossification within the mesenchyme which is of neural crest origin. Derivatives of the pharyngeal apparatus are presented in Table 19.1.

The second or hyoid arch develops a cartilaginous core, referred to as Reichert's cartilage, remnants of which give rise to the stapes. Some bones of the hyoid apparatus derive from mesenchyme of the second pharyngeal arch. Derivatives of the third pharyngeal arch give rise to the other bones of the hyoid apparatus and the stylopharyngeus muscle, a dilator of the pharynx.

Arches four and six, which are less prominent than the preceding arches, merge forming a fourth–sixth complex. These arches give rise to the laryngeal cartilages which surround the developing laryngo-tracheal groove.

Pharyngeal pouch derivatives

The endodermal epithelium of the pharyngeal pouches differentiates into a number of important structures including components of the lymphatic and endocrine system (Table 19.1). Development of the endocrine organs is described in Chapter 20. The first pharyngeal pouches give rise to the auditory tubes and tympanic cavities. In horses, ventral diverticula of the auditory tubes give rise to the guttural pouches.

Pharyngeal clefts

The ectoderm of the first pharyngeal cleft forms the epithelial lining of the external auditory meatus. In mammals, the second arch extends caudally over the second, third and fourth clefts. An ectodermally-lined transient structure, the cervical sinus, is formed by an outgrowth of the second pharyngeal arch which overlies the second and third pharyngeal clefts (Fig. 19.2). Mesenchymal tissue from the first and second arches surrounds the first pharyngeal cleft and proliferates, forming the auricle of the external ear.

Table 19.1 Derivatives of pharyngeal arches, pouches and clefts and their associated cranial nerves.

Pharyngeal arch	Muscles	Bone and cartilage	Other connective tissues	Pouch derivatives	Cleft derivatives	Cranial nerve
First (mandibular)	Muscles of mastication, mylohyoid, rostral belly of digastricus, tensor tympani, tensor veli palatini	Mandible, maxilla, pre-maxilla, zygomatic, auricle of ear, malleus, incus	Ligament of malleus, spheno-mandibular ligament, tympanic membrane (from first pharyngeal membrane)	Auditory tube, guttural pouch	External auditory meatus	Trigeminal (V)
Second (hyoid)	Muscles of facial expression, stapedius, stylohyoid, caudal belly of digastricus	Auricle of ear, stapes, stylohyoid, ceratohyoid, part of basihyoid	Stylohyoid ligament	Palatine tonsils	None	Facial (VII)
Third	Stylopharyngeus	Part of basihyoid bone, thyrohyoid cartilage	None	Parathyroids III, stroma of thymus	None	Glossopharyngeal (IX)
Fourth and sixth	Cricothyroid, levator veli palatini, constrictors of pharynx, intrinsic muscles of larynx	Cricoid, thyroid, arytenoid, corniculate and cuneiform cartilages of larynx.	None	Parathyroids IV, stroma of thymus, ultimobranchial bodies	None	Cranial and recurrent laryngeal branches of vagus (X)

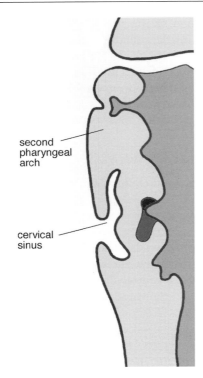

Figure 19.2 Cervical sinus formed by proliferation of the second pharyngeal arch which overgrows the second and third pharyngeal clefts.

Aortic arch artery derivatives

Each pharyngeal arch contains an artery, referred to as an aortic arch artery, which develops from mesoderm within the pharyngeal arch. The arteries form a vascular link between the aortic sac and the paired dorsal aortae. Differentiation of the aortic arch arteries is described in Chapter 11.

Muscles in the head which derive from somitomeres and somites

The muscles which derive from somitomeres include ocular muscles, muscles of mastication and muscles of facial expression. The constrictor muscles of the pharynx and extrinsic lingual muscles derive from somites one to five. Table 19.2 summarises the origin and innervation of muscles relating to the eye, muscles involved in mastication and facial expression and muscles relating to the pharynx and tongue.

Face

Development of the face, which includes the orbital, nasal and oral regions, involves the formation, fusion and patterning of five facial primordia during the embryonic period of development. These primordia, which result from proliferation of underlying neural crest-derived mesenchyme, include the single fronto-nasal prominence and the paired maxillary and mandibular prominences (Fig. 19.3). The paired maxillary prominences merge with the fronto-nasal prominence dorsal to the stomodeum, while the paired mandibular prominences merge ventral to the stomodeum. The fronto-nasal prominence, which develops in the region of the telencephalic bulges, forms two sets of bilateral ectodermal thickenings, the nasal and lens placodes. The nasal

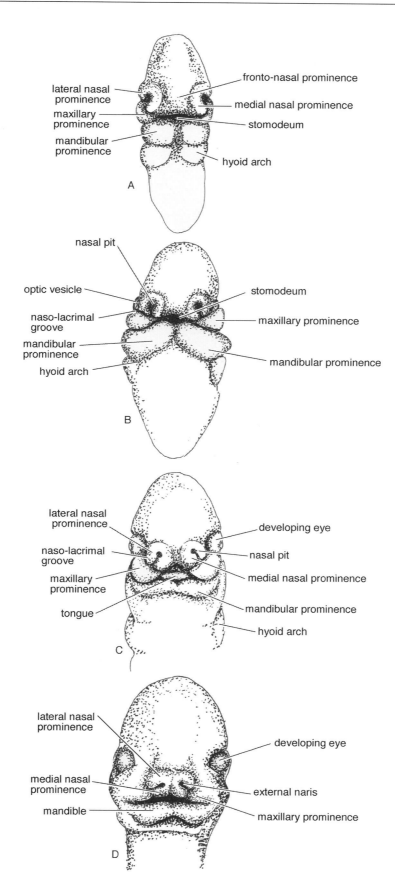

Figure 19.3 Sequential stages in the development of the porcine face.

Table 19.2 Muscles in the head region which derive from somitomeres and somites and their innervation.

Somitomeres or somites	Muscles	Cranial nerve innervation
Somitomeres 1 and 2	Dorsal, medial and ventral rectus muscles of eye	Oculomotor (cranial nerve III)
Somitomere 3	Dorsal oblique ocular muscle	Trochlear (cranial nerve IV)
Somitomere 4	Muscles of mastication	Trigeminal (cranial nerve V)
Somitomere 5	Lateral rectus and retractor bulbi muscles of eye	Abducens (cranial nerve VI)
Somitomere 6	Muscles of facial expression, caudal portion of digastricus	Facial (cranial nerve VII)
Somitomere 7	Stylopharyngeal muscle	Glossopharyngeal (cranial nerve IX)
Somites 1 and 2	Pharyngeal constrictor muscles	Vagus (cranial nerve X)
Somites 2 to 5	Extrinsic lingual muscles	Hypoglossal (cranial nerve XII)

placodes, the primordia of the nasal cavities, develop medially on the fronto-nasal prominence as oval swellings and are located dorsal to the maxillary prominences of the first pharyngeal arches. Lens placodes, which develop before the formation of the nasal placodes, are positioned lateral to the fronto-nasal primordia. Mesenchymal proliferations at the margins of the nasal placodes result in horseshoe-shaped medial and lateral nasal prominences. The nasal placodes occupy depressions, which, by a process of invagination, deepen, forming the nasal pits.

The major stages of facial development occur by growth and cytodifferentiation of the facial prominences and by fusion of segments of the prominences during the late embryonic period. The maxillary prominences increase in size and extend medially, fusing with the medial nasal prominences and forming the maxilla and incisive bones of the upper jaw and also the tissues of the upper lip. The final structural appearance of the upper lip is influenced by the form and extent of fusion of the maxillary and nasal prominences. In carnivores, sheep and goats, the line of fusion is marked by a medial groove, the philtrum. A well-defined plate or muzzle separates the nasal openings in horses and cattle. The mandibular prominences fuse, forming the lower jaw.

In the early stages of facial development, the maxillary and nasal prominences are separated by a deep naso-lacrimal groove which extends towards the nasal can-

thus of the developing eye. The ectoderm in the floor of the groove forms a solid cord of cells, which invaginates deeply into the underlying mesenchyme and loses its connection with the surface ectoderm. This solid cord of cells undergoes canalisation and forms the naso-lacrimal duct. The shape of the face in domestic animals varies not only between species but also within species. Large domestic animals have relatively long faces and elongated skulls referred to as dolicocephalic skulls. In contrast, primates have short faces and short or brachycephalic skulls. The skulls of dogs may be dolico-cephalic or brachycephalic, or have a shape intermediate between these two forms, termed mesocephalic.

Nasal cavities

The nasal pits, surrounded by the medial and lateral prominences, gradually invaginate into the underlying mesoderm of the fronto-nasal prominence at a position between the developing forebrain and the developing mouth. As the nasal pits deepen, they form nasal sacs. At first, the left and right nasal sacs are distinct structures separated from each other by a septum and separated from the oral cavity by a thin oro-nasal membrane which forms the primary palate (Fig. 19.4). Gradually, the caudal portion of the partition between the left and right medial walls of the primitive nasal sacs atrophies forming a common nasal cavity and, in addition, the caudal portion of the primary palate atrophies. The most rostral portion of the primary palate forms the maxillary process.

With the atrophy of the caudal portion of the septum between the left and right nasal sacs and of the caudal portion of the primary palate, there is direct communication between the caudal end of the nasal cavity and the oral cavity through an opening referred to as the choana. Later, processes referred to as the palatine processes grow ventrally from the lateral walls of the nasal cavity (Fig. 19.5). At this stage, the developing tongue not only fills the entire oral cavity but also projects into the nasal cavity. With the increase in growth and expansion of the oral cavity, the tongue no longer projects into the nasal cavity. Withdrawal of the tongue from the nasal cavity allows medial expansion of the palatine processes which meet and fuse in the midline, establishing a partition referred to as the secondary palate, between the oral and nasal cavities. The rostral area of the secondary palate fuses with the maxillary process (Fig. 19.6). Associated with the formation of the palatine processes, a nasal septum develops and grows ventrally from the dorsal wall of the nasal cavity. Fusion of the nasal septum with the secondary palate divides the common nasal cavity into left and right nasal cavities. At the site of fusion of the maxillary process with the secondary palate, small areas which fail to fuse form spaces in the palate between the mouth and nasal

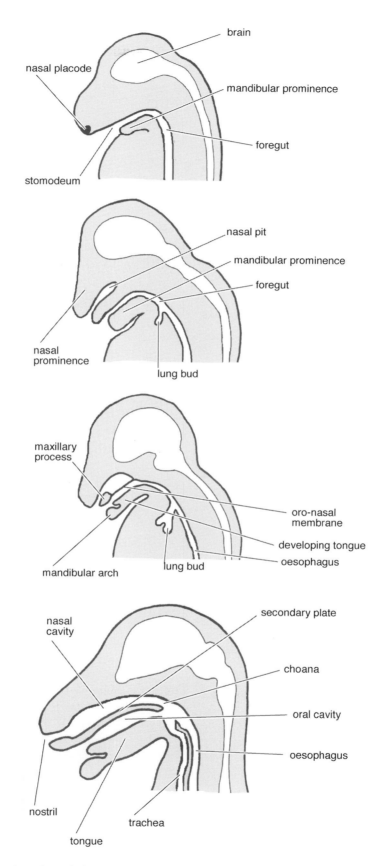

Figure 19.4 Longitudinal sections through the cranial regions of developing embryos at the level of the nasal pit showing progressive development of the nasal and oral cavities.

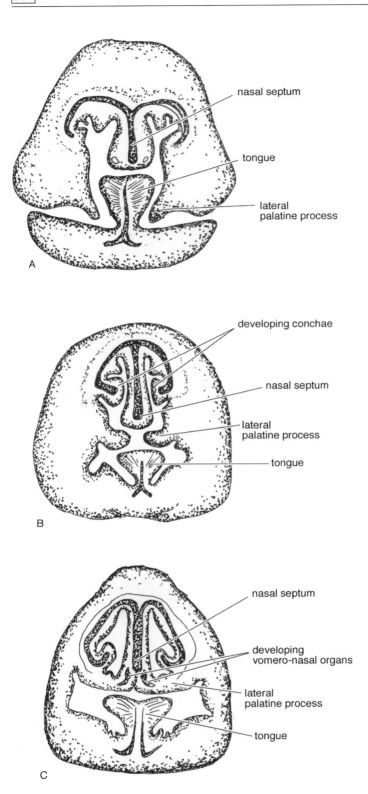

Figure 19.5 Cross-sections through the developing nasal and oral cavities in the pig showing the formation of the secondary palate, nasal septum and conchae.

cavities, the incisive foramina, through which the incisive ducts convey small amounts of fluid from the oral cavity to the vomeronasal organ and to the olfactory epithelium. Formation of the secondary palate does not completely separate the oral and nasal cavities. Caudally-located openings between the nasal cavities and the pharynx, the definitive choanae or posterior nares,

remain. The extent of fusion between the nasal septum and the secondary palate influences the form of communication between the pharynx and the nasal cavities. In horses, the nasal septum fuses with the secondary palate throughout its length so that each nasal cavity communicates with the pharynx by a separate opening. In the other domestic animals, the fusion of the nasal septum

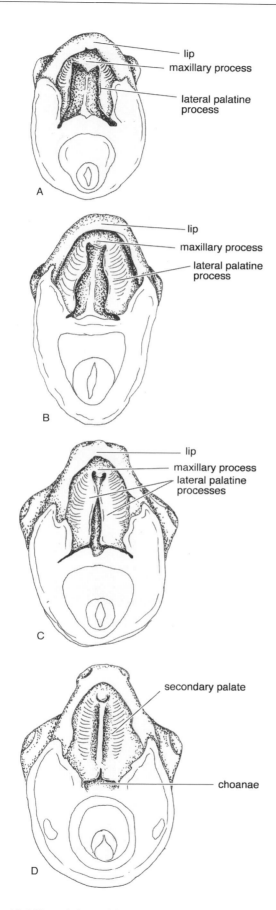

lip
maxillary process
lateral palatine process

A

lip
maxillary process
lateral palatine process

B

lip
maxillary process
lateral palatine processes

C

secondary palate

choanae

D

Figure 19.6 Ventral views of the developing porcine palatine processes showing progressive formation of the secondary palate.

with the secondary palate does not extend to the caudal end of the secondary palate and both nasal cavities share a common opening to the nasopharynx. The secondary palate is initially a membranous structure. Later, bone develops by intramembranous ossification in the rostral two-thirds, forming the hard palate, while the portion which projects into the pharynx, dividing it into oral and nasal spaces, remains membranous, forming the soft palate. In domestic animals, the hard palate, which forms the roof of the oral cavity, develops convex ridges or rugae. The convexity of these ridges, which project rostrally, may assist in the guidance of food caudally to the pharynx. The soft palate is long in domestic animals, especially in horses, a consequence of the dolicocephalic nature of their facial structures. In brachycephalic animals there is a tendency for the long soft palate to intermittently obstruct the entrance to the larynx causing periodic respiratory distress.

Conchae

Longitudinal laminae, which arise from the lateral walls of the nasal cavities, form shelf-like projections into these passageways. Later, when these laminae adapt a scroll-like conformation, they are referred to as conchae. The laminae consist of a core of mesoderm covered by an ectodermal lining. Gradually, a thin layer of endochondral bone develops in the original mesodermal core. The thin scroll-like bones formed in this manner are referred to as the turbinate bones. A dorsal and a ventral concha develop from the lateral wall of the nasal cavity, dividing the original large single nasal passageway into three narrow passageways, each referred to as a meatus (Fig. 19.7). A dorsal meatus, which is formed between the roof of the nasal cavity and the dorsal concha, leads into the caudal region of the nasal cavity. The middle meatus, which is formed between the dorsal and ventral conchae, also leads into the caudal region of the nasal cavity. The ventral nasal meatus, positioned between the middle meatus and the floor of the nasal cavity, is the largest meatus and leads into the nasopharynx through a choana. For clinical purposes, a nasogastric tube is passed along this meatus through the nasopharynx into the oesophagus. Smaller conchae, which arise from the tissue of the developing ethmoid bones of the skull, form the ethmoidal conchae.

With the exception of an area of the lateral walls of the nasal cavities and the ethmoidal conchae, which are covered by olfactory epithelium, the original ectodermal cells lining the developing nasal cavities give rise to pseudostratified ciliated columnar epithelium. The pseudostratified columnar olfactory epithelium contains sensory bipolar neurons, the dendrites of which extend to the epithelial surface. The axons of the bipolar neurons pass into the lamina propria forming non-myelinated

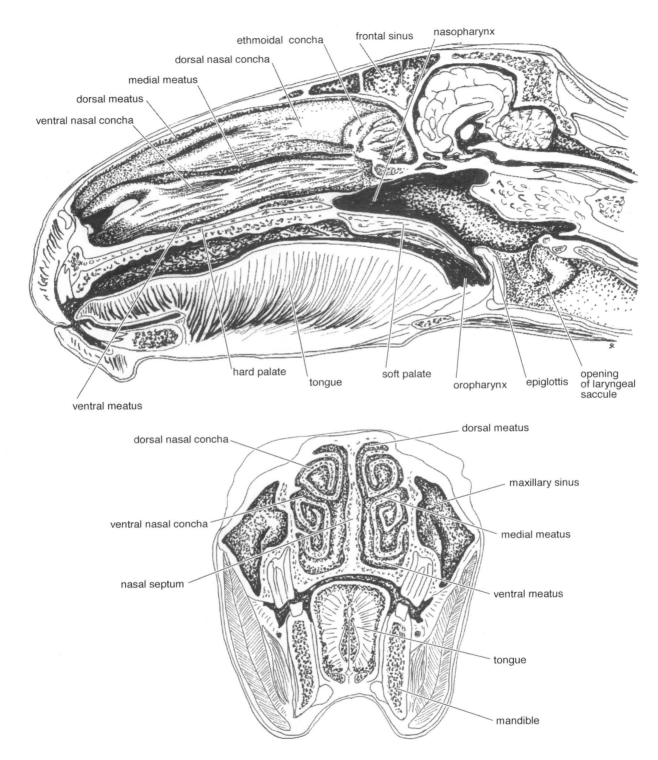

Figure 19.7 Longitudinal section through the equine head and cross-section through the fully-formed nasal and oral cavities showing prominent structures in this region.

bundles. These bundles converge giving rise to the first cranial nerve, the olfactory nerve. Glands which develop from the epithelium grow into the underlying lamina propria–submucosa of the olfactory mucosa. Through their secretions, these glands add moisture to the inhaled air post-natally. The mucosa of this olfactory region is highly vascular. The size and shape of the nasal

conchae, which vary greatly within and between species, are also influenced by age.

Vomeronasal organ

Lateral to the nasal septum, left and right vomeronasal organs develop in the floor of the rostral region of the nasal cavities. These organs, which arise as tube-like invaginations into the developing hard palate, contain elements of both respiratory and olfactory epithelium. The caudal ends of the tube-like organs are blind while the cranial ends open rostrally into the incisive ducts. In all domestic animals, with the exception of horses, the incisive ducts connect the nasal cavity with the oral cavity.

Paranasal sinuses

Epithelium which lines the nasal cavities invaginates into particular bones of the skull and contributes to the formation of paranasal sinuses. The epithelial invaginations extend into the diploë, the space occupied by spongy bone between internal and external compact laminae of flat bones. These epithelial ingrowths form cavitations which expand and gradually encroach into the diploë until the internal region of the bone is an air-filled space lined by respiratory epithelium. In domestic animals, the paranasal sinuses, which include the frontal, maxillary, palatine, sphenoidal and lacrimal sinuses, retain their connection with the nasal cavities (Fig. 19.7). Because they are prone to infection, the frontal and maxillary sinuses in domestic animals are of clinical importance. Apart from the frontal and maxillary sinuses which are present in all domestic mammals, species variation relating to the presence or absence of other paranasal sinuses is observed. At birth, the paranasal sinuses are poorly developed and most of their development takes place post-natally. Because the frontal sinuses in ruminants and pigs extend throughout the frontal bones, they overlie the cranium. The frontal sinuses of horned ruminants extend into the horn cores.

Oral cavity

The oral cavity develops initially from the stomodeum. However, with atrophy of the oro-pharyngeal membrane a portion of the foregut contributes to the formation of the oral cavity. Structures associated with the rostral region of the stomodeum are lined by ectoderm. Thus, the epithelium of the rostral portion of the tongue and the vestibule are ectodermal in origin. Although the exact demarcation between ectodermally-derived and endodermally-derived epithelium is not obvious in the fully-formed oral cavity, the derivatives of these embryonic tissues can be identified.

Up to the end of the embryonic period, the prominences from which the maxilla and mandible arise are masses of undifferentiated tissue. A thickened band of ectoderm on the occlusal surfaces of the developing jaws forms labio-gingival laminae on each developing jaw. These laminae, which follow the jaw contours, form deep plates. Gradual disintegration of the more central cells of the plate forms the labio-gingival groove which

divides each plate into two, giving rise to the primordia of the lips and gums. An epithelial thickening on the lingual surface of the gums gives rise to the dental lamina. The labio-gingival groove in both the upper and lower jaws deepens, forming the vestibule. Cheeks, the structures which form the lateral walls of the oral cavity, arise from the progressive fusion of the maxillary and mandibular prominences. In association with the lips, the cheeks define the limits of the opening into the oral cavity.

Tongue

During the fourth week of gestation in domestic animals, the tongue develops from the floor of the primordial pharynx. Due to the proliferation of the underlying mesoderm, three elevations occur at the level of the first pharyngeal arch, which give rise to two lateral lingual swellings and a medial lingual swelling, the tuberculum impar (Fig. 19.8). In the region of the second pharyngeal arch, an elevation referred to as the copula develops, while an additional swelling, the hypopharyngeal eminence, forms in a medial position in the region of the third and fourth arches. The two lateral lingual swellings extend toward the midline and fuse with the medial swelling, forming the rostral two-thirds or body of the tongue. In humans and carnivores, the medial lingual swelling contributes minimally to tongue development. However, in ungulates, the medial lingual swelling is considered to make a significant contribution to the dorsal prominence of the body of the tongue. In cattle, the dorsal prominence, which is especially large, is called the torus linguae. The line of fusion of the lateral lingual swellings can be recognised on the surface of the tongue in humans and carnivores by a medial groove. The caudal third or root of the tongue forms by the gradual proliferation of the hypopharyngeal swelling over the copula, a structure which subsequently atrophies. The epithelium covering the rostral two-thirds of the tongue is of ectodermal origin while that of the caudal third is endodermally derived. Towards the end of the embryonic period, lingual papillae develop on the surface of the tongue. Filiform papillae arise from slender outgrowths of proliferating epithelium induced by the underlying mesoderm. These papillae contain nerve endings which are sensitive to mechanical pressure. Vallate papillae develop by differential epithelial proliferation at the boundary between the body and root of the tongue. Their characteristic morphology includes a deep groove around their circular base. Epithelial foldings on the lateral aspect of the root of the tongue form foliate papillae. In ruminants, foliate papillae are not formed. Taste bud development is promoted by the interaction between the epithelial cells of the papillae and the gustatory neurons of cranial nerves VII, IX and X. Taste buds are associated with both vallate and foliate papillae.

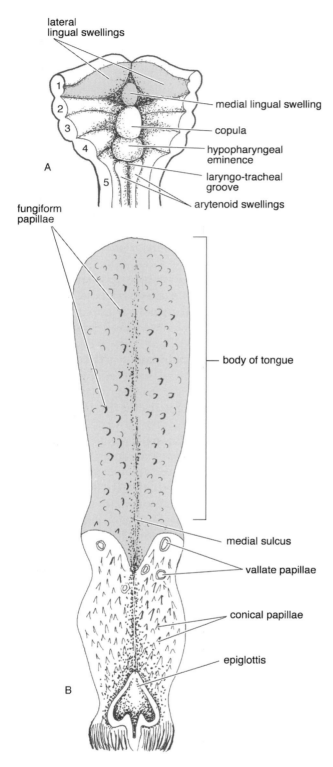

Figure 19.8 A, Early stage in the development of the canine tongue, showing the major structures which contribute to its formation and some associated structures. B, Fully-formed canine tongue.

The musculature of the tongue derives from myoblasts which migrate from the occipital myotomes. The connective tissue and vasculature of the tongue are formed from pharyngeal mesenchyme. As the epithelium of the

rostral two-thirds of the tongue covers the mandibular arch, its somatic sensory innervation is from the mandibular branch of cranial nerve V. The epithelium of the caudal third of the tongue derives from the third pharyngeal arch, and its sensory somatic innervation is from cranial nerve IX. The rostral two-thirds of the tongue receives its visceral taste sensation from the chorda tympani branch of cranial nerve VII. The caudal third receives its gustatory innervation from cranial nerve IX. Myoblasts, which migrate from the occipital somites innervated by cranial nerve XII, form the extrinsic lingual muscles. Consequently, the extrinsic muscles of the tongue are innervated by cranial nerve XII. Initially, the root of the tongue grows faster than the body of the tongue. As the oral cavity enlarges, the body of the tongue also enlarges and extends rostrally, filling the oral cavity.

Salivary glands

The salivary glands develop as solid ingrowths of the epithelium in the oral cavity during the later stages of embryonic development. The club-shaped epithelial buds grow into the underlying mesenchyme where they branch and sub-branch with their terminal branches forming secretory units or alveoli. The ducts and glandular tissue are derived from the oral epithelium while the connective tissue stroma and capsule of the gland are of neural crest-derived mesenchymal origin. Due to the loss of tissue demarcation following breakdown of the oro-pharyngeal membrane and the pattern of growth leading to the formation of the oral cavity, it is difficult to establish with certainty whether the epithelial ingrowths which give rise to the salivary glands are endodermal or ectodermal in origin. However, the position of the openings of salivary gland ducts in the newborn is considered to represent the site of the original epithelial ingrowth in the embryo.

The paired parotid, mandibular and sublingual glands are the major salivary glands in domestic mammals. The parotid gland arises from ingrowths of epithelium, probably ectodermal in origin, in the labio-gingival groove. The duct of the canine parotid gland opens into the vestibule of the mouth at the level of the fourth upper cheek tooth. The mandibular gland arises from an epithelial groove located near the ventral surface of the linguo-gingival space. The edges of the caudal end of the groove fuse, forming a solid cord which becomes detached from the surface. This cord extends caudally into the mesenchyme around the developing mandible, where it branches, forming the primordium of the gland. The other end of the groove closes and extends rostrally where it opens beneath the tongue. The epithelium of the ducts and parenchyma of the mandibular gland is considered to be endodermal in origin. The sublingual gland and its ducts are also considered to be of endodermal origin. The duct of the sublingual gland is located rostrally on the lower jaw near the frenulum of the tongue. Based on its mode of formation as already described, the sublingual gland, in common with the parotid and mandibular salivary glands, has only one excretory duct opening and, accordingly, is referred to as a monostomatic gland. In some species, sublingual salivary glands develop with multiple duct openings and are referred to as polystomatic glands. Up to ten small independent epithelial ingrowths from the linguo-labial groove give rise to polystomatic sublingual salivary glands. The secretory tissue of these separate glands coalesces forming a defined gland within a connective tissue capsule with the individual ducts opening into the oral cavity. Polystomatic sublingual salivary glands are considered to be endodermal in origin. Both monostomatic and polystomatic sublingual salivary glands are present in most domestic animals. In horses, however, only polystomatic sublingual salivary glands develop.

Clusters of oral epithelial ingrowths give rise to a number of diffuse salivary glands which open into the oral cavity. These glands, which are usually named according to their location, include labial, buccal, lingual, palatine and pharyngeal salivary glands. In carnivores, the dorsal buccal salivary glands become organised into compact salivary glands referred to as the zygomatic glands.

Teeth

Although there is considerable variation in the morphology and number of teeth present in mammals, all teeth have the same basic structure consisting of enamel, dentin and cementum. Because most mammals, including domestic mammals, have two forms of dentition, deciduous teeth and permanent teeth, they are described as diphyodonts. Deciduous teeth, which are fewer in number than permanent teeth, are formed early in development and, post-natally, they are replaced by permanent teeth at particular time intervals.

Based on their morphology, function and location in the jaws, the teeth of mammals are classified as incisor, canine, premolar and molar. Individual teeth may also be classified as either brachyodont or hypsodont. A brachyodont tooth consists of a crown, the free portion of the tooth which projects above the gum, a root, the embedded portion in the jaw, and a constricted neck at the gum line between the crown and the root. Hypsodont teeth have a body and a root. The body has a portion which protrudes above the gum and an embedded portion which is long in young animals. As animals age and the occlusal surface of the tooth wears, the embedded portion of the tooth moves towards the

surface of the gum and becomes progressively shorter. The roots of hypsodont teeth are short.

Development of a brachyodont tooth

The morphogenic and inductive processes in tooth development in mammals follow similar general developmental stages irrespective of the type of tooth or the species of animal. Teeth develop following interaction between the ectoderm of the dental lamina and the underlying neural crest-derived mesenchyme (Fig. 19.9). Ectodermal proliferations along the length of the dental lamina give rise to dental buds which project into the mesenchyme. The buds represent the ectodermal primordia of individual teeth and their number corresponds to the number of deciduous teeth for a given species. As the dental buds extend into the mesenchyme, they become cap-shaped and consist of an inner and outer layer of epithelial cells with a layer of loose reticular cells, the stellate reticulum, interposed between them. The mesenchyme beneath the concavity of the dental cap forms the dental papilla, the mesenchymal component of the developing tooth. As the dental cap grows deeper into the mesenchyme of the jaw, it acquires a bell-shaped appearance and remains connected to the oral epithelium by a cord of cells from the dental lamina. Buds of permanent teeth, which arise as outgrowths of these cords of cells, remain dormant until the commencement of permanent tooth development. Due to atrophy of the cords of cells, the connection between the surface epithelium and the bell-shaped component of the developing tooth, usually referred to as the enamel organ, gradually breaks down.

Because of the inductive influence of cells in the underlying reticular layer, the epithelial cells of the inner layer of the enamel organ elongate and differentiate into ameloblasts which are responsible for the production of enamel. One of the hardest substances in the body, enamel is composed of crystals of hydroxyapatite and has a low protein content. With the development of ameloblasts, the underlying mesenchymal cells of the dental papilla are induced to differentiate into tall columnar cells which form odontoblasts.

Under the inductive influence of the dental papilla, a small group of ectodermal cells of the inner epithelial layer of the enamel organ, located at the apex of the dental papilla, cease to divide and form a clump of cells referred to as the enamel knot. The cells of the enamel knot act as a signalling centre which regulates the shape of the developing tooth and specifies the site of cusp formation. With molar teeth, which may have a number of cusps, secondary enamel knots give rise to additional cusps. The ameloblasts first develop at the tip of the dental papilla and gradually extend to the sides and base of

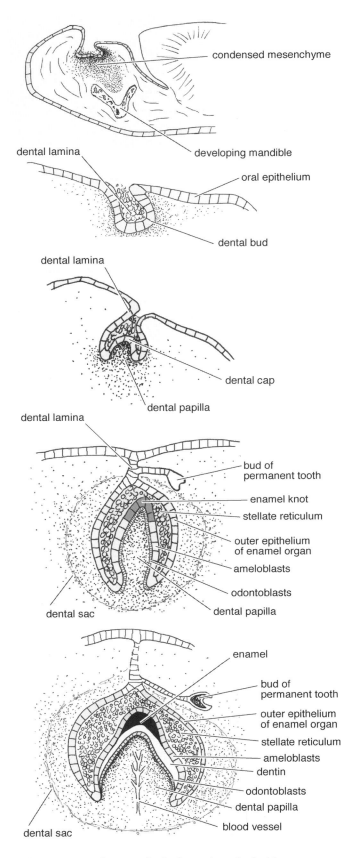

Figure 19.9 Early stages in the formation of a deciduous brachyodont tooth, showing the development of the dental bud, dental cap and dental papilla, and formation of the dental crown.

the developing crown. Associated with this change, odontoblasts form predentin at the tip of the papilla. Subsequently, with the deposition of crystals of hydroxyapatite and fluoroapatite, the matrix of the predentin becomes mineralised forming dentin. The core of the dental papilla gives rise to the pulp cavity of the tooth. Under the inductive influence of dentin, ameloblasts at the tip of the papilla produce enamel. Odontoblasts and ameloblasts move away from the dentin and enamel which they produce. Ameloblasts move towards the tooth surface while odontoblasts migrate into the pulp cavity. Unlike bone formation where the osteoblasts become trapped within the matrix becoming osteocytes, odontoblasts and ameloblasts do not become encased within the matrix which they produce, but remain on its surface. As dentin and enamel are formed, the shape of the tooth crown becomes established with development proceeding from the apex to the base of the enamel organ. The base of the enamel organ demarcates the junction between the crown and the root of the tooth. The inner and outer epithelial layers of the bell-shaped enamel organ which are in direct contact at the rim of the base, proliferate and extend into the underlying mesenchyme forming a tube-like structure, referred to as the epithelial root sheath (Fig. 19.10). This sheath contributes to root formation by inducing the mesenchymal cells of the dental papilla to develop into odontoblasts and form dentin. This dentin is continuous with the dentin produced by the odontoblasts during the formation of the crown. Due to the absence of the reticular layer, ameloblast differentiation does not occur during root formation. The root, therefore, is not covered by an enamel layer. As the increase in dentin production continues, the pulp cavity is gradually reduced in size to a narrow root canal. The root sheath slowly becomes detached from the developing root, and epithelial remnants which remain may give rise to a dental cyst at a later stage in development.

During the bell-shaped stage of development, the mesenchyme surrounding the developing tooth condenses, forming a vascular mesenchymal layer, the dental sac. The inner layer of cells of the dental sac, adjacent to the developing root, differentiate into cementoblasts which produce the bone-like connective tissue, cementum, covering the root of the tooth. Like developing osteoblasts, cementoblasts entrapped within their matrix become cementocytes. From the mesenchyme in the outer layer of the dental sac, osteoblasts arise. These osteogenic cells give rise to bone which forms the dental alveoli, structures which anchor the teeth in the jaws. Mesenchyme of the middle layer of the dental sac gives rise to tough collagenous fibres, the periodontal ligament, which becomes anchored to the bone of the alveolus and in the cementum covering the root. The periodontal ligament, which allows a slight degree of tooth movement

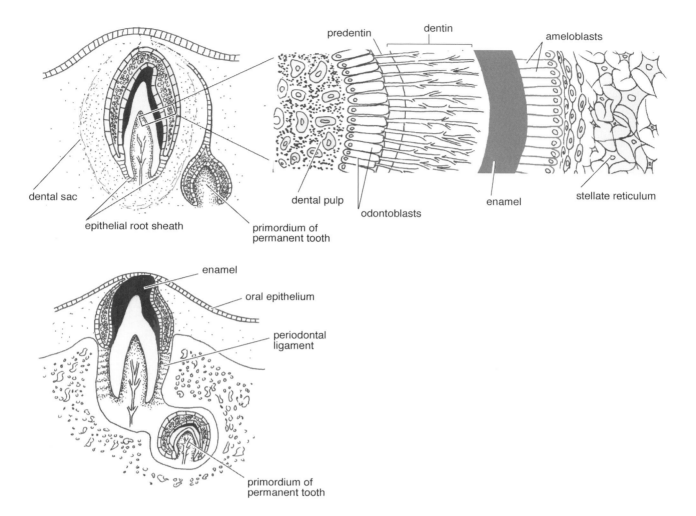

Figure 19.10 Final stage in the development of a deciduous brachyodont tooth, showing the structures which contribute to its formation.

within its alveolus, also functions as a shock-absorbing mechanism.

Although eruption of teeth through the gums occurs in association with root development, the factors which control this process are not known. As teeth develop, they grow towards the surface and the crown gradually erupts through the oral epithelium. Enamel production ceases when the crown of the tooth is formed and subsequently, the remnants of the enamel organ are shed. Odontoblasts, however, continue to produce dentin throughout the life of the tooth and, if damaged, enamel is replaced by dentin.

Permanent teeth develop in a manner similar to deciduous teeth. As permanent teeth grow, the roots of the deciduous teeth are resorbed, their attachment is loosened and they are shed.

Development of a hypsodont tooth

The development of hypsodont teeth is similar in most respects to that described for brachyodont teeth.

However, due to their morphological and functional characteristics, there are a number of obvious differences between these two types of teeth. A basic difference which distinguishes a hypsodont tooth from a brachyodont tooth is that the enamel organ is longer in the former and may exhibit foldings on its occlusal surface. In addition, folding of the enamel organ of a hypsodont tooth results in the formation of vertical ridges on its lateral and medial surfaces. Eruption, which is a slow process, occurs before root formation is complete. During formation, a hypsodont tooth is surrounded by a dental sac for a longer time than a brachyodont tooth. Accordingly, the enamel layer of a hypsodont tooth becomes coated with cementum.

Comparative aspects of dentition

Comparative features of an equine hypsodont incisor tooth and a canine brachyodont incisor tooth are illustrated in Fig. 19.11. The teeth of humans and carnivores are all brachyodont teeth. Apart from their canine teeth which are hypsodont, all porcine teeth are brachyodont in nature. Ruminant incisor teeth, which are present in

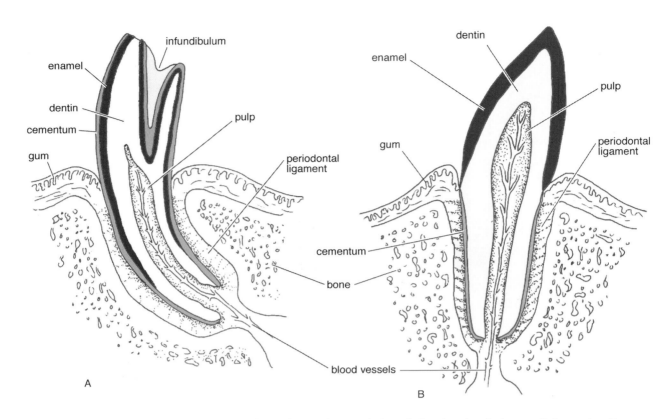

Figure 19.11 Comparative features of an equine hypsodont incisor tooth, A, and a brachyodont incisor tooth from a dog, B.

the lower jaw only, are brachyodont; their cheek teeth are hypsodont. The region occupied in other species by the upper incisor teeth is covered by a fibrous dental pad in ruminants. It is usual to describe teeth numbers in individual species by a dental formula which specifies the number of each type of tooth in the upper jaw and in the lower jaw.

Molecular aspects of tooth development

The arrangement of mammalian teeth, which are distributed along the parabolic curves of the jaw, is partly determined by a range of homeodomain-containing gene families including Dlx, Lhx and Gsc. A number of morphogenic signalling molecules including Shh, Fgf, Bmp and Wnt also play a role in the formation of teeth. Variations in the timing and intensity of these signalling molecules contribute to differences in the size and form of individual teeth. Signals from early epithelium, such as Fgf-8 and Bmp-4, regulate the expression of mesenchymal transcription factors such as Msx-1 and Msx-2, Dlx-1 and Dlx-2 and Gli-2 and Gli-3. It has been proposed that these transcription factors regulate signals which stimulate formation of the dental buds.

The dental bud functions as a transient epithelial centre which expresses a range of signalling molecules such as Bmp-2 and Bmp-4, Fgf-8, Shh, Wnt-10b, Msx-2, Lef-1 and P-21. Experimental evidence suggests that the

signalling molecules expressed in the dental bud are highly conserved across species. Signals from the epithelial cells induce the condensation of mesenchymal cells around the bud. Once the epithelial dental bud has reached its full size, a new signalling centre which regulates tooth morphology becomes established in the enamel knot. A number of signalling molecules including Shh, Edar, Msx-2, Lef-1, P-21 and members of the Fgf, Bmp and Wnt families of signalling molecules, are expressed locally in the enamel knot.

Development of the skull

The bones of the skull develop from mesenchyme which surrounds the developing brain. The skull may be considered as consisting of two major subdivisions, the neuro-cranium which surrounds the brain, and the viscero-cranium which constitutes supportive structural components of the oral cavity, pharynx and upper respiratory system. The neuro-cranium and viscero-cranium are composed of bones which develop by endochondral ossification and by intramembranous ossification from mesenchyme derived from neural crest cells and axial mesoderm.

Membranous neuro-cranium

Intramembranous ossification centres develop in the mesenchyme surrounding the dorsal surface and sides of the developing brain, giving rise to the primordia of the paired parietal and frontal bones and to the interparietal part of the occipital bone. During foetal life, these flat bones, which are separated by dense connective tissue, form fibrous joints referred to as sutures. Where more than two bones meet, the sutures are referred to as fontanelles. Both during foetal life and post-natal development, the bones formed by intramembranous ossification increase in size by appositional growth and the amount of connective tissue between them decreases.

Cartilaginous neuro-cranium

Initially, the cartilaginous neuro-cranium consists of a number of separate components which later fuse, forming the cartilaginous base of the developing skull. The neuro-cranium also contributes to the formation of the capsular structures which support the olfactory organs, eyes and inner ears. The cartilaginous neuro-cranium includes the paired parachordal, hypophyseal and prechordal cartilages (Fig. 19.12). The cartilaginous templates of the occipital, sphenoid, temporal and ethmoid bones develop from the cartilaginous base of the neuro-cranium, formed by fusion of individual cartilages. Later in development, the cartilaginous templates of these bones undergo endochondral ossification.

Membranous viscero-cranium

Intramembranous ossification centres which develop in the maxillary prominences of the first pharyngeal arches give rise to the squamous, frontal, maxillary and zygomatic bones. The squamous and frontal bones also contribute to the formation of the neuro-cranium.

Mesoderm of the mandibular prominence which surrounds Meckel's cartilage undergoes intramembranous ossification, forming the mandible.

Cartilaginous viscero-cranium

The viscero-cranial elements of the skull are derived from the cartilaginous templates of the paired mandibular and hyoid pharyngeal arches. The dorsal region of Meckel's cartilage gives rise to the malleus and incus, ossicles of the middle ear, while the stapes of the middle ear, together with the styloid process of the temporal bone, develop from the hyoid arch (Table 19.1).

Congenital malformations of face and oral cavity

Cleft lip and palate

Clefts in the face and palate arise from disturbances in the developmental processes which lead to the formation of the jaws and face. Both of these conditions are rare in domestic animals with a slightly higher incidence of palatine than labial anomalies. Cleft lip results from the failure of fusion between the maxillary and medial nasal prominences. This condition, which may be unilateral or bilateral, complete or incomplete, is often associated with cleft palate. Medial cleft lip, which is very rare, results from incomplete merging in the midline of the two medial nasal prominences.

Cleft palate can be classified as primary or secondary. Primary cleft palate is due to incomplete fusion of the fronto-nasal prominence with the maxillary prominences.

Figure 19.12 Dorsal view of the cartilages from which bones of the cranium derive by endochondral ossification.

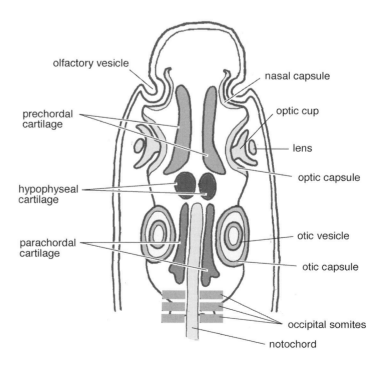

Secondary cleft palate results from incomplete fusion or failure of fusion between the lateral palatine processes, resulting in an opening between the nasal and oral cavities. These anomalies, which are considered to be multifactorial in origin, are often associated with developmental defects in other organs. Clinical signs include difficulty in sucking, with milk dripping from the nostrils, and at a later stage, dysphagia.

Agnathia

Developmental failure of the mandible results in the condition referred to as agnathia. This condition, which is reported in lambs, is rare in cattle.

Brachygnathia

An anomaly in which the mandible is markedly shorter than the maxilla is referred to as brachygnathia. This condition, which is commonly referred to as overshot jaw or 'parrot mouth', occurs in all species of animals. The severity of the condition can vary widely. Brachygnathia, which is considered to be hereditary, is often associated with other anomalies.

Prognathia

The term prognathia is used to describe the condition in which the mandible is longer than the maxilla with the mandibular incisors markedly rostral to the maxillary incisors. In brachycephalic dogs and Persian cats, this condition is accepted as a normal characteristic of these animals.

Choanal atresia or stenosis

Failure in the development of the caudal opening between the nasal cavity and pharynx gives rise to choanal atresia. This condition, although rare, occurs more frequently in foals than in other domestic animals. Foals with choanal atresia may die due to respiratory distress. A constricted opening between the nasal cavity and the pharynx, referred to as choanal stenosis, results in dyspnoea during exercise.

Atresia of the naso-lacrimal duct

Failure in canalisation of the naso-lacrimal duct, which usually occurs at its opening from the lacrimal sac, results in lacrimal secretions flowing over the surface of the face from the medial canthus of the eye.

Anomalies of the tongue

Developmental lingual defects in domestic animals are rare. An uncommon condition in pups, referred to as 'bird tongue', is characterised by a small pointed tongue resembling a chicken's tongue. This condition is considered to be due to failure of the lateral lingual processes to develop, with the body of the tongue developing solely from the medial lingual swelling. Affected pups are unable to suck, and die from dehydration and starvation. 'Bird tongue' in dogs is attributed to a recessive autosomal gene.

Pharyngeal cysts

Cyst-like structures found subcutaneously in the pharyngeal region are referred to as pharyngeal cysts. True pharyngeal cysts are due to failure of the second pharyngeal arch to overgrow the second and third pharyngeal clefts and obliterate the cervical sinus. The epithelium of the persisting cervical sinus becomes secretory forming a fluid-filled cyst. The majority of cysts in the pharyngeal region of dogs are not, in reality, cervical sinus-derived cysts, but are cysts associated with salivary glands.

Abnormal dentition

Anodontia, absence of teeth, which is rare in domestic mammals, results from failure of either the dental lamina or the dental papillae to develop and produce inductive factors. Developmental failure which results in a reduction in the number of teeth normally present, oligodontia, occurs sporadically in horses, dogs and cats. In brachycephalic breeds the cheek teeth numbers are reduced, while in toy breeds the incisor teeth are reduced in number. Polyodontia, excessive numbers of teeth, occurs in brachycephalic dogs, with an increase in the number of incisor teeth present. This condition has also been reported in horses and cats. Heterotopic polyodontia is a condition in which an extra tooth or teeth are located outside the normal dental arcade. A classical example of this condition is the so-called 'ear tooth' of horses which develops in a pharyngeal cyst. Such cysts may contain a number of teeth.

Odontogenic cysts are epithelial-lined cysts which develop from cells derived from degenerating root sheaths, dental laminae or malformed enamel organs. Dentigerous cysts may contain all or part of a malformed tooth. These cysts, which occur occasionally in young horses and ruminants, can cause distortion of the maxilla or mandible.

Further reading

Butler, A.B. and Hodos, W. (2005) Segmental organization of the head, brain and cranial nerves. In *Comparative Vertebrate Neuroanatomy*, 2nd edn. John Wiley and Sons, Hoboken, NJ, pp. 157–172.

Gans, C. and Northcutt, R.G. (1983) Neural crest and the origin of vertebrates: a New Head. *Science* **220**, 268–274.

Gerneke, W.H. (1963) The embryological development of the pharyngeal region of the sheep. *Onderstepoort Journal of Veterinary Research* **30**, 191–250.

Graham, A. (2001) The development and evolution of the pharyngeal arches. *Journal of Anatomy* **199**, 133–141.

Hatt, S.D. (1967) The development of the deciduous incisors in the sheep. *Research in Veterinary Science* **8**, 143–149.

Helms, J.A., Corders, D. and Tapadia, M.D. (2005) New insights into craniofacial morphogenesis. *Development* **132**, 851–861.

Hendrick, A.G. (1964) The pharyngeal pouches of the dog. *The Anatomical Record* **149**, 475–483.

Jacobson, A.G. (1993) Somitomeres: mesodermal segments of the head and trunk. In *The Skull, Vol. 1, Development.* Eds. J. Hanken and B.K. Hall. The University of Chicago Press, Chicago, pp. 42–76.

Kuatani, S. (2005) Craniofacial development and the evolution of the vertebrates: the old problems on a new background. *Zoological Science* **22**, 1–19.

Latshaw, W.K. (1987) Face, mouth, and pharynx. In *Veterinary Developmental Anatomy.* B.C. Decker, Toronto, pp. 87–112.

McCollum, M. and Sharpe, P.T. (2001) Evolution and development of teeth. *Journal of Anatomy* **199**, 153–159.

Pispa, J. and Thesleff, J. (2003) Mechanisms of ectodermal organogenesis. *Developmental Biology* **262**, 195–205.

Sack, O.W. (1964) The early development of the embryonic pharynx of the dog. *Anatomischer Anzeiger* **115**, 59–80.

Weinreb, M.M. and Sharon, J. (1964) Tooth development in sheep. *American Journal of Veterinary Research* **25**, 891–908.

20 Endocrine System

Organs located in different parts of the body contain specialised secretory cells which produce hormones. These specialised secretory cells may form defined endocrine organs, the endocrine glands, or they may occur as organised clusters within organs which do not have a solely endocrine function. In addition, endocrine cells may be present as solitary cells distributed in many tissues throughout the body. Collectively the organs, clusters of cells and individual cells with specialised secretory activity constitute the endocrine system. Unlike the products of exocrine glands which are conveyed through ducts, endocrine secretions diffuse into the bloodstream and are carried to target cells, tissues or organs. Endocrine secretions play a central role in regulating and coordinating the normal physiological activities of the body. The functioning of some endocrine organs may be stimulated or inhibited by hormones secreted by other endocrine organs. The defined endocrine glands include the pituitary gland, the pineal gland, the adrenal glands, the thyroid gland and the parathyroid glands. Organs which contain groups of endocrine cells include the pancreas, the testes and ovaries, and, in pregnant females, the placenta. The endocrine cells of the placenta and gonads and the functional roles of the hormones they produce are briefly reviewed in Chapters 10 and 18 respectively. Because thymic epithelial reticular cells secrete hormones which contribute to the maturation of T lymphocytes, the thymus can be considered as having an endocrine function. Cells of the diffuse endocrine system are found in gastrointestinal tract epithelium, the conducting airways of the respiratory system, the juxta-glomerular apparatus of the kidney, atrial myocardium and hepatic tissue. There is a close interrelationship in the functioning of the endocrine system and the nervous system, not only through internal signalling but also from environmental stimuli.

Pituitary gland

Ectoderm of both oral and neural origin contributes to the formation of the pituitary gland (hypophysis cerebri). That portion of the pituitary gland which develops from an upward evagination of oral ectoderm in the midline from the roof of the stomodeum, immediately rostral to the oro-pharyngeal membrane, is referred to as the adenohypophysis (Fig. 20.1). The primordial structure from which the adenohypophysis develops is known as the adenohypophyseal pouch or Rathke's pouch. A second component of the pituitary gland, the neurohypophysis, develops from a ventral diverticulum in the floor of the diencephalon known as the infundibulum. In domestic mammals, the two primordial structures meet and fuse forming the pituitary gland.

The adenohypophyseal pouch grows dorsally towards the infundibular downgrowth and gradually loses its connection with the oral ectoderm forming the adenohypophyseal vesicle. Cells of the rostral wall of the vesicle proliferate at a higher rate than cells of the caudal wall. The space remaining following mural proliferation is referred to as the adenohypophyseal cleft. Proliferating cells from the dorsal aspect of the rostral wall surround the stalk of the infundibulum, forming the pars tuberalis. The remaining cells of the rostral wall proliferate forming aggregations of cells which give rise to the pars distalis. The infundibulum gives rise to the hypophyseal stalk and an enlarged distal area, the pars nervosa of the pituitary. Cells of the pars distalis differentiate into endocrine cells, which, on the basis of their staining characteristics, can be classified as acidophils, basophils and chromophobes. The acidophils are the source of growth hormone and prolactin while the basophils give rise to the trophic hormones, adrenocorticotrophic hormone (ACTH), thyroid-stimulating hormone (TSH), follicle-stimulating hormone (FSH), and luteinising hormone (LH). Chromophobes are considered to be either stem cells or non-secreting stages of acidophils or basophils. In the pars distalis, acidophils, basophils and chromophobes are not evenly distributed and show species variation both in their numbers and in their distribution. The cell types in the pars tuberalis are similar to those present in the pars distalis.

The caudal wall of the adenohypophyseal vesicle which undergoes little proliferation and forms the pars intermedia comes in direct contact with the infundibulum. The extent of fusion of these two structures accounts for the anatomical relationship of the different regions of the pituitary gland in domestic animals. In humans, following fusion of the pars intermedia with the rostral

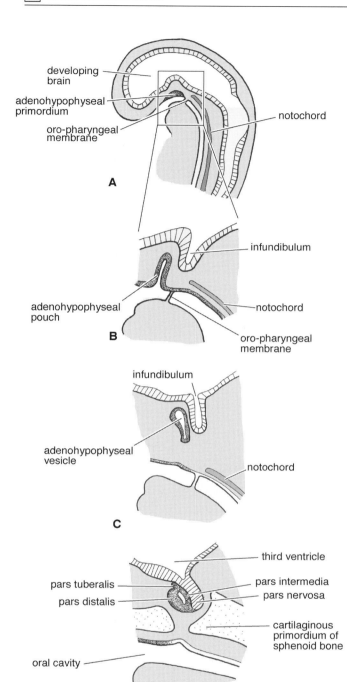

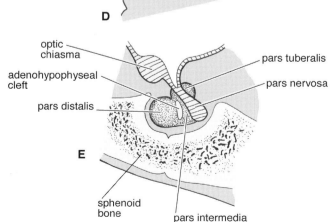

Figure 20.1 Sequential stages in the formation of the pituitary gland.

surface of the neural lobe, continued proliferation of the pars distalis obliterates the adenohypophyseal cleft. Because of limited proliferation of the pars distalis in ruminants, the cleft persists. An unusual feature of the pituitary gland in ruminants is the presence of a small segment of pars distalis-like tissue attached to the rostral surface of the pars intermedia. In horses, pigs and carnivores, the pars intermedia encloses the infundibulum so that the pars intermedia is in direct contact with the surface of the pars nervosa. The hypophyseal cleft, which persists in carnivores and pigs, is obliterated in horses. The most abundant cell type of the pars intermedia is a large, round, pale-staining cell which produces melanocyte-stimulating hormone. These large cells may sometimes form colloid-filled follicles (Fig. 20.2).

Processes of neurons from the supraoptic and paraventricular nuclei of the hypothalamus project into the infundibular stalk and extend into the developing pars nervosa. Neurosecretions from the supraoptic and paraventricular nuclei, antidiuretic hormone and oxytocin, are transported along axons to the pars nervosa where they are stored. The majority of glial cells of the pars nervosa are modified astrocytes and are referred to as pituicytes. The functioning of the adenohypophysis is under the control of hypothalamic neurohormones which either stimulate or inhibit secretions of particular cell types of the pars distalis. These hypothalamic neurohormones are carried to the pars distalis through the hypophyseal vascular portal system. Release of the hypothalamic neurohormones is influenced by feedback mechanisms from target organs acted on by hormones of the pars distalis.

Molecular regulation of pituitary gland development

The earliest transcription factors expressed in the pituitary primordium include Six-3, Pax-6 and Rathke's pouch homeobox (Rpx). Subsequently, Shh, Pitx, Ptx and P-Otx are expressed continuously throughout the oral ectoderm. By excluding Shh from the Rathke's pouch region, Bmp-4 signals from the ventral diencephalon suppress the expression of Shh creating a molecular border between oral and pouch ectoderm. Subsequently, expression of Bmp-2 can be detected at the oral ectoderm–Rathke's pouch boundary. Concurrently, Fgf-8 and Wnt-5a are expressed within the ventral region of the diencephalon. Fgf-8 is also expressed in the infundibulum. Based on the expression levels of Fgf-8 and Bmp-2, gradients of transcription factors Six-3, Nkx-3.1 and Prop-1 are expressed dorsally and Brn-4, Isl-1, P-Frk and GATA-2 are expressed ventrally. This variable expression of transcription factors along the dorsal–ventral axis not only establishes pituitary commitment but also induces the determination, formation

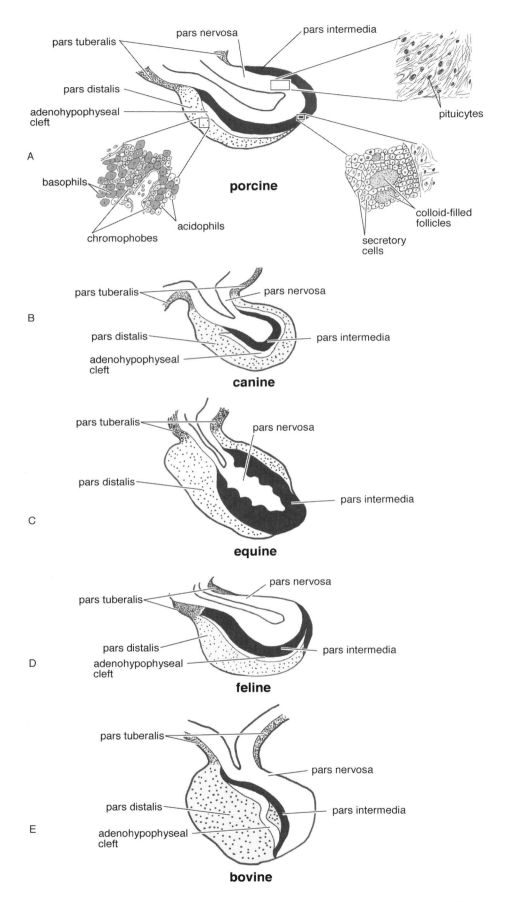

Figure 20.2 A, Relationships of the components of the fully formed porcine pituitary gland and histological features of the pars distalis, pars intermedia and pars nervosa. The relationships of the components of the canine, equine, feline and bovine pituitary glands are shown in B, C, D and E respectively.

and differentiation of the pituitary gland. Development and differentiation of pituitary gland cells is also specified by the homeodomain transcription factors Rpx, Ptx, Lhx-3, Prop-1 and Pit-1.

Pineal gland

The pineal gland (epiphysis cerebri) develops as a dorsal neuro-epithelial diverticulum of the caudal part of the roof of the diencephalon (Fig. 13.21A). After its formation, the gland remains attached to the diencephalon by a stalk. The neuro-epithelial cells differentiate into pinealocytes and glial cells. The developing gland is surrounded by a thin layer of pia mater-derived connective tissue. This connective tissue, which extends into the substance of the gland, subdivides it into lobules and also provides a blood supply. The pinealocytes develop processes which release their secretion, melatonin, into either capillaries derived from the vascular pia mater or into the cerebrospinal fluid of the third ventricle. The functioning of the pineal gland, including the synthesis and secretion of melatonin, is related to the duration of exposure of an animal to light and to darkness. Increased length of exposure to daylight activates sensory neurons in the retina for sustained periods. As a consequence of this exposure, impulses are relayed by nervous pathways to excitatory neurons, which in turn stimulate inhibitory neurons in the pineal gland, with the release of inhibitory neurotransmitters. Under the influence of these inhibitory neurotransmitters, the pinealocytes synthesise and release only low levels of melatonin. In contrast, when an animal is exposed to short periods of daylight, inhibitory neurons in the pineal gland are stimulated to a lesser extent. As a result, increased amounts of melatonin are synthesised and released. Accordingly, the rate of synthesis and release of melatonin is promoted by exposure to darkness and is decreased by exposure to light. Melatonin, by its action on the hypothalamus, promotes the secretion of gonadotrophin releasing hormone (GnRH), which in turn acts on the pars distalis of the pituitary gland, causing release of gonadotrophic hormones. Thus, photoperiodicity influences the onset of the breeding season in many species.

Adrenal glands

The paired mammalian adrenal glands develop from two distinct embryological tissues, neural crest ectoderm and intermediate mesoderm. The two components of the adrenal glands exhibit different histological features and have distinct physiological roles. In reality, the mammalian adrenal gland is composed of two conjoined endocrine organs which, during embryonic development, fuse forming a single anatomical structure. Studies of the comparative development and anatomical features of adrenal tissues in vertebrates illustrate the dual origin of the mammalian adrenal gland. In fish, the two tissues which are the counterpart of the adrenal gland in mammals exist as two separate endocrine organs, while in amphibians the two tissues are in direct contact. The two tissues which constitute the adrenal glands in reptiles and birds are randomly integrated. In mammals, the neural-crest-derived tissue occupies a central position, surrounded by the tissue derived from intermediate mesoderm. Thus, the typical histological appearance of the mammalian adrenal gland consists of an inner medulla and an outer cortex.

The cortical tissue of the mammalian adrenal gland, which forms towards the end of the embryonic period, first occurs as aggregations of mesodermal tissue derived from the regressing mesonephric tubules. These aggregations, which are located along the ventro-medial border of the mesonephros, become organised into cord-like structures. Later in development, neural crest cells migrate to a central position within the mesodermal mass forming the adrenal medulla (Fig. 20.3). Proliferation of the mesodermal cells in the outer layer forms the cortex. At this stage of development, the large adrenal cortex is referred to as the foetal cortex. Subsequently, a second proliferation of mesodermal cells surrounds the foetal cortex and post-natally becomes the definitive cortex as the foetal cortex regresses. After birth, the definitive cortex differentiates into three zones, the zona glomerulosa, the zona fasciculata and the zona reticularis. In utero, the foetal cortex produces higher levels of steroid hormones than the definitive cortex post-natally. The functioning of the foetal adrenal cortex is dependent on the secretion of the foetal pituitary hormone, ACTH. The maturation of the foetal lungs, liver and the epithelial cells of the digestive tract is influenced by hormones secreted by the foetal adrenal gland. In a number of mammalian species, initiation of parturition correlates with increased levels of the foetal adrenocortical hormone, cortisol. When the definitive cortex develops into the zona glomerulosa, the zona fasciculata and the zona reticularis, each zone produces specific steroid hormones. The zona glomerulosa produces the mineralocorticoid hormone, aldosterone, which has a role in electrolyte and water balance. The zona fasciculata secretes glucocorticoids which have a major role in carbohydrate, protein and fat metabolism. Cells of the zona reticularis produce low levels of sex hormones, mainly androgens.

The adrenal medulla resembles a modified ganglion of the sympathetic nervous system but with cell bodies devoid of axons. Neurosecretions of the cells of the adrenal medulla are released directly into the blood. Due to their affinity for chromium compounds, which stain the cells brown, the cell bodies of the adrenal medulla are called chromaffin cells. In response to activation of

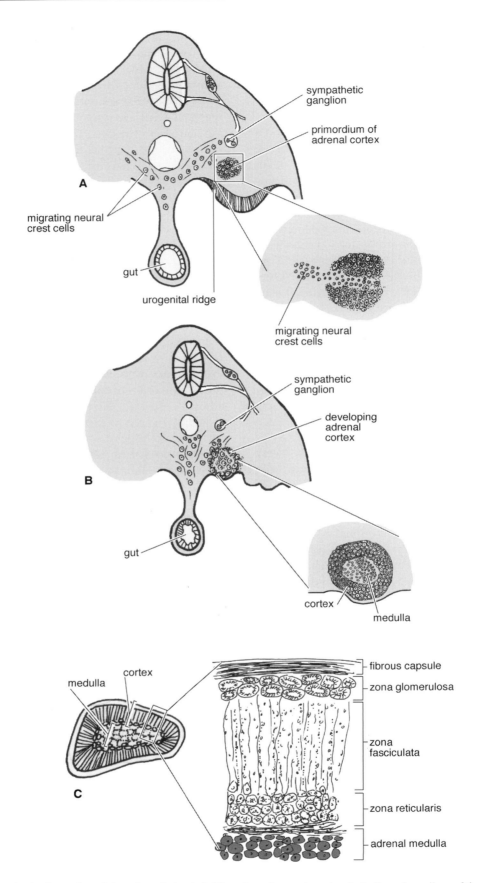

Figure 20.3 Stages in the formation of the adrenal gland. A, Migration of neural crest cells to the primordium of the adrenal cortex. B, Formation of adrenal medulla by neural crest cells. C, Fully formed adrenal gland showing the medulla, cortical zones and capsule.

the sympathetic nervous system, cells of the adrenal medulla secrete epinephrine and nor-epinephrine, with epinephrine produced in greater amounts.

Thyroid gland

The thyroid gland develops as a ventral midline endodermal diverticulum from the floor of the foregut at a level between the first and second pharyngeal arches. The caudal end of this primordial structure extends ventrally and caudally into the underlying mesoderm. Initially, it remains attached to the foregut by a duct, the thyro-glossal duct. The blind end of the primordial structure becomes bilobar and extends caudally to a position ventral to the commencement of the developing trachea (Fig. 20.4). During its caudal elongation, the thyroid primordium loses its connection with the foregut and occupies a position on the ventral aspect of the developing trachea where it forms two distinct lobes which remain attached by an isthmus of glandular tissue. Initially, the isthmus extends across the ventral aspect of the trachea connecting the laterally positioned lobes. The amount of glandular tissue which persists in the isthmus is not constant in all species. In humans and pigs, the amount of glandular tissue in the isthmus is substantial and forms a medial lobe, while in cattle, glandular tissue in the isthmus forms a well-defined band between the two lobes. The isthmus in horses is poorly defined, while in small ruminants it consists of a band of connective tissue. In dogs and cats, the connection between the lobes is lost and the thyroid gland consists of two distinct lobes of secretory tissue. The site of origin of the thyroid primordium in mammals persists post-natally as a shallow depression on the surface of the tongue referred to as the foramen caecum. The endodermal cells of the thyroid diverticulum differentiate into cuboidal epithelial cells which, when organised into follicles, synthesise the thyroid hormones thyroxine (T_4) and tri-iodothyronine (T_3). Thyroid hormone synthesis and release are under the control of thyroid stimulating hormone produced by the pars distalis of the pituitary gland. The hormones secreted by the thyroid gland have a central role in the control of the metabolic activity of organs and tissues throughout the body.

As the thyroid primordium migrates caudally close to the pharyngeal pouches, ventral components of the fourth pharyngeal pouches, the ultimo-branchial bodies, become incorporated into the thyroid tissue and contribute to its formation. The cells of the ultimo-branchial body include cells derived from the neural crest which give rise to the C-cells or parafollicular cells of the thyroid gland. Parafollicular cells secrete calcitonin, a hormone which regulates blood calcium levels in a number of ways. Calcitonin suppresses osteoclast activity, thereby decreasing the availability of calcium ions from bone; it also stimulates calcium deposition in bone and promotes calcium ion excretion by the kidneys. The regulatory influence of calcitonin on blood calcium levels also involves its antagonistic action on parathyroid hormone secretion by the parathyroid glands.

Molecular regulation of thyroid gland development

From the beginning of differentiation of the thyroid follicular cells, the simultaneous expression of thyroid-specific transcription factors Ttf-1 and Ttf-2, together with Pax-8, persists throughout development. In *Ttf-1* knockout mice, thyroid follicular cells and C-cells are absent. In homozygous *Ttf-2* knockout mice, the thyroid bud does not migrate to its usual site, leading to either ectopy or failure of thyroid development. C-cells, however, develop normally. *Pax-8* knockout models have a complete absence of thyroid follicular cells, but their C-cells are normal. Production of TSH by the pituitary gland and the presence of its receptor on target cells are required for the proliferation and maintenance of differentiated thyroid follicular cells.

Parathyroid glands

The parathyroid glands develop from the dorsal segments of the third and fourth pharyngeal pouches. The name assigned to each parathyroid gland relates to the pharyngeal pouch from which it derives. The dorsal part of the left and right third pharyngeal pouches gives rise to an external parathyroid or parathyroid III gland. The primordium of each gland loses its connection with the pharyngeal wall and is drawn caudally by the developing thymus (Fig. 20.4). The dorsal segment of the left and right fourth pharyngeal pouches gives rise to an internal parathyroid or parathyroid IV gland, which also loses its connection with the pharyngeal wall. Because they are drawn caudally by the developing thymus, the parathyroid III glands occupy a final position caudal to the parathyroid IV glands. As a consequence of caudal migration of the thyroid gland, the parathyroid IV glands usually become attached to or embedded within the substance of the thyroid gland. Due to the influence of thymic migration on parathyroid III glands, they are usually located caudal to the thyroid close to the bifurcation of the carotid artery. Unlike other domestic species, the equine parathyroid III glands are drawn more caudally by their attachment to the migrating thymus. In their final position they are located close to the thoracic inlet. Because the primordia of porcine parathyroid IV glands regress, only parathyroid III glands develop in pigs.

The cells of the parathyroid glands differentiate into cords of cells referred to as chief cells, which secrete

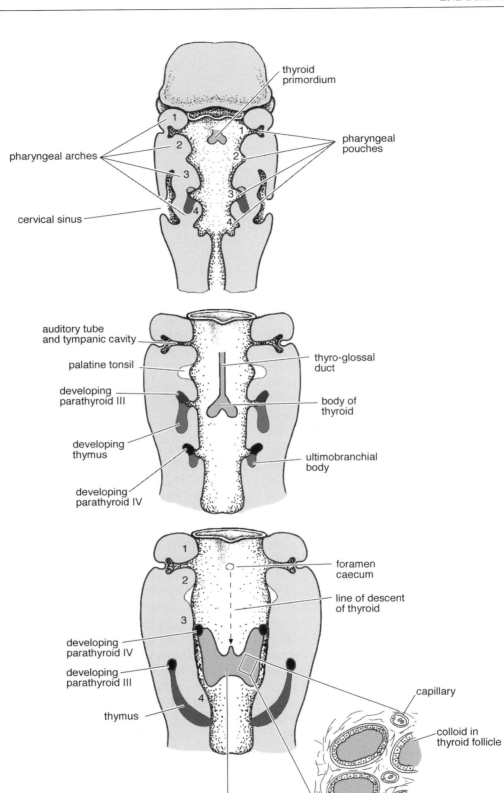

Figure 20.4 Sequential stages in the formation of the thyroid and parathyroid glands, the thymus, palatine tonsil and associated structures. Details of the histological structure of the developing thyroid gland are shown.

parathyroid hormone or parathormone. Parathyroid hormone increases blood calcium levels by stimulating osteoclasts to release calcium ions from bone, by inhibiting calcium deposition in bones, by promoting calcium absorption from dietary sources and by decreasing renal excretion of calcium. In humans, horses and ruminants, a second cell type, referred to as an oxyphil cell, with an undetermined function, contributes to the parenchyma of the parathyroid glands.

Thymus

The thymus develops from the ventral portion of the left and right third pharyngeal pouches, with a minor contribution in some species from the fourth pharyngeal pouches (Fig. 20.4). The cells of the thymic primordia proliferate and extend caudally, initially as two tubular structures. Continued cellular proliferation causes elimination of the cavities of these tubular structures resulting in the formation of solid structures. As they extend caudally, the caudal ends of the primordia meet and fuse in the mid-line and become attached to the developing pericardium. Associated with the caudal migration of the heart to the thoracic cavity, the caudal end of the thymus is drawn into the thoracic cavity to a position in the cranial mediastinum. At this stage of development, the embryonic thymus is Y-shaped with its bifid cranial end attached to the wall of the developing pharynx and with the caudal end of the fused portion located in the thoracic cavity. In ruminants and pigs, this embryonic shape persists with the neonatal thymus consisting of pharyngeal, cervical and thoracic regions. In horses, the left and right connection of the thymus with the pharynx is lost and each paired cranial portion, together with a segment of the fused cranial cervical portion, regresses. A small component of the fused cranial cervical part persists together with the thoracic part. In carnivores and humans, the complete cervical portion of the thymus regresses and only the thoracic part remains as a bilobed structure.

During its caudal migration, the thymus becomes surrounded by neural crest-derived mesenchymal cells which form a connective tissue capsule. This capsule forms septa which extend into the endodermal mass of the developing thymus. During the early embryonic period, cells derived from bone marrow migrate to the epithelial thymus. These cells, pro-thymocytes, occupy positions between the epithelial cells causing them to form an endodermally-derived, spongy, reticular network containing a diverse range of epithelial reticular cells. Responding to inductive factors from the epithelial reticular cells, the thymocytes proliferate and become organised on the periphery, forming a densely cellular cortex and a less dense medulla. Some medullary epithe-

lial cells form concentric layers of squamous cells around individual enlarged endodermal cells. Subsequently, the central cells degenerate and the surrounding cells accumulate kerato-hyalin granules, giving rise to structures known as thymic or Hassall's corpuscles. Under the influence of hormones produced by the epithelial reticular cells, including thymosin and thymopoietin, the pro-thymocytes become competent T lymphocytes. On leaving the thymus, mature T lymphocytes seed other lymphoid organs with subsets which are responsible for cell-mediated immune responses.

A special barrier, referred to as the blood–thymus barrier, serves to isolate T lymphocytes from antigenic challenge. In the thymus, cortical capillaries have a continuous endothelium, perivascular connective tissue and a sheath composed of the processes of epithelial cells. This barrier minimises the entry of foreign antigens into the cortical parenchyma. The thymus, which is particularly prominent in young animals, undergoes gradual involution with the onset of sexual maturity. Involution is characterised by the gradual reduction in thymocyte numbers with enlargement of the epithelial reticular cells and replacement of the lymphatic tissue by adipocytes.

Pancreatic islets

Within the developing pancreas, clusters of cells bud off from the developing exocrine component of the pancreas forming endocrine structures referred to as the pancreatic islets or islets of Langerhans. Cells within these islets differentiate into particular cell types each with the capability of producing a specific endocrine secretion. These endocrine cells, which are designated as α-cells, β-cells and δ-cells, produce glucagon, insulin and somatostatin respectively. Glucagon raises blood glucose levels by increasing the rate of glycogen breakdown and promoting glucose release from hepatocytes. In contrast, insulin increases the rate of glucose uptake and utilisation by binding to cell surface insulin receptors, principally on myocytes and hepatocytes, thereby lowering blood glucose levels. Somatostatin has a local inhibitory effect on the release of insulin and glucagon. Two other cell types, G cells and PP cells, secrete gastrin and pancreatic polypeptide respectively. Within the pancreatic islets, β-cells are the predominant cell type present. The next most numerous cell type is the α-cell, followed by the δ-cell. The G cells and PP cells form a minority of cell types in the pancreatic islets. The distribution of cell types among pancreatic islets is not always uniform. Within the different anatomical regions of the pancreas, there is a lack of uniformity in the distribution of islets, with species-associated variation also observed.

Further reading

Cohen, H., Radovick, S. and Wondisford, F.E. (1999) Transcription factors and hypopituitarism. *Trends in Endocrinology and Metabolism* **10**, 326–332.

Eiler, H. (2004) Endocrine glands. In *Duke's Physiology of Domestic Animals*, 2nd edn. Ed. W.O. Reece. Comstock Publishing Associates, Cornell University Press, Ithaca, NY, pp. 621–669.

Godwin, M.C. (1936) The early development of the thyroid gland in the dog with special reference to the origin and position of accessory thyroid tissue. *Anatomical Record* **66**, 233–251.

Godwin, M.C. (1937) The development of the parathyroid in the dog with emphasis upon the origin of accessory glands. *Anatomical Record* **68**, 305–325.

Hullinger, R.L. (1993) The endocrine system. In *Miller's Anatomy of the Dog*, 3rd edn. Ed. H. Evans. W.B. Saunders, Philadelphia, PA, pp. 559–585.

Kingsbury, B.F. and Roemer, F.J. (1940) The development of the hypophysis in the dog. *American Journal of Anatomy* **66**, 449–481.

Mullis, P.E. (2001) Transcription factors in pituitary development. *Molecular and Cellular Endocrinology* **185**, 1–16.

Shanklin, W.M. (1944) Histogenesis of the pig's neurohypophysis. *Journal of Anatomy* **74**, 327–353.

Sjaastad, O.V., Hove, K. and Sand, O. (2003) The endocrine system. In *Physiology of Domestic Animals*. Scandinavian Veterinary Press, Oslo, pp. 199–234.

Vliet, G.U. (2003) Development of the thyroid gland: lessons from congenitally hypothyroid mice and men. *Clinical Genetics* **63**, 445–455.

21 Eye and Ear

Eye

The embryonic tissues which contribute to the formation of the eye include neural and surface ectoderm and neural crest-derived mesoderm. Ocular development and differentiation rely on sequential interaction between these basic tissues. The primordia which initiate ocular development can be identified first as a pair of shallow grooves on either side of the folding prosencephalon (Fig. 21.1). These structures can be recognised towards the end of neurulation prior to the closure of the rostral neuropore. Formation of these grooves is induced by factors from adjacent pharyngeal endoderm and mesoderm. Following closure of the rostral neuropore, the grooves form diverticula, the optic vesicles, the cavities of which are initially continuous with the cavity of the forebrain (Fig. 21.2). As the optic vesicles grow laterally and their lateral walls make contact with the surface ectoderm, the neuroepithelium of the optic vesicles induces the surface ectodermal epithelium to proliferate and form the lens placodes (Fig. 21.3). Following formation of the lens placodes, the lateral walls of the optic vesicles begin to flatten and become concave. This results in the conversion of the optic vesicles into double-walled optic cups. The inner and outer walls of each optic cup are initially separated by a space. The walls of the cup become apposed resulting in the gradual disappearance of the intervening space. Narrowing of the stem of the optic vesicle leads to formation of the optic stalk. Because the invagination which shapes the optic cup occurs at the ventral margin of the vesicle, the rim of the optic cup is not continuous at its ventral aspect. This invagination results in the formation of a groove in the ventral rim of the cup which extends along the ventral surface of the optic stalk. This groove, referred to as the choroid fissure, provides access for the hyaloid blood vessels which supply the developing retina and lens (Fig. 21.4). Associated with closure of the choroid fissure towards the end of the embryonic period, the hyaloid vessels become enclosed within the optic stalk (Fig. 21.5), and the rim of the optic cup becomes a continuous structure enclosing a rounded space, the primordium of the pupil. With the development of the optic cup, the lens placode invaginates into the rim of the optic vesicle

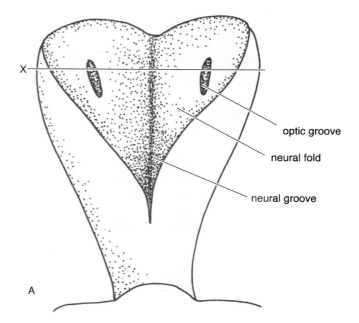

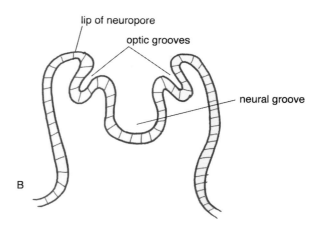

Figure 21.1 Dorsal view of forebrain, A, prior to closure of the rostral neuropore showing the optic grooves and a cross-section, B, through the forebrain at the level of the optic grooves (X).

and forms the lens vesicle (Fig. 21.6). The lens vesicle subsequently loses contact with the surface ectoderm, is surrounded by mesenchymal tissue and becomes positioned at the opening of the optic cup (Fig. 21.7).

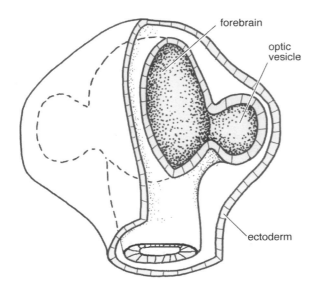

Figure 21.2 Developing forebrain showing the optic vesicles.

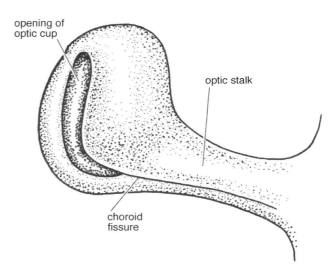

Figure 21.4 Ventro-lateral view of the optic cup and optic stalk showing the ventral choroid fissure.

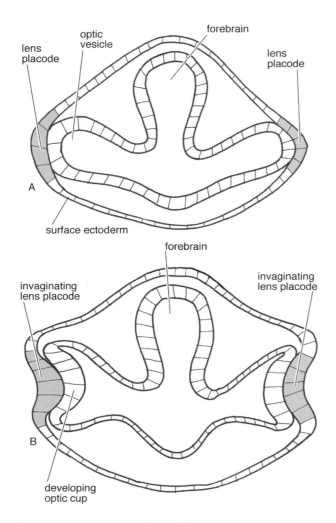

Figure 21.3 Cross-section through forebrain at the level of the optic vesicles showing contact between the neuroepithelium of the optic vesicles and the surface ectoderm, A. Early stage in the formation of the optic cups and lens placodes, B.

Molecular aspects of development of the eye

Initially, the transcription factor Pax-6 is expressed in a region in the anterior neural ridge prior to neurulation. For normal eye development, a high and continuous level of expression of the transcription factor Pax-6 is required in cells which derive from the surface ectoderm and optic cup. In these cells, Pax-6 up-regulates genes encoding Six-3, c-Maf and Prox-1, and genes encoding structural proteins such as crystallins, cell adhesion molecules and molecules essential for the morphogenesis of ectodermally-derived ocular tissues. A low and transient expression of Pax-6 is required for the differentiation of the epithelial layers of the cornea. Humans heterozygous for mutations in *Pax-6* develop defects of the iris, corneal opacity, cataracts and foveal dysplasia.

Conversion of the single zone specified for ocular development into bilateral zones is dependent on the secretion of Sonic hedgehog. Absence of Shh expression in this region results in a condition known as cyclopia, the formation of a single eye in the midline of the cranial region. The plant *Veratrum californicum* contains the alkaloids jervine and cyclopamine, which, if ingested by ewes in early pregnancy, induces cyclopia in their lambs. Shh up-regulates *Pax-2* in the centre of the eye field and down-regulates *Pax-6*. Later, *Pax-2* is expressed in the optic stalks and *Pax-6* in the optic cups and overlying ectoderm.

The process of optic cup formation is regulated by interactive signals between the optic vesicle, the surrounding mesenchyme and the overlying surface ectoderm in the lens-forming region. Fibroblast growth factors from the surface ectoderm support differentiation of the neural

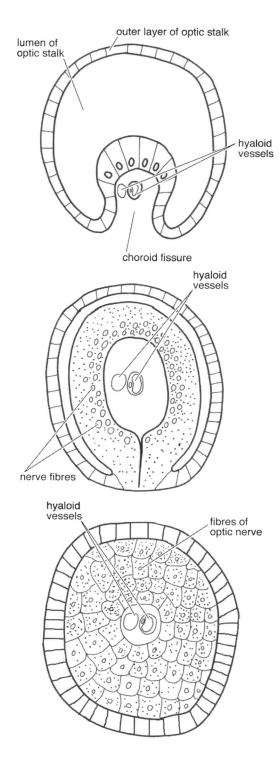

Figure 21.5 Sequential stages in the closure of the choroid fissure in the optic stalk showing the incorporation of the hyaloid vessels into the optic stalk and subsequent development of the optic nerve.

retina. Tgf-β, secreted from the surrounding mesenchyme, directs formation of the outer retinal layer. These signals cause regionalisation of the inner and outer layers of the optic cup and up-regulate transcription factors such as Mitf and Chx-10 which, in turn, promote the differentiation of the pigmented and neural layers respectively.

Experiments with avian embryos suggest that early differentiation of the mesenchymal cells in the cornea and in associated structures depends on signals arising from the lens placode. Similar inductive influences may apply to the development of the mammalian eye. Mutations in a number of genes encoding transcription factors expressed in the lens placode result in malformation of the lens and structures anterior to the lens. These transcription factors include Maf, Foxe-3 and Pitx-e.

It is probable that the various transcription factors which control eye morphogenesis do so by modulating signalling molecules. These signalling molecules, which include Bmp-4 and Tgf-β2, are directly involved in the formation of the mesenchymally-derived structures in the anterior region of the eye. Bmp-4 is expressed in the iris, the ciliary body and retinal pigmented epithelium of both the embryonic and post-natal murine eye. Mice heterozygous for a null allele of *Bmp-4* show a variety of ocular abnormalities in the iris, cornea and anterior chamber of the eye.

Tgf-β2 is expressed during both pre-natal and post-natal ocular development in the anterior portion of the eye. In homozygous *Tgf-β2* knockout mice, the cornea is thinner than normal, the corneal endothelium is completely absent and the lens and iris are in direct contact with the corneal stroma.

Differentiation of the optic cup

The retina derives from the apposed walls of the optic cup. The outer wall of the optic cup, which initially is separated from the inner wall by a space referred to as the intra-retinal space, remains thin and becomes pigmented forming the pigmented layer of the retina (Fig. 21.7). It also contributes to the formation of the ciliary body and iris. Differentiation of the inner wall of the retina involves a series of developmental changes. Two distinct areas of differentiation develop in the inner layer of the retina. A narrow region close to the rim of the optic cup, the blind area of the retina, remains thin-walled and subsequently contributes to the formation of the ciliary body and iris. The remainder, referred to as the visual area of the retina, develops in a manner analogous to the stages of neural tube differentiation. The neuroepithelial cells of the inner wall of the cup proliferate and differentiate giving rise to the specialised layers of the visual retina which include the light-sensitive rods and cones, the bipolar and ganglion cells and the supportive glial cells (Fig. 21.8). As the optic vesicle invaginates and forms the optic cup, its light-sensitive photoreceptors are positioned adjacent

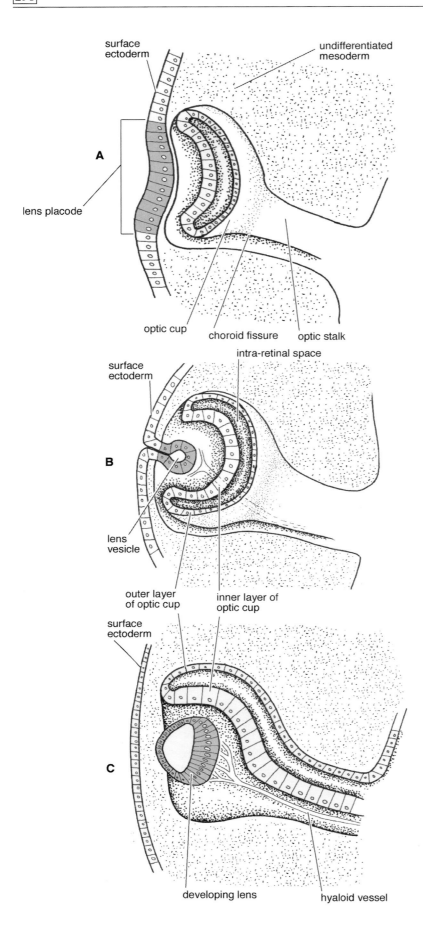

Figure 21.6 Sequential stages in the development of the lens vesicle and its invagination into the optic cup. A, Initial stage in the formation of the lens vesicle. B, Invagination of the lens vesicle into the optic cup. C, Longitudinal section through the optic stalk showing the position of the developing lens, which has lost contact with the surface ectoderm, within the optic cup.

Figure 21.7 Differentiation of the cells in the inner and outer walls of the optic cup. The position of the developing lens in relation to the optic cup and the early stages of eyelid formation are also shown.

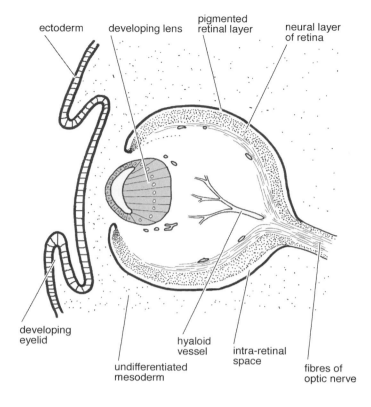

ectoderm   developing lens   pigmented retinal layer   neural layer of retina

developing eyelid

undifferentiated mesoderm

hyaloid vessel

intra-retinal space

fibres of optic nerve

to the pigmented retinal layer. The cellular layers constituting the inner wall of the optic cup are designated according to their positions relative to the outer wall. Accordingly, the cells of the inner wall which are immediately adjacent to the pigmented retinal layer are called the outer visual layer of the retina, and the retinal layer most distant from the pigmented layer is referred to as the inner layer. Thus, light passes through the inner layers of the retina before reaching the visual receptors. The impulses generated in the rods and cones are relayed to the overlying bipolar neurons and thence to the ganglion cells. The axons of the ganglion cells enter the optic stalk and signals are relayed via the optic nerve to the visual cortex of the brain. With the proliferation of nerve fibres, the structure of the optic stalk changes. The axons of the ganglion cells infiltrate the optic stalk and form the optic nerve which surrounds the remnants of the hyaloid artery within the optic stalk, termed the central artery of the retina. Prior to entering the brain, the optic nerves from each side meet and form an X-shaped structure, the optic chiasma. At the optic chiasma, some fibres from each optic nerve cross to the opposite side and accompany the fibres from that side to the brain. Some optic nerve fibres terminate in the rostral colliculus while others synapse with neurons in the lateral geniculate body of the thalamus. From the geniculate body, information is conveyed to the visual cortex.

During their development, the optic cup and lens vesicle become surrounded by neural crest-derived mesoderm. The mesoderm surrounding the optic cup differentiates

into an inner pigmented vascular layer and an outer fibrous layer. The inner pigmented layer, the choroid, is in direct contact with the outer pigmented layer of the optic cup. The outer fibrous layer forms the sclera. These layers, which have a protective role, correspond to the meningeal layers of the central nervous system. The sclera is continuous with the dura mater which ensheaths the optic nerve at the point where the nerve enters the optic foramen of the skull. With the exception of the porcine eye, a reflective structure, the tapetum lucidum, is present in the choroidal layer of the eyes of domestic animals. In carnivores the tapetum lucidum consists of several layers of flat cells packed with parallel crystalline rods. In herbivores it consists of collagen fibres and fibrocytes. The collagen fibres or intracellular crystalline rods are thought to improve low-light vision by reflecting incoming light.

During early development, some loose mesenchymal tissue which surrounds the optic cup migrates to a position between the retina and the lens. These mesenchymal cells contribute to the formation of the vitreous body and derive their blood supply from branches of the hyaloid artery. Later, when the hyaloid artery within the vitreous body atrophies, the space which it occupied is referred to as the hyaloid canal. Mesenchymal cells in the region between the lens and the surface ectoderm become arranged into two layers and the resultant cavity between them forms the anterior chamber of the eye. The outer wall of this chamber is continuous with the sclera and the inner wall is continuous with the

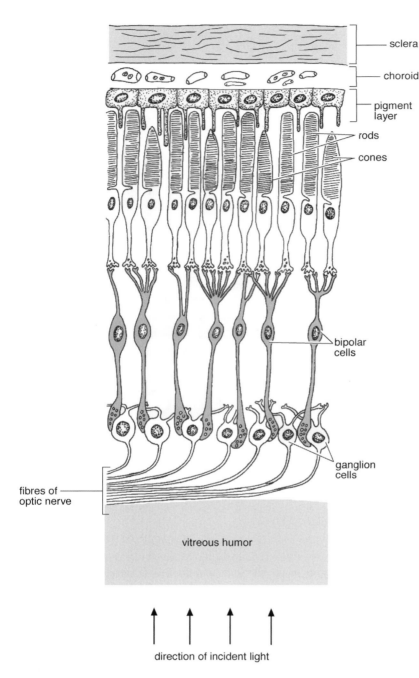

Figure 21.8 The cellular layers of the fully differentiated retina.

sclera

choroid

pigment layer

rods

cones

bipolar cells

ganglion cells

fibres of optic nerve

vitreous humor

direction of incident light

choroid. The outer layer gives rise to the substantia propria and the mesothelium of the cornea. The outer epithelial layer of the cornea derives from surface ecto-derm. The inner wall of the anterior chamber forms the irido-pupillary membrane which, in its central part, is in contact with the anterior surface of the lens (Fig. 21.9).

Mesenchymal tissue on the outer surface of the blind portion of the retina contributes to the formation of the connective tissue elements of the iris and the dilator and sphincter muscles of the pupil. The region of the non-visual retina between the iris and the visual retina becomes folded forming the ciliary processes (Fig. 21.10). The ocular mesenchyme covering the non-visual retina provides a vascular supply to the ciliary processes.

Mesenchymal cells between the ciliary processes and the lens form radially-arranged fibres, the suspensory ligament of the lens. During the late foetal period, the irido-pupillary membrane breaks down and the space bounded by the lens, suspensory ligament and iris forms the posterior chamber of the eye. Ciliary muscles which develop in the outer mesenchymal layer control the tension of the suspensory ligament. This ligament, in turn, regulates the shape of the lens and thereby visual accommodation.

Lens

Shortly after the formation of the lens vesicle, the epithelial cells of its posterior wall begin to elongate and

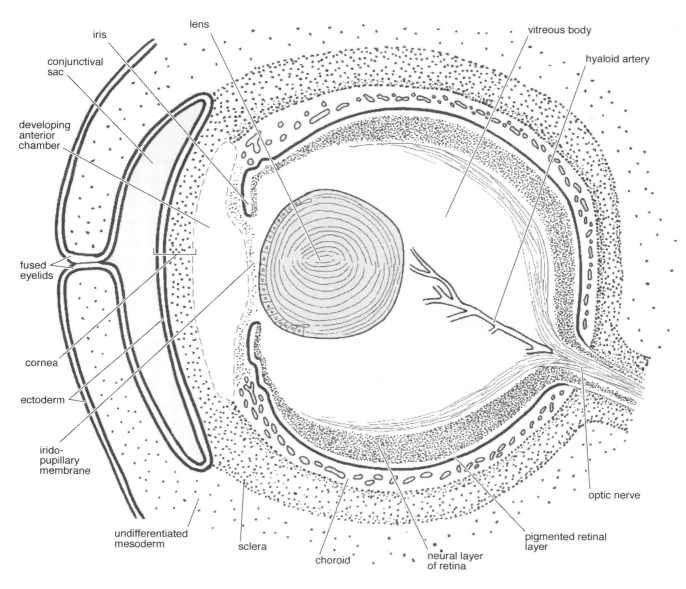

Figure 21.9 Section through the developing eye showing the relationships of its structures.

grow forwards towards the thinner anterior wall of the vesicle (Fig. 21.11). During growth and elongation, these epithelial cells undergo profound transformation into transparent, elongated cells which contain large quantities of specialised proteins called crystallins. A unique feature of lens cell differentiation is that the cells, which initially contain normal cell organelles, undergo a special form of apoptosis which does not go to completion. The cell organelles gradually disappear leaving living fibres with intact outer membranes, an inner cytoskeleton of proteins and transparent cytoplasm composed of crystallins. The mechanism which prevents complete cellular destruction is not known. Differentiation followed by transformation of the cells of the deep wall of the vesicle form a rounded lens body or embryonic nucleus. Later, the primary lens fibres are augmented by a new population of secondary lens fibres. These fibres arise from the epithelium which differentiates from cells of the anterior wall of the lens vesicle and proliferates forming concentric layers around the primary fibres of the lens nucleus.

Formation of the eyelids

Towards the end of the embryonic period, two folds of ectoderm with mesodermal cores grow towards each other over the developing cornea. Subsequently, the edges of the ectodermal layers meet and become attached to each other by the epithelial lamina between them. Adhesion of the eyelids is a temporary union as they separate again before or shortly after birth. Separation of the eyelids occurs around the seventh month of gestation in humans, about the eighth day post-natally in pups and about the tenth day post-natally in kittens.

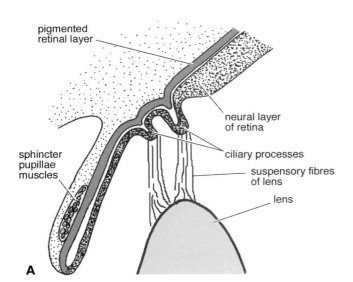

Figure 21.10 Development of iris and ciliary body.

pigmented retinal layer

neural layer of retina

ciliary processes

suspensory fibres of lens

lens

sphincter pupillae muscles

A

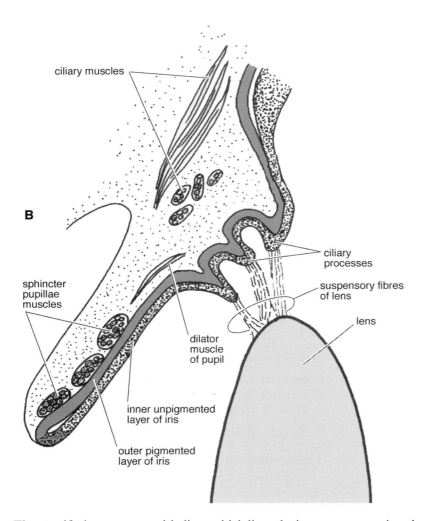

ciliary muscles

B

sphincter pupillae muscles

dilator muscle of pupil

inner unpigmented layer of iris

outer pigmented layer of iris

ciliary processes

suspensory fibres of lens

lens

The stratified squamous epithelium which lines the inner surface of the eyelids and continues over the anterior surface of the sclera is called the conjunctiva. The space enclosed by the conjunctiva when the eyelids are shut is the conjunctival sac. The conjunctiva lining the eyelids is referred to as the palpebral conjunctiva and that covering the sclera is known as the bulbar conjunctiva. In the medial angle of the eye of domestic animals, a fold of mesenchyme covered by conjunctiva gives rise to the third eyelid. Subsequently, the mesenchymal tissue forms a cartilaginous core which imparts rigidity to the third eyelid. Eyelashes develop in a linear manner from

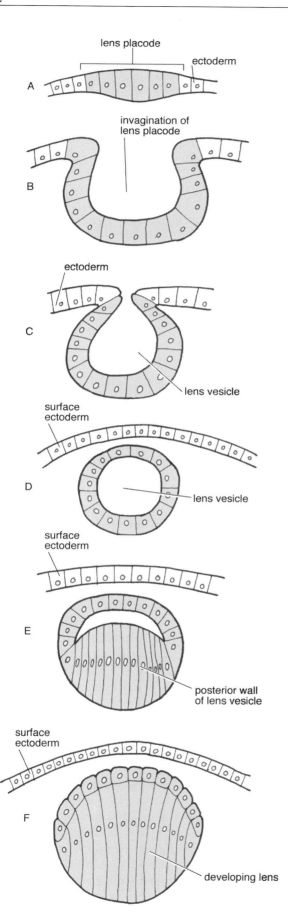

follicles along the margins of the eyelids. Each lash has associated sebaceous glands and modified sweat glands. In dogs, eyelashes develop only on the upper eyelids. The tarsal (meibomian) glands of the eyelids, which are large modified sebaceous glands, open on to the margins of the eyelids.

The lacrimal gland develops from epithelial proliferations of the conjunctival sac which fuse and give rise to a glandular structure with acini and ducts (Fig. 21.12). Soon after birth, the lacrimal gland begins to secrete a watery fluid into the conjunctival sac which lubricates the cornea. Both deep and superficial lacrimal glands may develop in association with the third eyelid.

Superficial rod-like cords of ectoderm extend from the medial canthi of the eyelids to the developing nasal pits which are the primordia of the nasal cavities. As these cords lose their contact with the surface and move deeper into the underlying mesenchyme, they become canalised forming the membranous naso-lacrimal duct. The rostral end of each duct opens into the corresponding developing nasal cavity while its proximal part bifurcates at the medial canthus giving a branch to each eyelid. These ducts become the lacrimal canaliculi. The openings of these canaliculi on the eyelids are named the lacrimal puncta. A dilatation of the naso-lacrimal duct close to its bifurcation forms the lacrimal sac. The lacrimal glands and their associated duct systems constitute the lacrimal apparatus.

Muscles of the eye

The extrinsic muscles of the eye develop from head somitomeres (Table 19.2). The intrinsic muscles, the ciliary and pupillary muscles, develop from neural crest-derived mesenchyme. A section through a fully developed eye is shown in Fig. 21.13.

Anomalies of the eye

Congenital ocular anomalies occur in domestic animals, especially in purebred dogs. Many of these defects involve the eyelids.

Entropion, a condition in which all or part of the margin of the eyelid is turned inwards, may involve one or both eyelids. This common ocular condition is reported in pedigree dogs and sporadically in lambs.

Figure 21.11 Sequential stages in the formation of the lens. A, Formation of lens placodes from surface ectoderm. B and C, Stages in the invagination of the lens placodes leading to formation of the lens vesicle. D, Separation of the lens vesicle from the surface ectoderm. E, Elongation of cells in the posterior wall of the lens vesicle. F, Obliteration of the cavity within the developing lens.

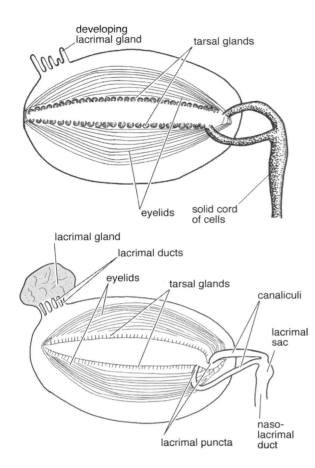

Figure 21.12 Stages in the development of the lacrimal apparatus.

Ectropion, an everted margin of the eyelid with a large palpebral fissure, is reported in several breeds of dogs including Bloodhound, Great Dane, St. Bernard and several spaniel breeds. As a consequence of ectropion, conjunctival exposure to environmental irritants and bacterial infections may result in chronic conjunctivitis in affected animals.

The absence of an eye, anophthalmos, due to developmental failure of the optic vesicle, is rare in animals. Microphthalmos, an abnormal reduction in ocular size affecting one or both eyes, sometimes occurs in association with other ocular abnormalities.

Non-closure of the lips of the choroid fissure results in a defect on the ventral surface of the eyeball referred to as coloboma. Failure of the fissure to close may occur anywhere along its length. The condition, which occurs in all domestic species, is especially prevalent in collie dogs as one of the manifestations of the collie eye anomaly, a consequence of defective growth of the optic cup.

Corneal opacity, which results from persistent pupillary membranes, is due to persistence of some of the meso-

derm covering the anterior surface of the lens during early development. During the formation of the anterior chamber of the eye, mesoderm which fails to undergo apoptosis may persist as a partial sheet of cells on the anterior surface of the lens. This condition, which occurs as a hereditary defect in the Basenji breed, also occurs in Welsh Corgi, Chou Chou and some other dog breeds.

Congenital cataract, an opacity of the lens or its capsule, is a condition which is reported sporadically in animals. The condition, although usually genetically determined, may result from environmental factors. A higher incidence of congenital cataracts is reported in horses than in other domestic animals.

Ear

The ear, the special sensory organ of the body associated with hearing and equilibrium in vertebrates, has three distinct sub-divisions referred to as the external, the middle and the inner ear. Each of these sub-divisions has a separate embryological origin. The external ear, which directs sound towards the middle ear, is formed from the first pharyngeal cleft and its surrounding mesoderm. This part of the ear consists of the auricle, the external auditory meatus and the outer lining of the tympanic membrane. The middle ear, which conducts sound from the external to the inner ear, is derived from the first pharyngeal pouch and its surrounding mesoderm. This segment of the ear is composed of the auditory tube, the tympanic cavity and its associated auditory ossicles. The inner ear, also referred to as the vestibulocochlear organ, includes the utricle, the semicircular ducts and the saccule. This sub-division of the ear develops from the otic placode. The vestibular apparatus is the sensory transducer for balance, while the cochlear apparatus contains auditory sensory receptors. Impulses sensed by these organs are relayed to the brain by cranial nerve VIII.

In an evolutionary context, vestibular function, which precedes hearing, is one of the earliest special senses to evolve. Fish, which lack both an external and middle ear, have a sensory organ which corresponds to the vestibular component of the inner ear of mammals. Thus, the piscine inner ear serves primarily as an organ of balance. In amphibians, reptiles, birds and mammals, hearing became a vital sense as these diverse animals evolved from an exclusively aquatic to a terrestrial environment. Accordingly, auditory function, which became as important as that of equilibrium, is related to the evolution of the external and middle ear, structures associated with the reception of sound waves and their transmission to the inner ear.

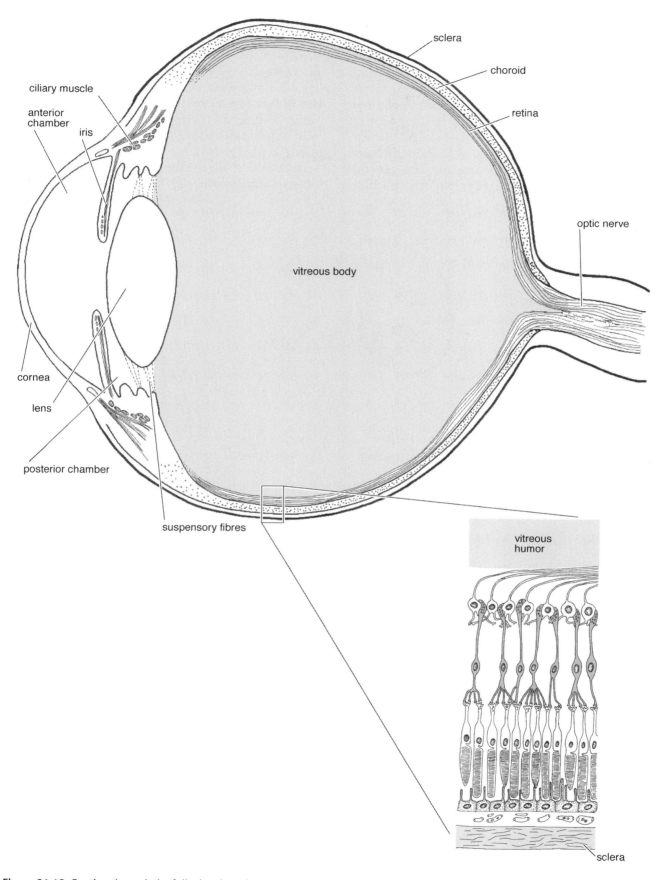

Figure 21.13 Section through the fully developed eye.

Inner ear

Bilateral ectodermal thickenings, the otic placodes, which develop in a position lateral to the rhombencephalon give rise to the inner ears (Fig. 21.14). The diverse membranous structures which develop from the otic placodes are collectively referred to as the membranous labyrinth of the inner ear. Invagination of the otic placode forms the otic pit, which, for a short time, retains its connection with surface ectoderm and then separates forming the otic vesicle. The cavity of the otic vesicle fills with fluid, referred to as the endolymph. Some cells which bud from the vesicle give rise to the sensory ganglia of cranial nerve VIII. An evagination from the dorso-medial region of the otic vesicle elongates forming the endolymphatic duct. Subsequently, the terminal end of this duct dilates forming the endolymphatic sac which occupies a position beneath the dura mater. The otic vesicle differentiates into two distinct regions, a dorsal expanded part referred to as the utricle, and a ventral portion, the saccule (Fig. 21.15). Two flat structures, which subsequently develop surface depressions,

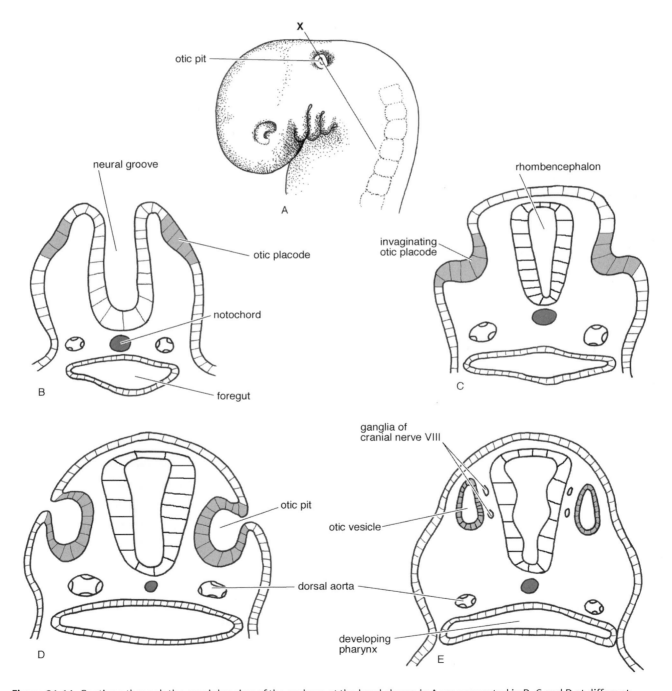

Figure 21.14 Sections through the cranial region of the embryo at the level shown in A are presented in B, C and D at different stages of development, leading to the formation of the otic vesicles, E.

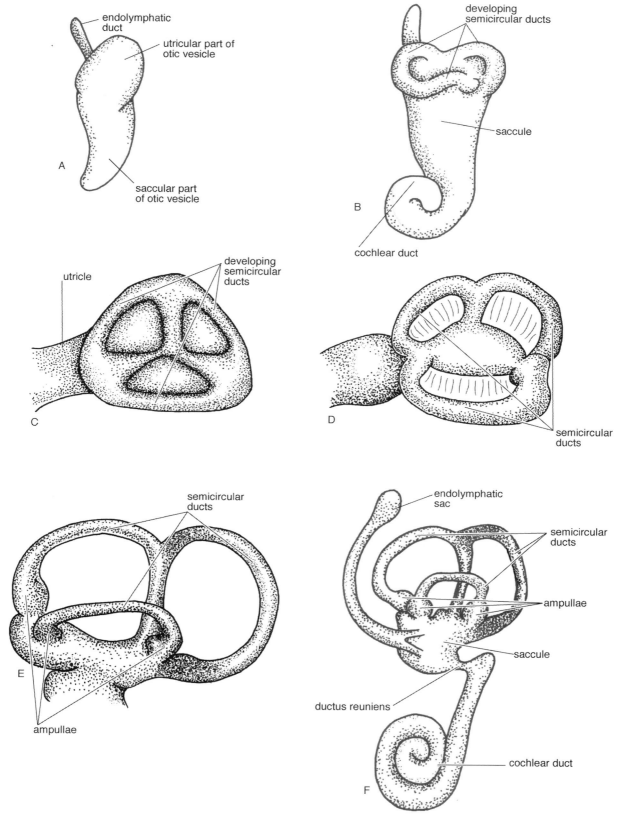

Figure 21.15 Stages in the formation of the membranous components of the inner ear. A, Development of the utricle and the saccule from the otic vesicle. B, Early stage in the formation of the semicircular ducts from the utricle and of the cochlear duct from the saccule. C and D, Intermediate stages in the formation of the semicircular ducts. E, Fully-differentiated semicircular ducts. F, Membranous components of the inner ear.

extend from the utricle. One of these structures occupies a vertical position parallel to the medial plane. The second is positioned at right angles to the first, in a horizontal position parallel to the lateral plane and located lateral to the first (Fig. 21.15). Division of the first structure which occupies a position parallel to the medial plane gives rise to anterior and posterior semicircular structures. Subsequently, the central portion of these divisions undergoes apoptosis and two tubes referred to as the anterior and posterior semicircular ducts are formed. In their final position relative to each other, these two semicircular ducts form a 90° angle. The medial portions of the two primordia persist as the common trunk of these two ducts. The central portion of the diverticulum, which occupies a position parallel to the lateral plane, also undergoes apoptosis and the residual tissue forms the lateral semicircular duct. In its final position, this semicircular duct is at right angles to the two vertically positioned ducts. Dilatations at the end of each semicircular duct, referred to as ampullae, contain the sensory organs of balance (Fig. 21.15).

The saccule forms a ventral evagination, the cochlear duct, which first tapers and then adopts a spiral configuration (Fig. 21.15). A narrow duct which maintains communication between the cochlear duct and the saccule is referred to as the ductus reuniens. The mesenchyme surrounding the membranous labyrinth differentiates into cartilage. The inner lining of this cartilaginous shell undergoes vacuolation resulting in a space between the outer shell of the cartilaginous and membranous labyrinth, the perilymphatic space. This space becomes filled with fluid referred to as perilymph. The perilymphatic space which surrounds the cochlear duct becomes sub-divided into two spaces, the scala tympani and the scala vestibuli (Fig. 21.16). The cochlear duct is separated from the scala vestibuli by a vestibular membrane and from the scala tympani by the basilar membrane. The lateral wall of the cochlear duct is attached to the cartilaginous shell by the spiral ligament, while its medial angle is connected to and supported by a cartilaginous process, the modiolus. Later, the cartilaginous capsule surrounding the membranous labyrinth of the inner ear is replaced by bone, forming the osseous labyrinth within the petrous temporal bone of the skull.

A group of cells which migrate from the medial wall of the otic vesicle to a more medial position contribute to the formation of the stato-acoustic ganglion. Some components of this ganglion also derive from neural crest cells. Later, the ganglion divides into cochlear (spiral) and vestibular portions which relay impulses to the brain from the sensory cells of the organ of Corti, the saccule and the semicircular ducts via the fibres of cranial nerve VIII.

Middle ear

The first pharyngeal pouch, which develops as an endodermal out-pouching of the foregut between the first and second pharyngeal arches, gives rise to the auditory tube and primitive tympanic cavity of the middle ear. The definitive tympanic cavity is formed from the dorsal blind end of the first pharyngeal pouch which grows towards the first pharyngeal cleft. The inner ectodermal wall of the first cleft and the endodermal wall of the tympanic cavity are separated by a layer of mesenchyme. Later, the mesodermal layer decreases in depth and forms a thin connective tissue layer interposed between the outer ectodermal layer of the first pharyngeal cleft and the inner endodermal layer of the tympanic cavity. The membrane formed from the fusion of these three tissues is the tympanic membrane. This structure forms a partition between the external ear and the middle ear. In *Equidae*, a large ventral diverticulum develops from each auditory tube, the guttural pouches. These large mucus-secreting sacs communicate with the pharynx via the auditory tube. While the functional significance of these pouches is uncertain, they may have a role in controlling blood pressure in the internal carotid arteries or they may act as a cerebral blood-cooling system in times of exercise stress. Because of their vulnerability to infection and their proximity to vital vascular and nervous structures, the guttural pouches are of clinical importance.

The ossicles of the middle ear are formed from the mesoderm of the first and second pharyngeal arches (Fig. 21.17). The malleus and incus are formed from mesoderm of the first pharyngeal arch while the stapes is formed from mesoderm of the second arch. At first, the ossicles are composed of mesenchyme; later they become cartilaginous and finally, the cartilage is replaced by bone. The ossicles, which are initially embedded in loose mesenchymal tissue, later become suspended within an air-filled cavity as the mesenchyme is resorbed. The endodermal epithelium which lines the tympanic cavity extends into the newly formed cavity and both surrounds and suspends the ossicles. The malleus, which becomes anchored to the tympanic membrane, articulates with the incus, which in turn articulates with the stapes. The oval-shaped footplate of the stapes fits into a corresponding oval opening in the osseous labyrinth, the vestibular window, where it is held in position by a flexible annular ligament. Two muscles, both mesodermal in origin, which assist in the transmission of auditory stimuli, develop within the middle ear. The tensor tympani muscle, which develops from the first pharyngeal arch, is innervated by cranial nerve V, and the stapedius muscle, which arises from the second pharyngeal arch, is innervated by cranial nerve VII.

Figure 21.16 Sequential stages in the formation of the structures of the inner ear. A, Cochlear duct surrounded by cartilage. B, Further development of the cochlear duct and development of the perilymphatic space. C, Formation of the scala tympani and scala vestibuli, the cochlear duct and the spiral ganglion in the osseous labyrinth.

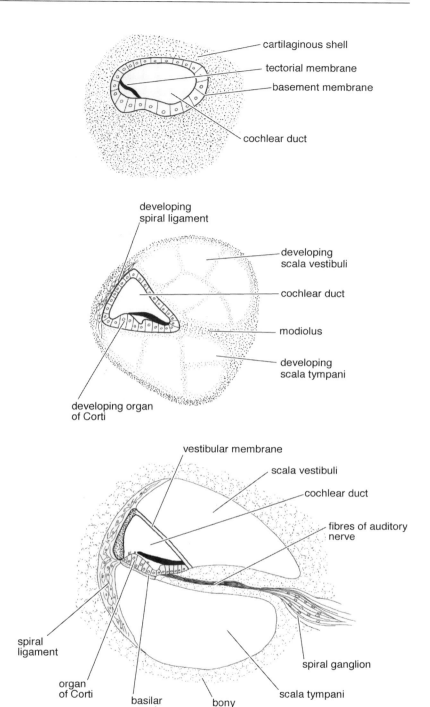

External ear

The auditory meatus of the external ear develops from the first pharyngeal cleft. Ectodermal cells at the blind end of the first pharyngeal cleft proliferate forming a solid epithelial mass, the meatal plug (Fig. 21.17). The plug, which persists for most of the foetal period, undergoes lysis in the peri-natal period. The ectoderm of the expanded auditory meatus comes in close contact with the endodermal wall of the tympanic cavity separated only by a thin layer of mesoderm. Collectively, these three layers form the tympanic membrane. The structures of the auricle of the external ear which surround the entrance of the external auditory meatus derive from mesenchymal proliferations around the first pharyngeal cleft.

The anatomical arrangements of the external ear, middle ear and inner ear of the dog and their associated structures are shown in Fig. 21.18.

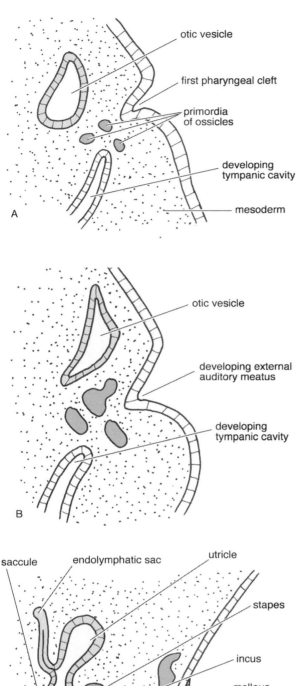

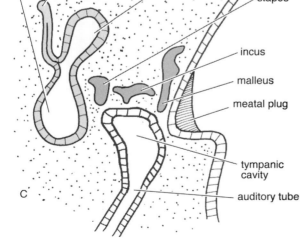

Figure 21.17 Stages in the formation of the middle and external ear.

Otic induction

The inductive mechanisms which relate to the development of the ear are gradual processes involving a number of interactions between different tissues. Both the hindbrain and the cranial mesoderm have been implicated as signalling sources for otic placode induction. At a stage related to somitogenesis, different regions of ectoderm have the capacity to respond to otic inductive signalling to varying degrees, with the head ectoderm adjacent to the otic placode the most receptive to induction. Studies have highlighted members of the fibroblast growth factor family, Fgf-3, Fgf-8, Fgf-10 and Fgf-19, as important otic inducers. In the species studied, Fgf-3 expression is found in the hindbrain primordium by the end of gastrulation and its expression is maintained as the otic placode forms. Across species, Fgf-3 is the most widely conserved otic inducer. A number of other otic inducers including Wnt-8 are recognised. It is uncertain, however, if Wnt-8 induces otic development directly in association with Fgf, or indirectly by up-regulating *Fgf* gene expression.

A number of genes are expressed in the early stages of otic development and serve as molecular markers for this process. The transcription factor Pax-8, which is the earliest marker of otic fate, is expressed in the pre-otic cells of vertebrates during the latter half of gastrulation. A closely related homologue, Pax-2, has also been identified as a regulator of otic development and is expressed in pre-otic cells by the early stage of somitogenesis. Although *Pax-2* is not required for otic induction in murine models, it is required for development of the cochlea. Because members of the Pax family of transcription factors are closely related in molecular structure, redundancy in genes encoding these factors may compensate in part for any disruption in the function or expression of these genes, making it difficult to elucidate the precise role of specific Pax genes in otic development.

Members of the distal-less (Dlx) and eyes-absent (Eya) family of transcription factors are expressed in the pre-placodal domain and play critical roles in pre-otic development in vertebrate models. Targeted disruption of the murine *Eya-1* gene results in developmental failure of the otic vesicle following its formation. Although *Dlx-5* does not alter placodal development, *Dlx-5* mutants do not develop anterior and posterior semicircular ducts. In double murine mutants for *Dlx-5* and *Dlx-6*, otic placode development is impaired. Dlx genes function in concert with another gene family, the muscle segment homeobox, Msx, genes. Dlx proteins act as transcriptional activators, regulating differentiation and positional identity, while Msx proteins are transcriptional repressors which inhibit cellular differentiation and promote cellular proliferation. The co-expression of Dlx and

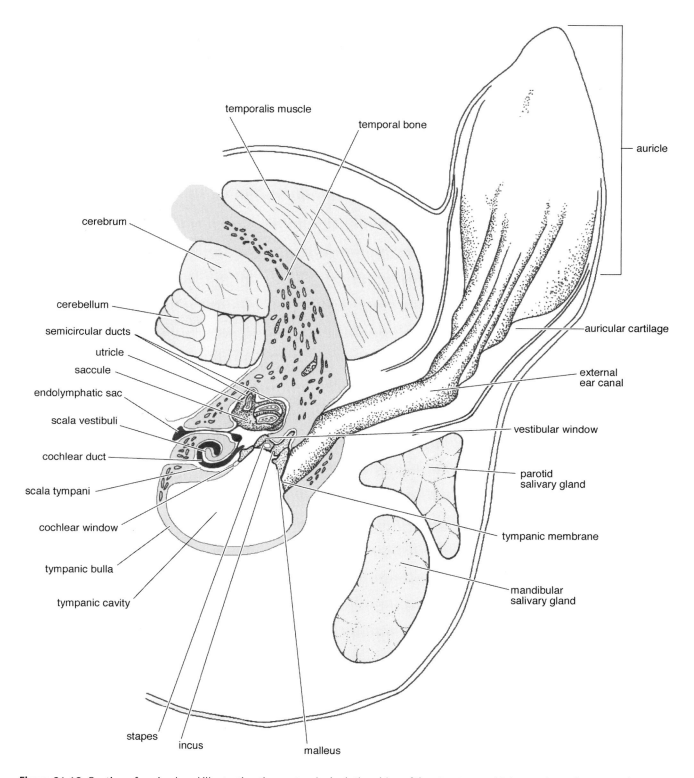

temporalis muscle

temporal bone

auricle

cerebrum

cerebellum

semicircular ducts

utricle

saccule

endolymphatic sac

scala vestibuli

cochlear duct

scala tympani

cochlear window

tympanic bulla

tympanic cavity

auricular cartilage

external
ear canal

vestibular window

parotid
salivary gland

tympanic membrane

mandibular
salivary gland

stapes

incus

malleus

Figure 21.18 Section of canine head illustrating the anatomical relationships of the structures which constitute the external ear, middle ear and inner ear of the dog. Other cranial structures are also shown.

Msx genes probably maintains an equilibrium between proliferation and differentiation in otic development.

Patterning of the otic placode

Alterations in the levels and regions of expression of some genes relevant to otic development, such as *Dlx* and *Pax-2*, are regulated by Shh. Retinoic acid produced by cells in the developing otic vesicle is required for normal patterning of this structure.

Further reading

Aguirre, G., Rubin, L.F. and Bistner, S.I. (1972) The development of the canine eye. *American Journal of Veterinary Research* **33**, 233–241.

Baptiste, K.E. (1998) A preliminary study on the role of the equine guttural pouches in selective brain cooling. *Veterinary Journal* **155**, 139–148.

Bistner, S.I., Rubin, L.F. and Aguirre, G. (1973) The development of the bovine eye. *American Journal of Veterinary Research* **34**, 7–12.

Cvekl, A. and Tamm, E. (2004) Anterior eye development and ocular mesenchyme: new insights from mouse models and human diseases. *BioEssays* **26**, 374–386.

Jean, D., Ewan, K. and Gruss, P. (1998) Molecular regulators involved in vertebrate eye development. *Mechanisms of Development* **76**, 3–18.

McConaghy, F.F., Hales, J.R.S., Rose, R.G. and Hodges, D.R. (1995) Selective brain cooling in the horse during exercise and environmental heat stress. *Journal of Applied Physiology* **79**, 1849–1854.

Myers, L.J. and Coulter, D.B. (2004) Vision. In *Dukes' Physiology of Domestic Animals*, 2nd edn. Ed. W.O. Reece. Comstock Publishing Associates, Cornell University Press, Ithaca, NY, pp. 843–851.

Priester, W.A. (1972) Congenital ocular defects in cattle, horses, cats and dogs. *Journal of the American Veterinary Medical Association* **160**, 1504–1511.

Riley, B.B. and Phillips, B.T. (2003) Ringing in the new ear: resolution of cell interactions in otic development. *Developmental Biology* **261**, 289–312.

Samuelson, D.A. (1991) Ophthalmic embryology and anatomy. In *Veterinary Ophthalmology*, 2nd edn. Ed. K.N. Gelatt. Lea and Febiger, Philadelphia, pp. 3–123.

Strain, G.M. and Myers, L.J. (2004) Hearing and equilibrium. In *Dukes' Physiology of Domestic Animals*, 2nd edn. Ed. W.O. Reece. Comstock Publishing Associates, Cornell University Press, Ithaca, NY, pp. 852–864.

Szabo, K.T. (1989) *Congenital Malformations in Laboratory and Farm Animals*. Academic Press, San Diego.

Wilcock, B.P. (1993) The eye and ear. In *Pathology of Domestic Animals*, 4th edn. Eds. K.V.F. Jubb, P.C. Kennedy, and N. Palmer. Academic Press, San Diego, pp. 441–529.

22 Integumentary System

The integumentary system comprises the skin, hair, skin glands, hooves, claws, digital pads, horns and feathers. Although the mammary gland is a skin-derived organ which is sometimes considered with the integumentary system, because of its close association with female reproduction it is included in Chapter 18. The skin, the body's external covering, is a complex structure which functions as a protective layer against physical, mechanical, chemical and biological injury. In addition, it has a role in body temperature regulation, reception of external sensory stimuli, secretion, immune responses, vitamin D synthesis and body surface pigmentation.

The skin consists of two layers: a superficial layer, the epidermis, which is derived from ectoderm, and a deeper layer, the dermis, which develops from mesoderm.

Epidermis

The epidermal layer covering the embryo initially consists of a single layer of cuboidal cells resting on a basal lamina (Fig. 22.1A). Shortly after neurulation, these ectodermally-derived cells divide and give rise to a superficial layer of flattened cells, the periderm, and an underlying layer of cuboidal cells, the basal layer (Fig. 22.1B). Further proliferation of the cells of the basal layer gives rise to an intermediate layer resulting in a multi-layered covering, the epidermis (Fig. 22.1C and D). The exchange of water, sodium and glucose between amniotic fluid and the epidermis probably involves peridermal cells. Close to mid-pregnancy, the basal epidermal cells under the periderm undergo differentiation, giving rise to the typical epithelial layers characteristic of post-natal stratified squamous epithelium consisting of a stratum basale (stratum germinativum), stratum spinosum, stratum granulosum and stratum corneum (Fig. 22.1E). The cells in these epithelial layers which synthesise the scleroprotein keratin are termed keratinocytes. Transforming growth factor-α (Tgf-α) is one of a number of factors which promote the differentiation of the epidermal cells. This factor is synthesised in the basal epidermal cells and acts as an autocrine growth factor, stimulating proliferation of these cells. Keratinocyte growth factor, otherwise known as Fgf-7, which is produced by the fibroblasts of the underlying mesenchymally-derived dermis, regulates the growth of the basal cells

of the epidermis. As the epithelium differentiates into its characteristic layers, the peridermal cells, which undergo apoptosis, are shed into the amniotic fluid. Loss of the peridermal layer and formation of the stratum corneum of the stratified squamous epithelium coincide with cessation of exchange of water and electrolytes between amniotic fluid and epidermis. This loss of exchange may also be related to the commencement of kidney function and the passing of urine into the amniotic cavity with its accumulation within the amniotic sac. In some areas of the body, proliferation of the cells of the basal layer gives rise to epidermal papillae which extend into the underlying developing dermis. During the period of epidermal proliferation, cells of neural crest and mesodermal origin also contribute to the population of cells found in the skin. Melanoblasts, derived from the neural crest, migrate to the underlying mesoderm and later move to the basal layer of the epithelium where they differentiate into melanocytes, cells which synthesise melanin pigment. Melanin is stored intracellularly as granules referred to as melanosomes. These pigment granules, which are moved to the tips of dendritic processes of melanocytes, are transferred to adjacent keratinocytes by a process referred to as cytocrine secretion. Within keratinocytes, melanosomes become strategically positioned where they act as a barrier to solar radiation. Melanosomes also impart pigmentation to the skin, hair, hooves, horns and a number of ocular structures.

Langerhans cells, which derive from the bone marrow, are of the monocyte–macrophage lineage. These cells, which are more numerous in the stratum spinosum than in other layers of the epithelium, are present in the epidermis from an early stage in embryonic development. Langerhans cells, which act as antigen-presenting cells for T lymphocytes, are a peripheral component of the immune system.

A third cell type, the Merkel cell, which migrates to the basal layer of the epidermis, functions as a sensory cell through its interaction with free nerve endings. Although the origin of Merkel cells is unresolved, there is convincing evidence that they derive from the neural crest. These cells can detect tactile stimuli and changes in contact pressure.

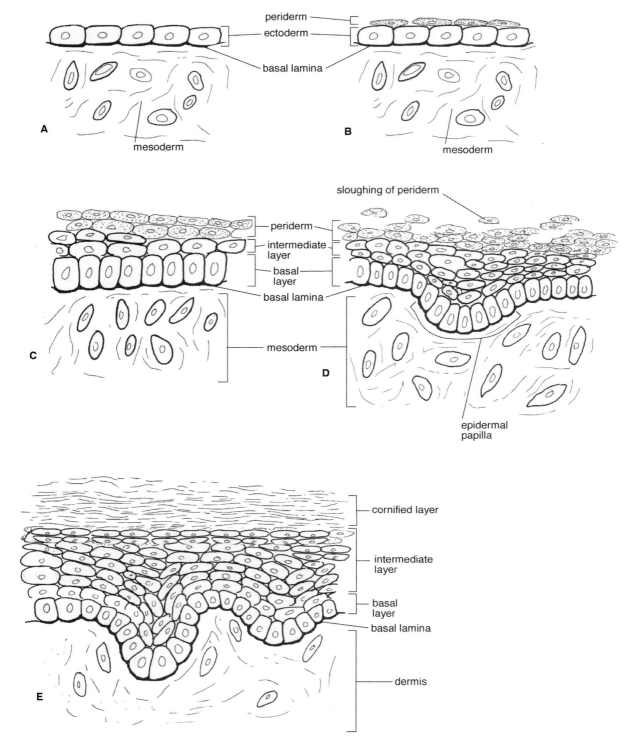

Figure 22.1 Successive stages in the development of the epidermis and dermis. A, Ectoderm composed of a single layer of cells with underlying mesoderm. B, Development of periderm. C, Formation of a multi-layered epidermis. D, Foetal epidermis showing the formation of an epidermal papilla. E, Development of the epidermis at the late foetal stage showing the typical layers of stratified squamous epithelium.

Dermis

The dermis, which develops during the late embryonic period, arises from mesenchymal cells derived in part from dermatomal cells and also from somatopleural mesoderm. The mesenchyme differentiates into the connective tissue cells which give rise to collagenous and elastic fibres. The dermis, which is located immediately beneath the epidermis, projects between the epidermal papillae. The superficial papillary layer of the dermis is composed of loose connective tissue, while the thicker underlying reticular layer contains dense irregular connective tissue. Afferent nerve fibres, which grow into the dermis, innervate the dermis and epidermis.

Hypodermis

Beneath the dermis in most regions of the body, mesenchymal cells form a layer of loose connective tissue, the hypodermis, consisting of irregular bundles of collagen fibres interspersed with elastic fibres and adipocytes. This layer of loose connective tissue anchors the skin to underlying structures. Hypodermis is not present in particular regions such as the lips, cheeks, eyelids, auricles of the ears, and anus, and in its absence the dermis attaches to the underlying structures. The hypodermis is usually referred to as subcutaneous connective tissue in histology, whereas in gross anatomy it is referred to as the superficial fascia. Bundles of skeletal muscle, the subcutaneous muscle, develop in the hypodermis in specific regions of the body, such as the thoracic and cervical regions. The nature and depth of the hypodermis vary considerably with species. Because the hypodermis is less dense in carnivores and sheep than in other domestic species and contains a high proportion of elastic fibres, the skin in these animals can be easily raised by grasping. In pigs, the hypodermis, which is a comparatively thick layer, attaches the skin firmly to the underlying structures. Porcine fat in the hypodermis forms a well-defined layer, the panniculus adiposus, which may be up to 5 cm thick. In horses, cattle and goats, which have a thin layer of hypodermis, the skin closely follows the outline of the underlying structures. The presence of fat in the hypodermis contributes to insulation against heat loss.

The skin contains a variety of nerve endings which are more numerous in hairless areas than in hair-covered areas. While sensory fibres are prominent in the dermis and hypodermis, they also extend to the external root sheaths of hair follicles and between the cells of the deeper layers of the epidermis. Nerve endings in the skin can morphologically be divided into free nerve endings and encapsulated nerve endings. Free nerve endings, which are found principally in the epidermis, detect stimuli associated with pain, heat and cold. Structures with diverse morphology, referred to as encapsulated nerve endings, are located in the dermis or hypodermis and serve as mechanoreceptors. Innervation of blood vessels and sweat glands is supplied principally by the sympathetic division of the autonomic nervous system.

Three vascular plexuses parallel to the skin surface, the subcutaneous, cutaneous and superficial plexuses, provide the arterial blood supply to the skin. The subcutaneous plexus derives from arterial branches to superficial cutaneous structures. The cutaneous plexus, which supplies the hair follicles and sweat glands, arises from branches of the subcutaneous plexus. The superficial plexus, which derives from branches of the cutaneous plexus, supplies the papillary processes. The epidermis derives its nutrients and oxygen by diffusion from the capillary loops in the papillary processes. A network of veins corresponding to the arterial plexuses provides venous drainage. In superficial regions of the dermis, a lymphatic network which forms plexuses drains into cutaneous lymphatic vessels.

Hair

One of the features which distinguishes mammals from other vertebrates is the presence of hair. Slightly raised elevations on the smooth bare skin in areas around the lips, periorbita, cheeks and lower jaw of the foetus are the first macroscopic evidence of hair development. With the exception of notable anatomical regions, the entire body surface of domestic animals is covered by closely-spaced hairs. Areas devoid of hair include the muzzle, muco-cutaneous junctions, hooves and digital pads. Marked variation in hair density, type, distribution pattern and colour is evident among species, and, within species, hair characteristics are breed-related.

The primordial structures from which hairs develop arise during the early foetal period when the epidermis is composed of three layers. Solid proliferations from the basal layer of the epidermis which project into the underlying mesoderm, form hair buds or pegs (Fig. 22.2). As the hair bud extends into the dermis at an oblique angle, an aggregation of mesenchymal cells, known as the hair papilla, projects into the tip of the bud. The epidermal cells of the bud grow around the hair papilla like an inverted cup, forming the hair bulb. The structure formed from the epidermal ingrowth, together with the hair papilla, is referred to as a hair follicle. The inner layer of epidermal cells of the hair bulb which gives rise to the hair shaft and epithelial root sheaths is known as the germinal matrix.

The formation of hair follicles requires interactions between cells in the basal layers of the epidermis and the underlying mesoderm. It has been postulated that the relative concentrations of the transcription factors Tcf-3 and Lef-1 regulate the ability of stem cells to differentiate and form hair. A Wnt family signal is required in the dermis for generation of the first dermal signal which directs the formation of a hair follicle. The dermal signal activates ectodysplasin synthesis in the ectoderm, which, together with Wnt signals from the buds themselves, contributes to the initiation of hair bud formation. These Wnt signals regulate expression of *Shh* and *Bmp* genes. The signalling molecule Shh induces the aggregation of

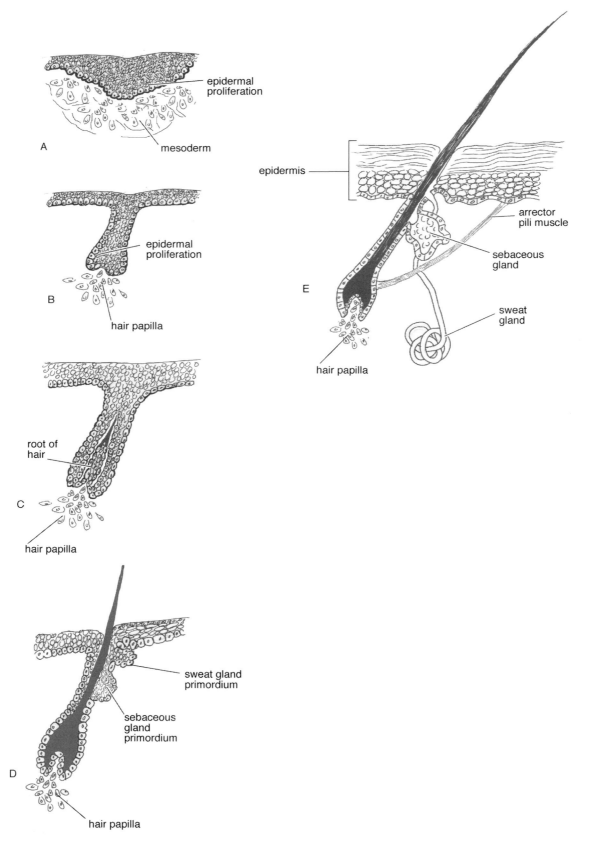

Figure 22.2 Stages in the development of a simple hair follicle. A, Primordium of hair follicle. B, Hair bud. C, Bulbar stage of follicle formation. D, Projection of hair shaft from the follicle and formation of primordium of a sebaceous gland and a sweat gland. E, Mature hair follicle showing arrector pili muscle, sebaceous gland and apocrine sweat gland.

mesenchymal cells in the dermis and promotes the development of individual hair follicles. The Bmp signals suppress hair follicle development in regions of the dermis immediately adjacent to an existing hair follicle primordium, thus regulating the spacing of hair follicle formation.

The developing hair follicle which connects the germinal matrix with the surface becomes canalised and the layer of epidermal cells surrounding the newly-formed space gives rise to the external root sheath of the follicle. Cells in the centre of the germinal matrix adjoining the hair bulb proliferate and are displaced into the lumen of the external root sheath, forming the hair shaft. Continued proliferation of the basal cells of the matrix force the hair shaft towards the surface of the skin from which it subsequently projects. As cells of the hair are pushed towards the surface and move further away from the papilla, their source of nutrients, they undergo keratinisation. Cells at the periphery of the germinal matrix proliferate and grow between the hair shaft and the external root sheath forming the internal root sheath. This internal root sheath, which extends halfway along the follicle, produces soft keratin. Melanocytes present in the hair bulb impart pigmentation to the developing hair.

Hair keratin expression has a distinct pattern along the length of hair shafts. The keratins Ha-2 and Hb-2 are expressed specifically in the hair cuticle, the layer of cells on the surface of the hair shaft, while Ha-1 expression begins at the transitional region between the matrix and cortex and continues throughout the lower and middle portions of the cortex. Differential expression of these keratin proteins may influence hair texture.

Mesenchymal cells surrounding the developing hair follicle differentiate into a connective tissue sheath. A small band of smooth muscle, also derived from mesenchymal cells in the dermis, attaches this connective tissue sheath to the superficial layer of the dermis on the side of the hair follicle which forms the greater angle with the surface. On contraction, these muscle bands, known as arrector pili muscles, decrease the greater angle between the hair follicle and the skin surface, thereby moving the hair shaft into an erect position. Arrector pili muscles are especially well developed along the dorsal midline of dogs where they cause the hair to become erect in response to a threat of aggression.

Primordia of sebaceous glands form as cellular outgrowths from the basal layer of the walls of developing hair follicles at levels closer to the surface than the points of attachment of arrector pili muscles (Fig. 22.2D). Smaller epidermal outgrowths, superficial to sebaceous gland primordia, may develop from the follicular wall forming the primordia of sweat glands (Fig 22.2D).

Hair follicles are classified as either primary or secondary. Primary hair follicles have a large diameter and the bulbs are located deep in the dermis. Arrector pili muscles and both sebaceous and sweat glands are normally associated with primary follicles. A single hair which emerges from these follicles is referred to as a guard hair. Initially, primary hair buds tend to develop at closely-spaced time intervals and at even distances from each other. Subsequently, new primary follicles develop among those already established, resulting in groups of two, three or four follicles in close proximity to each other. Hair follicles which have a relatively small diameter and are located more superficially in the dermis than primary follicles are referred to as secondary follicles. Hairs which emerge from secondary follicles are referred to as secondary or under hairs. While secondary follicles have associated sebaceous glands, unlike primary follicles they lack sweat glands and arrector pili muscles.

Hair follicles may be described as simple, when a single hair is present, or compound, when two or more hairs project through a common pore (Fig. 22.3). In dogs and cats, compound hair follicles develop post-natally. In canine skin, up to 15 secondary buds develop from the primary follicles in a manner analogous to the development of primary buds, giving rise to hair shafts which project from the skin surface through a common pore.

There is wide variation not only in hair follicle types but also in their surface distribution among domestic

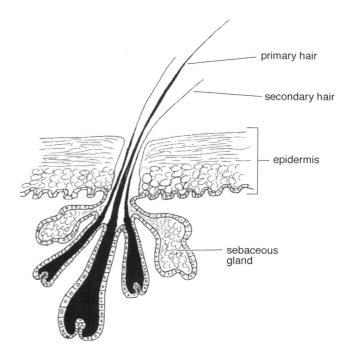

Figure 22.3 Compound hair follicle, which develops post-natally, showing the primary hair and associated secondary hairs.

animals. Only primary hair follicles, which are distributed evenly in rows over the body surface, are present in horses and cattle. In pigs, primary hair follicles occur in clusters with three or four primary hair follicles per cluster. From the compound follicles in canine skin which occur in clusters of three, a single large primary hair surrounded by a group of smaller secondary hairs emerges. In cats, single large primary follicles are surrounded by two to five compound follicles. Each compound follicle has three coarse primary hairs and from six to twelve secondary hairs.

In sheep, wool hair follicles occur in clusters. Typically, each cluster consists of groups of follicles composed of three primary follicles interspersed among secondary follicles. Although the ratio of secondary follicles to primary follicles varies in different locations of the body, there are up to six times the number of secondary follicles to primary follicles per group. The number of secondary follicles present in the skin of high-wool-producing sheep is greater than in mountain breeds.

Sinus hair follicle

Hairs which grow from special follicles, referred to as sinus hair follicles, have sensory or tactile functions. Such hairs are referred to as sinus, sensory or tactile hairs. Sinus hair follicles are distributed primarily in the head region, predominantly around the lips, cheeks and chin, and above the eyes. In cats, sinus hair follicles are also present in the carpal region. Although sinus hair follicles evolved later than other hair follicles, their appearance precedes other hair follicle types during foetal development. Sinus hair follicle development is initially similar to primary hair follicle development. Later, however, a sinus hair follicular bud enlarges and extends deep into the hypodermis. Sinus hair follicles have no related sweat glands and their associated sebaceous glands are poorly developed. The development of a blood-filled sinus which separates the dermal connective tissue sheath into an inner and outer layer is a characteristic feature of a sinus hair follicle. In ruminants and horses, trabeculae are present between the outer and inner layers of the dermal sheath. Skeletal muscle attached to the outer dermal sheath of sinus hair follicles permits a degree of voluntary control over tactile hair orientation. Free nerve endings, which are numerous within the inner dermal sheath and extend into the outer root sheath, are responsible for the exquisite sensitivity of tactile hairs.

Hair growth cycle

Post-natally, hair growth occurs cyclically with alternating periods of proliferation and quiescence. The hair growth cycle is divided into three phases: an actively growing stage, anagen, followed by a regressional stage, catagen, and a resting stage termed telogen (Fig. 22.4). During the anagen stage, cellular proliferation in the matrix of the follicular bulb results in active hair growth. With the regression which occurs in the catagen stage, hair follicle cell proliferation decreases. In this stage, the hair root becomes club-shaped, the hair follicle becomes shorter and the hair papilla enters a regressive phase. During telogen, the club-shaped hair root is surrounded by its external root sheath only and the follicle remains attached by a cord of epithelial cells to the regressing hair papilla. At this stage, the distal end of the hair follicle is at the level of the attachment of the arrector pili muscle. Subsequently, a renewed anagen stage commences which leads to the formation of a replacement hair. The epithelial cord gives rise to a new hair bulb which caps the newly-developing hair papilla. As the replacement hair extends towards the surface into the external root sheath, it gradually displaces the old hair on to the surface, where it is shed. In both humans and domestic animals, hormonal factors can markedly influence hair growth and hair loss.

The rate at which animals shed their hair varies with species. In rats and mice, the hair growth cycle lasts less than a month, unlike most other animals, which shed their coats seasonally, either once or twice a year. Domestic sheep shed only a small proportion of their wool hair fibres seasonally. However, in some sheep breeds, the hair growth cycle extends over several years.

Mammalian skin glands

Based on their morphology and secretions, two distinctly different types of glands, sweat glands and sebaceous glands, can be identified in mammalian skin. In particular species of animals, special skin glands located in different regions of the body develop either as a modification of one of these basic types or from a combination of both types.

Sebaceous glands

Glands referred to as sebaceous glands are distributed in the skin of domestic animals in association with hair follicles (Fig. 22.2). These glands usually develop later than sweat glands and arise as lateral outgrowths of the basal epithelium of the developing follicles below the level of sweat gland primordia. Sebaceous glands are numerous and prominent in cattle, dogs and cats but are generally sparse and inconspicuous in pigs. These glands develop as pear-shaped lobular structures with clusters of acini opening into a single short wide duct. As a consequence of repeated mitotic division within sebaceous glands, small basal cells give rise to cells which migrate into and fill the acinar lumen. As these cells enlarge, they accumulate lipid droplets and their nuclei become pyknotic and disappear. Subsequently, with the disintegration of

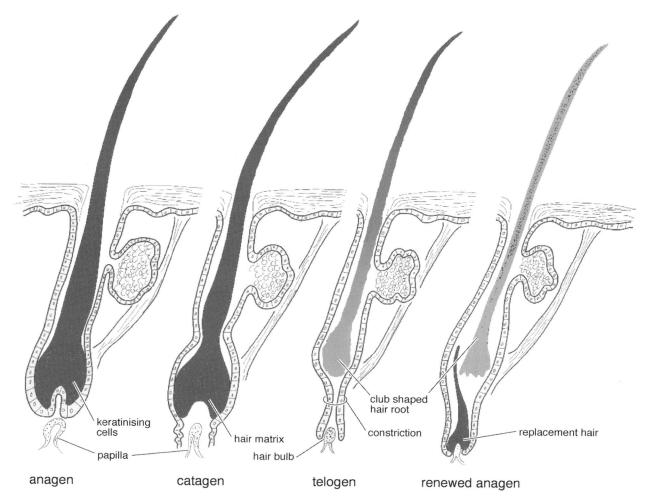

Figure 22.4 Sequential stages in the hair cycle, anagen, catagen, telogen and commencement of a new anagen stage.

these sebaceous gland cells, sebum, which consists of a mixture of lipid, keratohyalin granules, keratin and associated cellular debris, is produced. Sebum is discharged through short ducts into the lumen of the hair follicles. Because the entire sebaceous gland cell forms the material secreted by the gland, the mode of secretion of sebaceous glands is termed holocrine. Sebum, which has antibacterial and antifungal activity, lubricates the hair and skin and maintains the skin in a pliable state. In addition, sebum enhances the water-repelling properties of the integument and limits water loss through evaporation. Both gonadal and adrenal hormones influence sebaceous gland secretion.

In horses, the secretions of sebaceous glands, which are especially well developed and extensively distributed, in combination with the secretions of sweat glands which are rich in proteins, generate a profuse lather-like effect evident after sustained exercise. Some domestic species have especially well developed accumulations of sebaceous glands in defined regions of the body. These include glands in the infraorbital, inguinal and interdigital regions of sheep, base-of-horn glands in goats, and paranal sac glands and circumanal glands in carnivores.

Sebaceous glands are absent from the muzzles of cattle and the snouts of pigs, from footpads, hooves, claws and horns and also from the teats of cows.

Sweat glands

Based on their modes of secretion, mammalian sweat or sudiferous glands are considered to be of two types, apocrine and eccrine. Secretion from eccrine glands, merocrine secretion, is through exocytosis, a process whereby small secretory granules are discharged into the gland ducts. Apocrine glands discharge large granules within secretory vesicles which contain a portion of the cell's cytoplasm. This process of secretion is referred to as apocrine secretion.

Apocrine sweat glands develop as nodular outgrowths of the basal layer of the epithelium of the hair follicle closer to the skin surface than sebaceous glands (Fig. 22.2). The dense cellular proliferation extends into the connective tissue, and the base of the gland may be located below the level of the hair bulb. The distribution of apocrine sweat glands, although constant within a given species, varies among species. In addition, variation in the structural features of glands is evident. The distal end of the developing gland may be coiled into a spherical structure or may assume a spiral appearance. A lumen develops in the distal region of the apocrine gland and extends to the site of origin of the gland where it opens into the hair follicle as the gland duct. Following formation of the lumen, the gland is lined by a double layer of cells; the inner layer forms the secretory acini and the outer layer differentiates into myoepithelial cells located between the secretory cells and the basal lamina. The secretory acinus has a large lumen lined by cuboidal or columnar epithelium. The gland duct has a narrow lumen and is lined by a double layer of cuboidal epithelium. During development, some ducts open directly on to the skin surface, independent of hair follicles. Apocrine sweat glands are the principal sweat glands in those regions of the skin of domestic animals which are covered with hair. Secretions of apocrine sweat glands are viscous and contain a scent which is characteristic of the individual animal and of the species. In humans, apocrine sweat glands are confined to the eyelids and the axillary, pubic and perineal regions.

The openings of the ducts of eccrine glands are not usually associated with hair follicles. Where the ducts penetrate the cornified epithelium of the skin, they have a corkscrew-like appearance and their openings on the body surface can be seen as fine pores. In humans, eccrine sweat glands are the predominant sweat glands, while in domestic animals they are confined to the footpads of carnivores, the frog of equine hooves, porcine snouts and bovine muzzles.

The naming of sweat glands as apocrine or merocrine as used in this chapter conforms to conventional nomenclature which was based on their perceived modes of secretion. Current research findings question the validity of this nomenclature as there is a lack of conclusive evidence of cytoplasmic loss in so-called apocrine sweat gland secretion. Accordingly, it seems preferable to describe the mode of secretion of all sweat glands as merocrine. Nevertheless, the long-established terms apocrine and merocrine have been retained as a basis for naming these morphologically distinct glands.

Avian skin

The avian body is covered by thin, poorly keratinised skin composed of epidermis and dermis. The stratified squamous epithelium of the epidermis contains fewer layers than mammalian skin. The dermis consists of a superficial layer of loose connective tissue containing delicate collagenous fibres and a deeper layer of coarse interwoven fibres. The hypodermis contains an abundance of fat cells. Apart from the large, branched, alveolar, holocrine gland, the uropygial gland, the skin of birds contains no glands. The uropygial gland, which

resembles a sebaceous gland and is located at the base of the tail, is a bi-lobed structure. In domestic poultry, the gland is drained by a pair of ducts, each of which opens on to the skin surface through a single nipple-like papilla. This gland produces an oily secretion which the bird applies to its feathers during preening. Uropygial glands initially develop as paired glands which later unite, forming a single bi-lobed structure. These glands are more highly developed in aquatic than in non-aquatic birds. In a number of avian species, including pigeons, parrots and woodpeckers, a uropygial gland does not develop. Many epithelial cells in specific regions of avian skin have the ability to secrete lipid droplets which help to protect the skin and render it waterproof.

A unique feature of avian skin is its covering of feathers. In addition to their contribution to flight, feathers entrap air for insulation, help to maintain a constant high body temperature, and reduce water loss through evaporation.

Feathers

The first indication of feather development occurs in a chick embryo at approximately the eighth day of development. It is characterised by a concentration of dermal cells beneath an epithelial thickening. Further development results from an epithelio-mesenchymal interaction inducing the formation of cone-shaped papillae which displace the overlying epidermis outwards, forming feather buds (Fig. 22.5). The epidermal cells at the base of each bud sink into the dermis forming ectodermally-lined follicles. As the feather follicles elongate, the apices of the feather buds project from the openings of the follicles. The type of feather formed by a feather bud is influenced by the subsequent stages of development. The early stages of follicular development in down and contour feathers are similar (Fig. 22.5). In down feather formation, cells at the base of the circular feather papilla proliferate forming an epithelial collar from which a number of longitudinal columns of cells project into the dermal core of the papilla. The columns separate and become cornified, each giving rise to a barb ridge, a barb primordium (Fig. 22.5). The epidermal layer of the follicle forms an outer sheath which covers the circlet of developing barbs. When an individual feather reaches its maximum length, the outer sheath splits open, allowing its barbs to expand in a plume-like fashion, forming the definitive down feather. Regular branches, referred to as barbules, which are given off from barbs, contribute to the insulating properties of down feathers. The quill, that part of the feather from which barbs do not develop, arises from the follicle collar at the base of the follicle. The feather is anchored in the follicle by the cylindrical quill.

The early stages of contour feather development are similar to those described for down feathers. However,

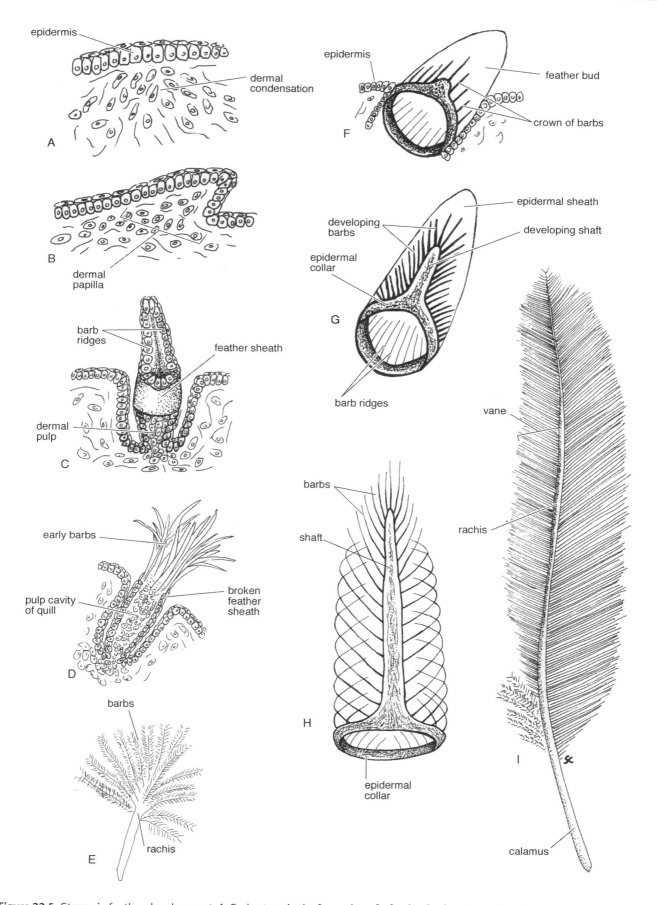

Figure 22.5 Stages in feather development. A, Early stage in the formation of a feather bud. B, Formation of a cone-shaped dermal papilla. C, Feather bud projecting from the skin surface at the stage of follicle formation. D, Feather barbs projecting through broken sheath. E, Down feather. F, Early stage in cell proliferation from the epithelial collar of a feather follicle. G, Formation of barbs from a developing rachis. H, Circular arrangement of feather barbs before they assume a flat form. I, Contour feather.

as contour feather development proceeds, proliferation of a discrete segment of the superficial portion of the epithelial collar occurs, forming a shaft or rachis ridge which elongates towards the apex of the feather follicle. Barbs, which project from either side of this shaft, grow in a circular fashion within the confines of the epidermal sheath. Subsequently, the outer sheath of the feather bud splits, the apical part of the shaft and barbs are freed from their conical encasement and the barbs straighten. The barbs, which project from either side of the fully formed rachis, collectively constitute a flattened structure referred to as the vane. The base of the feather shaft, which is located within the follicle and is devoid of barbs, is referred to as the quill or calamus (Fig. 22.5). Two signalling factors, Bmp-2 and Shh, are the principal regulators of feather morphogenesis. A distinct expression pattern of Shh and Bmp is established at each stage of feather development.

In the proximal region of the barb ridges, Shh promotes cell proliferation while in the distal regions of this structure, Bmp-2 suppresses Shh and promotes differentiation. A balance between the factors Bmp-4 and noggin determines the number, size and spacing of barb ridges, while Shh also influences the spacing between barbs by inducing apoptosis.

The first feathers formed by the embryo are down feathers, while the most prominent feathers formed in mature birds are the contour feathers. In addition, semiplume, filoplume and bristle feathers may be present in different avian species. Semiplumes insulate against heat loss, and in aquatic birds they increase buoyancy. Filoplumes are located very close to contour feathers. Their follicles have many associated free nerve endings and it is suggested that these feathers have a role in the proprioceptive sensation necessary for the optimal orientation of contour feathers. Bristle feathers, which are comparatively rigid, are located around the nostrils and eyes and may have tactile functions. Feathers normally develop along predetermined feather tracts or pterylae, with featherless apterylae arranged between feathered areas.

Congenital and inherited defects of the skin

Defects of the skin may be genetic in origin or may occur due to non-genetic factors during embryological development. Genetic mutations which cause skin anomalies may be evident at birth or may become apparent during post-natal development. Classification of defects is usually based on the cells or structures where the primary abnormality is expressed. Structures involved may include the epidermis, dermis, hair follicles or sweat glands.

Congenital absence of an area of epidermis, *epitheliogenesis imperfecta*, has been recorded in piglets, calves,

lambs and foals. Lesions are well demarcated and the exposed dermis is susceptible to trauma which predisposes to secondary bacterial infection.

A congenital condition characterised by abnormal and hypertrophic epithelial proliferation with accumulation of thick, horny scales, separated by fissures which follow the wrinkle lines of the skin, is referred to as congenital ichthyosis. The term is based on the similarity of the affected skin to fish scales. The condition has been reported in cattle and dogs. In cattle, the defect which has a hereditary basis, is attributed to a single recessive gene.

A group of skin conditions which result from defects in dermal-epidermal attachment structures are sometimes referred to as epidermolysis bullosa syndromes. These conditions, which have been reported in all domestic animals, predispose to dermal-epidermal separation following minor cutaneous trauma with the formation of flaccid bullae at the site of injury. Lesions may be present at birth or may develop post-natally.

With inherited epidermal dysplasia of calves, animals appear normal at birth but begin to lose condition between 4 and 8 weeks of age. The skin over most of the body becomes slightly thickened, relatively hairless and scaly. Affected calves become progressively emaciated within months. Histological skin changes include acanthosis and hyperkeratosis.

Absence of hair, alopecia, and the presence of less hair than normal, hypotrichosis, occur occasionally in domestic animals. Congenital hypotrichosis has been reported in cattle, sheep and pigs. Follicular dysplasia affects many dog breeds and some cat breeds. Skin and coat colour abnormalities are sometimes associated with hypotrichosis.

Hooves and claws

In regions of the skin which are constantly exposed to pressure and other forms of mechanical stress, the keratinised layer of the epidermis is thickened. A family of major structural proteins, α-keratins, present in the epidermis, are found in mammalian skin and some skin derivatives. In mammals, structures with high mechanical resistance such as hair, hooves, horns and claws contain α-keratins with a high content of trichohyalin together with sulphur-containing proteins. In quadruped mammals, the extremities of the digits are exposed to the greatest mechanical impact. Accordingly, over a long evolutionary period, the extremities of the limbs of mammals have become altered and modified in various ways for the protection of the underlying tissues. Thus, the feet of animals reflect evolutionary changes involving the epidermis, dermis and hypodermis and the bones, tendons and ligaments of the pedal region. The modified keratinised skin, together with those parts of the terminal phalanges, including supporting connective tissue and skeletal structures, enclosed by this modified skin, constitute the digital organ. These digital organs are suitably adapted to meet the locomotory needs of individual species. Based on the form of their digital organs, domestic mammals may be divided into two groups, the unguiculates, or clawed animals which include the carnivores, and the ungulates, or hoofed animals, including horses, ruminants and pigs. Hooves and claws are the modified keratinised epidermal capsules enclosing the underlying structures of the distal phalanges. In addition to their protective functions, hooves and claws are used for scratching or digging and also as weapons. Although the digital organs of different species are morphologically distinct, in reality they have many developmental features in common.

Equine hoof

The equine hoof has evolved from a four-toed foot in the oldest known ancestor of the horse, the *Eohippus*, to a single-toed foot, which illustrates the final stage of digitigrade evolution. Grossly, the equine hoof consists of the horny epidermal covering of the distal end of the digit, comprising the wall, sole and frog (Fig. 22.6).

During the early foetal period, the epidermis on the dorsal and lateral surfaces of the terminal region of the third digit proliferates. The thickened epidermis covers a thin layer of dermis up to the end of the second month of gestation, when the developing hoof is approximately 6–10 mm in length. Although the terms 'dermis' and 'corium' are sometimes used interchangeably, the term 'corium' is used here in relation to hoof and horn. During the third month, increased growth of the corium and hypodermis at the junction of the hair-bearing skin and hoof occurs, forming a proximal, slightly elevated perioplic cushion and a more prominent distal elevation, the coronary cushion. The hypodermis of the frog and bulbs increases in depth, giving rise to the shock-absorbing digital cushions. The tissues of the digital cushions consist of elastic, fibrous and adipose tissue which is especially abundant in the region of the bulbs where it forms shock-absorbing pads. At this stage of its development, the typical hoof-shaped structure with its wall, bars, sole, bulbs and frog has the morphological characteristics of the mature hoof.

The embryonic hoof wall is formed from up to 600 corium-derived primary vertically orientated folds referred to as laminae, which extend from the coronary groove to the weight-bearing surface of the hoof. Each lamina has a central dermal core covered by an epidermal layer. Between 100 and 200 secondary laminae extend at right angles from each primary lamina. The epidermal papillae, which arise from the inner layer of the coronary cushion, fuse forming coronary cushion-derived keratinised epidermal laminae which extend between the murally-derived epidermal laminae. Continued proliferation of the coronary cushion-derived epidermal laminae causes these laminae to move distally past the stationary cells of the non-keratinised epidermal laminae of the wall which are firmly anchored to the corium. The coronary cushion-derived laminae give rise to secondary laminae which also interdigitate with the secondary laminae derived from the hoof wall. This complex interdigitation anchors the keratinised hoof to the underlying connective tissue.

The outer layer of epidermis overlying the coronary cushion forms cone-shaped papillae which contain central cores of corium, the dermal papillae. Growth of the epidermal papillae is parallel to the long axis of the third phalanx, at an oblique angle to the sole. The basal epidermal cells located at the apex of the papillae proliferate and grow distally towards the ventral surface, forming epidermal tubules. Individual tubules, which may be round, oval or wedge-shaped in cross-section, consist of a hollow medulla containing cellular debris surrounded by a dense, lightly pigmented cortex of keratinised cells referred to as hoof horn. This tubular horn develops in a manner comparable to hair shaft development. The basal epidermal cells deep in the inter-papillary region proliferate and give rise to inter-tubular horn, which is relatively unstructured and fills the space between the horn tubules. Close to the eighth month of gestation, epidermal papillae on the surface of the periople proliferate and form a layer of soft tubular and inter-tubular horn, which extends over part of the surface of the hoof wall, imparting a glossy appearance to the wall. The perioplic epidermis also grows over the bulbs of the heel forming soft horn.

The horn of the hoof wall derives from three regions of epidermal growth. Proliferation of the epidermal cells of the periople gives rise to the outer layer, the stratum externum. The epidermal papillae of the coronary cushion give rise to tubular and inter-tubular horn which forms the intermediate layer, the stratum medium. The inner layer or stratum internum derives from the vertically orientated epidermal laminae. Post-natally, the wall of the hoof grows towards the ventral border at the rate of 4–6 mm per month, taking up to 12 months to grow from the coronary border to the weight-bearing ventral surface.

The horn of the hoof sole is formed from epidermal papillae. These papillae, which have dermal cores, grow towards the ventral surface forming tubular and inter-tubular horn in a manner similar to that described for the stratum medium (Figs. 22.6 and 22.7).

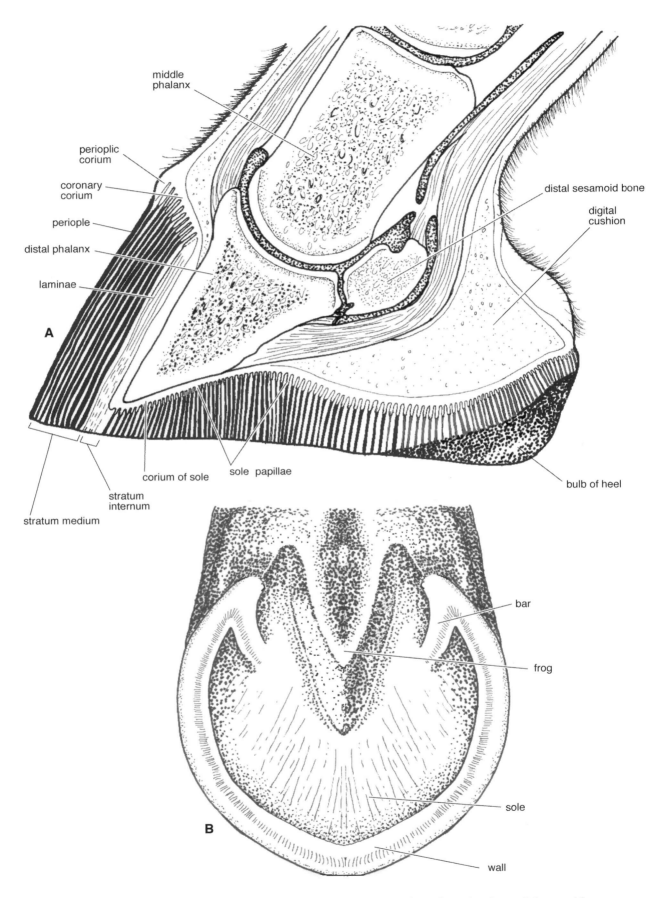

Figure 22.6 Equine hoof. A, Longitudinal section through the digital organ. B, Sole surface, showing wall, bars and frog.

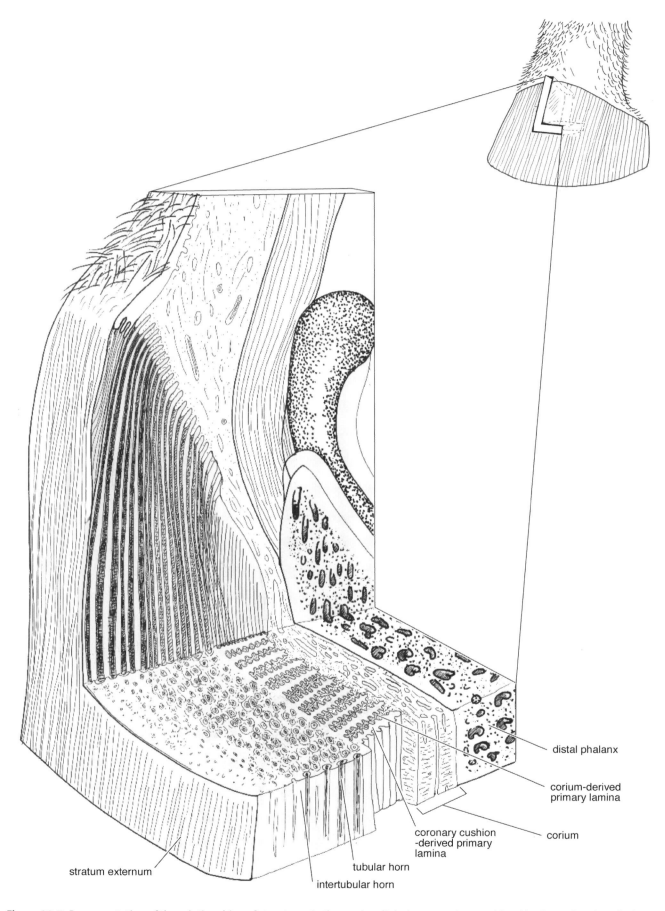

distal phalanx

corium-derived
primary lamina

corium

coronary cushion
-derived primary
lamina

tubular horn

intertubular horn

stratum externum

Figure 22.7 Representation of the relationships of structures in the equine digital organ using combined horizontal and vertical sections.

The horn of the frog, which has a soft texture, is formed from papillae in a manner similar to horn formation in the sole. The corium of the frog blends with the digital cushions. Secretions of branched eccrine glands in the digital cushions contribute to the frog's pliability.

Due to the persistence of the periderm in the developing hoof during gestation, the proliferating epidermis is initially soft and forms a cushion covering the tip of each hoof. This soft horn, referred to as the eponychium, prevents damage to the amnion during foetal movements in late pregnancy. Following parturition, the eponychium shrivels and wears off.

Chestnuts and ergots

The chestnut in the horse is a hairless horny protuberance of thickened keratinised tubular and inter-tubular horn with an underlying corium which is devoid of glands. On the forelimb the chestnut is located on the medial surface proximal to the carpus, while on the hind limb it is located on the medial surface distal to the tarsus (Fig. 22.8). There is wide variation in the size

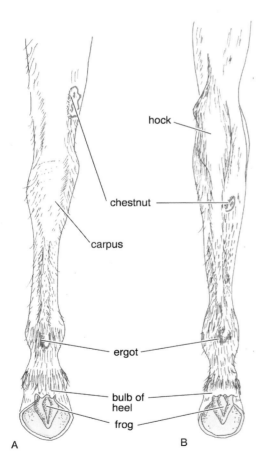

A   B

Figure 22.8 Caudal view of the left equine forelimb, A, and left equine hind limb, B, showing the positions of chestnuts and ergots.

and shape of chestnuts within horse breeds. Chestnuts, which are considered to be vestiges of carpal and metatarsal pads, are usually larger in forelimbs than in hind limbs. Occasionally, chestnuts are absent from the hind limbs.

Ergots, which appear as wart-like projections on the palmar and plantar surfaces of the fetlocks, consist of tubular and inter-tubular horn. These structures, which are hairless and thickly keratinised, are considered to be rudimentary sole pads of the third digits. Long hairs which grow around the ergots, and are particularly prominent in heavy draft horses, are referred to as feather.

Ruminant and porcine hooves

The pattern of development of the feet of even-toed ungulates resembles that of equine hooves but with some notable differences. Ruminant and porcine feet are composed of two weight-bearing hooves and two accessory, non-weight-bearing hooves (Fig. 22.9). The general structure of a hoof in ruminants and pigs closely resembles that of the equine hoof, consisting of a wall, sole and prominent bulb. The corium and hypodermis of ruminant and porcine hooves are also similar in structure and composition to the corium and hypodermis of an equine hoof; perioplic and coronary regions are also present. The epidermis of ruminant and porcine hooves consists of keratinised stratified epithelium. The periople and coronary epidermal papillae extend along a proximal–distal axis and form the tubular and inter-tubular horn of the wall. Ruminant and porcine hooves differ from equine hooves in that they have neither frogs nor bars, and, unlike equine hooves, do not have secondary laminae.

Canine and feline claws

In carnivores, the claw, which is composed of a hard keratinised layer of modified skin, encloses the distal phalanx. The claw, consisting of a wall and a sole, is conspicuously curved and corresponds to the shape of the enclosed phalanx (Fig. 22.10). The sole is formed from soft horn linking the thin lateral margins of the wall. The corium of the claw, which is composed of dense irregular connective tissue, forms a ridge over the dorsal surface of the distal phalanx. As the corium is highly vascular, damage to this structure from close clipping of the claws results in haemorrhage. A fold of skin referred to as the claw fold covers the proximal region of the claw. The outer surface of this fold has the typical features of normal skin, including hair cover. Proliferating epithelial cells of the inner surface of the fold, which is hairless, form a thin layer of keratinised cells which cover the proximal region of the claw in a

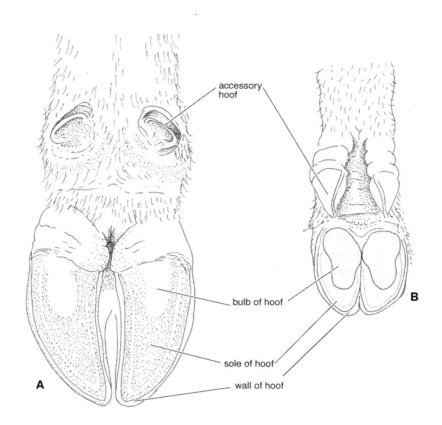

Figure 22.9 Caudal view of the distal end of the bovine forelimb, A, and porcine forelimb, B.

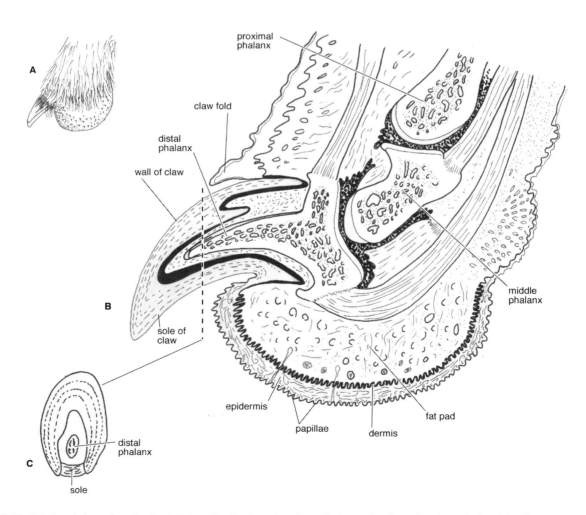

Figure 22.10 A, Lateral view of canine foot. B, Longitudinal section through the canine foot showing relationship of structures. C, Cross-section through claw at the level indicated.

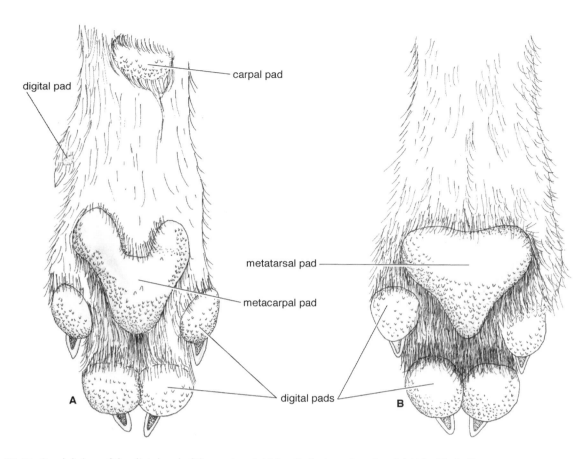

Figure 22.11 Caudal view of the distal end of the canine right forelimb, A, and canine right hind limb, B.

manner similar to the stratum externum of the equine hoof.

Footpads

Modified epithelial structures with a protective role, located on the palmar and plantar surfaces of canine and feline limbs, are referred to as footpads. In the forelimbs of carnivores, footpads include carpal pads, metacarpal pads and the pads of the second to the fifth digits. In the hind limbs, they include metatarsal pads and the pads of the second to the fifth digits (Fig. 22.11). Footpads are modified hairless regions of skin which offer protection during locomotion. They are covered by thick, keratinised, stratified, squamous epithelium containing all the layers present in the stratified epithelium of the skin, including a well-defined stratum lucidum. Because of the presence of keratinised papillae on the surface of the thick stratum corneum, the canine digital pad has a roughened surface. In contrast, the feline footpad has a smooth surface. The corium and hypodermis in footpads are well developed, particularly in the digital pads, where they form digital cushions. The digital cushions contain an abundance of adipose tissue and coiled tubular eccrine sweat glands.

Horns and related structures

The horns of domestic ruminants consist of bony cornual processes, covered by modified skin. The epidermal covering of horns, which is highly keratinised, is devoid of glands and hair. In domestic ruminants, horns, which are usually present in both sexes, are non-branching and have a conical shape. Bovine horn primordia are formed close to the end of the second month of gestation by cellular proliferation of the epidermis in the frontal region of the head. The primordia, which are surrounded by grooves, are covered by hair, with associated sweat and sebaceous glands. A delayed period of cornual development follows with no further epithelial proliferation occurring until after birth. The hair around these primordial structures, which grows longer than the hair in the surrounding areas, can be recognised by its whorl-like appearance post-natally.

At approximately one month of age, the hair and glands on the horn buds of calves atrophy and the epidermis proliferates forming conical horn buds. Soon afterwards, a bony outgrowth, which constitutes the osseous core of the developing horn, develops on each frontal bone. In succeeding months, the solid frontal cornual

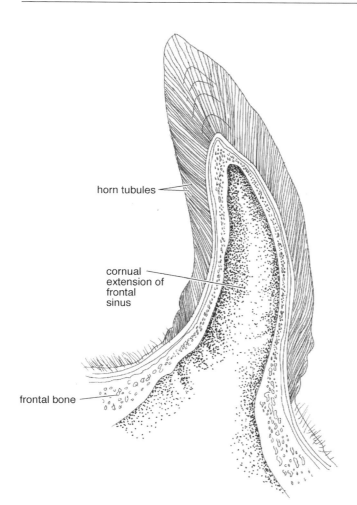

horn tubules

cornual
extension of
frontal
sinus

frontal bone

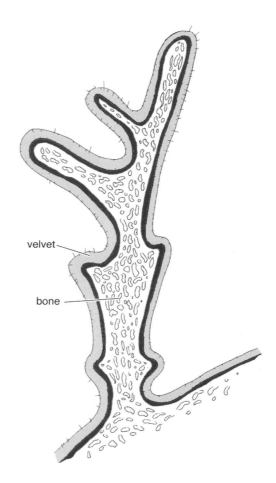

velvet

bone

Figure 22.13 Longitudinal section through velvet-covered antler of a deer.

Figure 22.12 Longitudinal section through a bovine horn.

process gradually becomes hollow. This process of cavitation continues in mature animals until only the tip of the frontal process remains solid. The space which constitutes the frontal sinus extends into the horn cavity (Fig. 22.12).

The corium covering the cornual process, which is fused with the periosteum, contains apically-directed papillae. The orientation of these apically-directed papillae ensures that as they proliferate, the horn increases in length as well as in thickness. The process whereby cornual epithelial proliferation gives rise to keratinised tubular and inter-tubular horn is similar to the process involved in hoof horn formation. Horn produced by the epidermis at the base of the cornual process is referred to as epiceras. This soft horn extends over the tubular and inter-tubular layer of horn and resembles the stratum externum produced by the periople in the equine hoof. Horn growth in bulls tends to occur evenly from the base of the horn to the apex, producing a uniformly smooth surface. In cows, and also in male and female small ruminants, periods of normal horn growth, followed intermittently by periods of less intense growth,

result in the formation of alternating ridges and grooves on the surface of the horn. During periods of stress, such as the increased nutritional and metabolic demands which occur in pregnancy and disease, a reduction in horn growth is reflected in groove formation on the horn. In cows, the period of reduced horn growth correlates with the late stage of pregnancy and high milk production. The associated horn depressions may be referred to as pregnancy grooves and can be used to estimate the age of cows which have had a number of calves. Assuming that a cow had her first calf towards the end of her second year, the cow's age is equivalent to the number of cornual grooves plus two additional years.

Antlers of deer and related species are branched outgrowths of bone from the skull which have a skin covering, referred to as velvet (Fig. 22.13). Among the Cervidae, these horn-like structures are usually present only in males, with the exception of caribou and reindeer, in which antlers are present in both sexes. Antlers undergo cyclical growth, maturation and shedding, a process which is associated with the breeding season.

The bone of antlers develops by a modified process of endochondral ossification during which cartilage at the tip of the branching antlers proliferates. The chondrocytes gradually cease to proliferate and the calcified cartilage is replaced by bone. At this stage, the antlers have achieved their maximum length. As the bone of the antler develops, it becomes covered by skin. Following cessation of antler growth, the blood supply to the velvet ceases, causing atrophy and ultimately sloughing of this tissue. At the end of the breeding season, constituents of the bone at the base of the antlers are resorbed and the structures break off, leaving bony pedicles, the sites of future antler re-growth.

The osseous processes of the frontal bones of giraffes are similar to antlers, but unlike antlers are not shed at the end of the breeding season. The so-called horn of the rhinoceros, which does not have a bony core, is composed of a solid mass of fused hair-like keratin fibres.

Further reading

Bragulla, H. (2003) Fetal development of the segment-specific papillary body in the equine hoof. *Journal of Morphology* **258**, 207–224.

Bragulla, H., Budras, K.-D., Mülling, C., Reese, S. and König, H.E. (2004) Common integument (integumentum commune). In *Veterinary Anatomy of Domestic Mammals*. Eds. H.E. König and H.-G. Liebich. Schattauer Publishers, Stuttgart, pp. 585–635.

Hamrick, M.W. (2001) Development and evolution of the mammalian limb: adaptive diversification of nails, hooves, and claws. *Evolution and Development* **3**, 355–363.

Jenkinson, D. (1967) On the classification of sweat glands and the question of the existence of an apocrine secretory process. *British Veterinary Journal* **123**, 311–316.

Pispa, J. and Thesleff, I. (2003) Mechanisms of ectodermal organogenesis. *Developmental Biology* **262**, 195–205.

Pollitt, C.C. (1992) Clinical anatomy and physiology of the normal equine foot. *Equine Veterinary Education* **4**, 219–224.

Pollitt, C.C. (1999) *Color Atlas of the Horse's Foot*. Mosby, Philadelphia, PA.

Prum, R.O. and Brush, A.H. (2003) Which came first, the feather or the bird? *Scientific American* **288**, 60–69.

Stump, J.E. (1967) Anatomy of the normal equine foot, including microscopic features of the laminar region. *Journal of the American Veterinary Medical Association* **151**, 1588–1598.

Wu, P., Hou, L., Plikus, M., Hughs, M., Scehnet, J., Suksaweang, S., Widelitz, R., Jiang, T. and Chuong, C. (2004) Evo-Devo of amniote integuments and appendages. *International Journal of Developmental Biology* **48**, 249–270.

Yu, M., Wu, P., Widelitz, R.B. and Chuong, C.M. (2002) The morphogenesis of feathers. *Nature* **420**, 308–312.

Yu, M., Yue, Z., Wu, P., Wu, D., Mayer, J., Widelitz, R.B., Jiang, T. and Chuong, C. (2004) The developmental biology of feather follicles. *International Journal of Developmental Biology* **48**, 181–191.

23 Age Determination of the Embryo and Foetus

The stages of *in utero* development which follow fertilisation and the formation of a zygote can be arbitrarily divided into two phases, the embryonic stage and the foetal stage. The embryonic period is defined as the interval from fertilisation to the development of organ primordia. This interval in sheep, pigs and dogs is approximately 30 days, whereas in humans, horses and cattle the interval extends up to approximately 56 days. Data related to the stages of development from zygote formation to implantation are presented in Table 23.1.

Developmental change during the embryonic period is rapid and by the end of this stage the primordia of most organs are established. The embryonic period is especially important as the differentiating cells which give rise to organ primordia are particularly susceptible to adverse genetic influences and deleterious external factors during this stage of development. The foetal period, which extends from the end of the embryonic period to parturition, is characterised by the growth and initiation of physiological functioning of body systems.

In order to compare the rate of development among different species and the effect of drugs, radiation and environmental factors on such development, it is necessary to record normal developmental features of the embryo and foetus for defined stages of gestation. Such information is of value for estimating the age of embryos collected from abattoirs for research purposes or of aborted foetuses. Data for domestic species have been compiled which record the stage of pregnancy coinciding with features such as total length, crown–rump length, somite count, presence of ossification centres and the appearance of external features such as eyes, ears, limbs, teeth and hair (Figs. 23.1 to 23.6). Data relating to numbers of somite pairs presented in Figs. 23.3 and 23.4 are derived from published sources. Limitations of these data relate to the fact that such information is based on mean values without regard for breed, litter size and the nutritional status of the dam. Recorded lengths of embryos of comparable ages may differ depending on whether the measurements are based on fixed or unfixed specimens, and in many

Table 23.1 Time in days, estimated from ovulation, at which early stages of embryological development occur in domestic animals, from zygote formation to implantation.

Species	Two-cell stage	Four-cell stage	Eight-cell stage	Morula formation	Blastocyst formation	Emergence of blastocyst from zona pellucida	Time interval during which implantation occurs
Cats	3	3.5	4	5	6 to 7	9	12 to 14
Cattle	1	1.5	2.6	6	7 to 8	9 to 11	17 to 35
Dogs	4	5	6	7	8	10	14 to 18
Goats	1.6	2.5	3.5	5	6 to 7	7 to 8	15 to 18
Horses	1	1.5	3.5	4.5	6 to 7	8 to 9	17 to 56
Pigs	1	2	3	4	6	6 to 7	12 to 16
Sheep	1.5	2	3	5	6	7 to 8	14 to 18

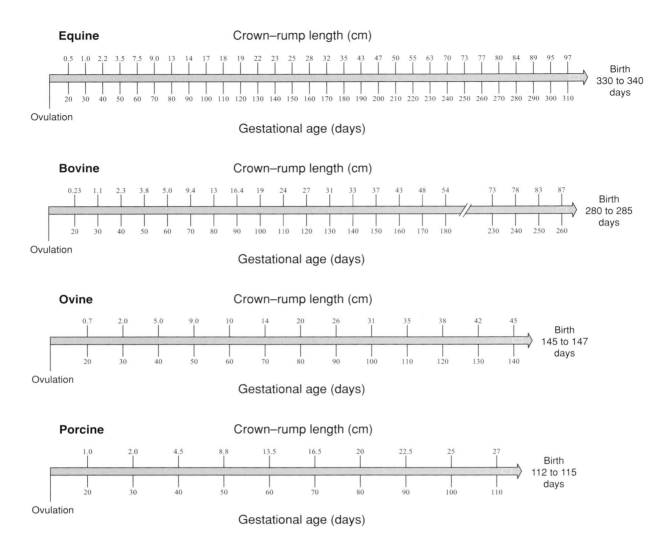

Figure 23.1 The relationship between crown–rump length and gestational age, measured from ovulation, at given times during *in utero* development in equine, bovine, ovine and porcine species. These measurements, which are compiled from published reports, are influenced by breed differences, genetic factors and nutritional influences and are intended as a guide to age determination.

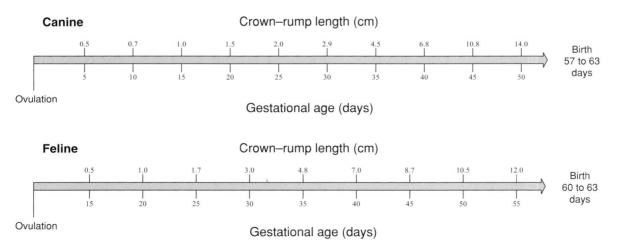

Figure 23.2 The relationship between crown–rump length and gestational age, measured from ovulation, at given times during *in utero* development in canine and feline species. These measurements, which are compiled from published reports, are influenced by breed differences, genetic factors and nutritional influences and are intended as a guide to age determination.

Equine

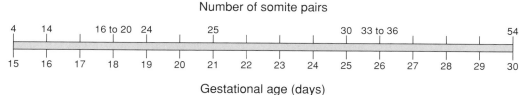

Bovine

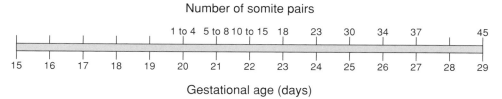

Ovine

Porcine

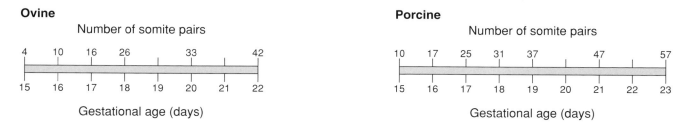

Figure 23.3 The number of somite pairs observed at different gestational ages, measured from ovulation, at given times during *in utero* development in equine, bovine, ovine and porcine species. To facilitate comparison of data, an arbitrary starting gestational age of 15 days has been selected for all species. These data, which are derived from published sources, are incomplete.

Canine

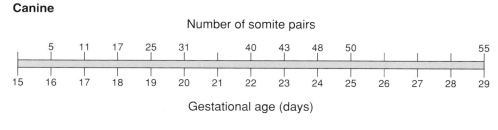

Feline

Figure 23.4 The number of somite pairs observed at different gestational ages, measured from ovulation, at given times during *in utero* development in canine and feline species. To facilitate comparison of data, an arbitrary starting gestational age of 15 days has been selected for both species. These data, which are derived from published sources, are incomplete.

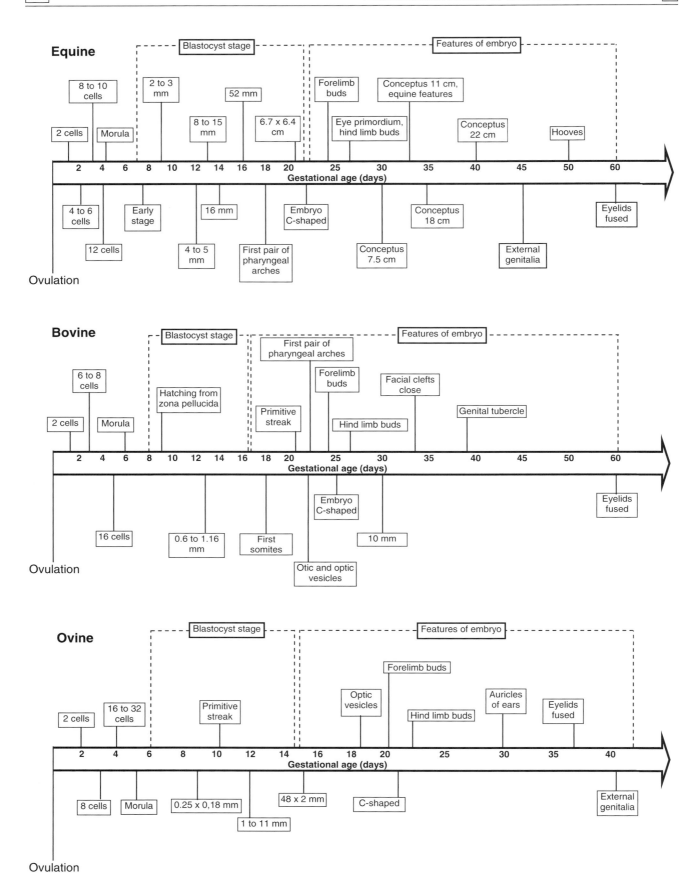

Figure 23.5 Developmental changes in equine, bovine and ovine embryos during early gestation. Measurements refer to approximate diameter of the blastocyst, the maximum length of the conceptus and the crown–rump length of the embryo. Some readily recognisable anatomical structures are listed.

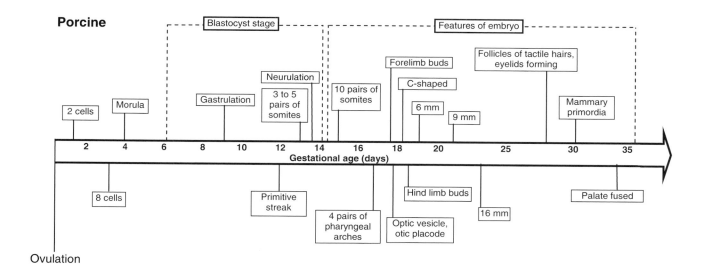

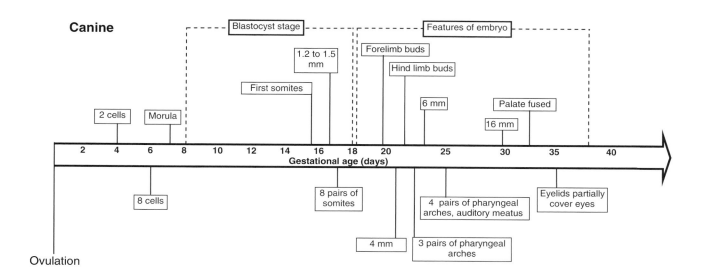

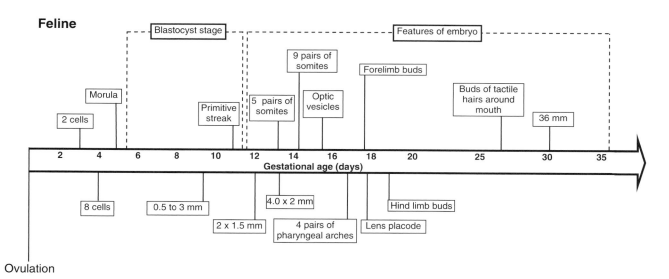

Figure 23.6 Developmental changes in porcine, canine and feline embryos during early gestation. Measurements refer to approximate diameter of the blastocyst, the maximum length of the conceptus and the crown–rump length of the embryo. Some readily recognisable anatomical structures are listed.

instances information on whether or not the embryos are fixed is not reported. As there are slight differences in the chronology and pattern of organ development in different species, measurement of length alone does not offer a valid comparison of the degree of development among different species. A more satisfactory method for studying inter-species differences is division of the period of development into a fixed number of stages, based on external features and organ development. Human embryonic development has been arbitrarily divided into 23 stages using similar criteria. While defined stages of development are documented for pigs and cats, a comparable system for other domestic animals has not yet been formulated. Because of the many factors which can influence *in utero* development, data presented in this chapter, which are compiled from published sources, should be considered only as an estimate of embryonic or foetal age.

Further reading

Bergin, W.C., Gier, H.T., Frey, R.A. and Marion, G.B. (1967) Developmental horizons and measurements useful for age determination of equine embryos and fetuses. Ed. F.J. Milne. In *Proceedings of the 13th Annual American Association of Equine Practice Meeting*. New Orleans, LA, pp. 179–196.

Butler, H. and Juurlink, B.H.J. (1987) *An Atlas for Staging Mammalian and Chick Embryos*. CRC Press, Boca Raton, FL.

Evans, H.E. (1974) Prenatal development of the dog. Gaines Veterinary Symposium, Cornell University, New York.

Evans, H.E. and Sack, W.O. (1973) Prenatal development of domestic and laboratory animals: growth curves, external features, and selected references. *Anatomia, histologia, embryologia* 2, 11–45.

Gjesdal, F. (1969) Age determination of bovine foetuses. *Acta Veterinaria Scandinavica* 10, 197–218.

Green, W.W. (1946) Comparative growth of the sheep and bovine animal during prenatal life. *American Journal of Veterinary Research* 7, 395–402.

Harris, H. (1937) The foetal growth of the sheep. *Journal of Anatomy* 71, 516–527.

Knospe, C. (2002) Periods and stages of the prenatal development of the domestic cat. *Anatomia, Histologia, Embryologia* 31, 31–51.

Lowrey, L.G. (1911) Prenatal growth of the pig. *American Journal of Anatomy* 12, 107–138.

Marrable, A.W. (1971) *The Embryonic Pig, a Chronological Account*. Pitman, New York.

Marrable, A.W. and Flood, P.F. (1975) Embryological studies on the Dartmoor pony during the first third of gestation. *Journal of Reproduction and Fertility Supplement* 23, 499–502.

Nichols, C.W., Jr. (1944) The embryology of the calf: fetal growth weights, relative age, and certain body measurements. *American Journal of Veterinary Research* 5, 135–141.

O'Rahilly, R. and Muller, T. (1987) *Developmental Stages in Human Embryos*. Carnegie Institution of Washington Publication.

Patten, B.M. (1948) *Embryology of the Pig*, 3rd edn. Blakiston, New York.

Rüsse, I. (1991) Frühgravidität, Implantation und Plazentation. In *Lehrbuch der Embryologie der Haustiere*. Eds. Rüsse, I. and Sinowatz, F. Paul Parey, Berlin, pp. 153–218.

Van Nierkerk, C.H. and Allen, W.R. (1975) Early embryonic development in the horse. *Journal of Reproduction and Fertility Supplement* 23, 495–498.

Warwick, B.L. (1928) Prenatal growth of the swine. *Journal of Morphology and Physiology* 46, 59–84.

24 Genetic, Chromosomal and Environmental Factors Which Adversely Affect Pre-natal Development

Abnormalities of the structure or function of cells, tissues or organs which are present at birth are termed congenital defects. These developmental defects can be caused by genetic, chromosomal or environmental factors.

Developmental defects in animals may result in early embryonic death, foetal death, mummification, abortion and stillbirths together with specific congenital defects relating to body systems. A congenital defect can be classified as a malformation, deformation or disruption. A malformation develops due to a defect which is intrinsic to the embryological differentiation or development of a structure. A deformation occurs due to an alteration in the shape or structure of a body part which had previously undergone normal differentiation. The term disruption refers to a structural defect which results from the destruction of a previously normal structure due to interruption of blood supply or to mechanical interference.

In both human and animal populations, reproductive failure encompasses sterility, infertility, abortions, stillbirths and malformations. Foetal growth retardation and prematurity at birth may also indicate interference with normal *in utero* development. Congenital defects can be caused by genetic factors and environmental influences; the aetiology of many is unknown. In the human population, it has been estimated that close to 70% of congenital defects are of uncertain or unknown cause; approximately 20% may be due to genetic factors such as mutations and chromosomal abnormalities, and 10% can be attributed to teratogenic environmental factors such as chemicals, therapeutic drugs, certain poisonous plants and infectious agents. Reliable data relating to the occurrence of congenital defects in animal populations are not readily available. Estimates

suggest that congenital defects in lambs, calves and foals occur to an upper limit of 3–4%. In dog populations developmental defects are reported to affect approximately 6% of pups. Congenital defects are reported infrequently in cats. Some developmental defects in animals can be related directly to nutritional deficiencies, consumption of toxic plants, exposure to environmental pollutants or injurious physical factors and to infections with pathogenic microorganisms. The frequency of defects varies with species, breed, season of the year, geographical location and the extent of the ingestion of toxic substances and of exposure to deleterious physical factors or infection with teratogenic pathogens. If infection occurs at an early stage of gestation, serious congenital defects may follow. Infection of the foetus with pathogenic agents before it becomes immunologically competent may result in immunotolerance to that pathogen. If such foetuses survive to birth, they remain infected for life and produce no immune response to the infectious agent which caused the congenital infection.

Mutations

Mutations, which can be defined as random changes in nucleotide sequences of genes, can occur spontaneously or may be induced by external influences. These changes can occur through the substitution, insertion or deletion of nucleotide bases. Genetic changes present in the gametes can be transmitted to future generations. The impact of a mutation on a developing animal depends on how the mutational change alters the conformation or function of a final gene product. Mutations which do not affect a coding region or do not alter the amino acid sequence of the final protein are referred to as silent mutations. Other mutations, however, can result in either complete loss of function or reduced activity in a specific gene product. In a given animal population, mutations

Table 24.1 Some animal diseases or conditions which result from dysfunction of a single gene.

Disease	Animal species	Affected gene product
Albinism	Cats, cattle, chickens, dogs, sheep	Tyrosinase
Dwarfism	Chickens	Growth-hormone receptor (GHR)
GM$_1$ gangliosidosis	Cats, cattle, dogs and sheep	β-Galactosidase
Goitre	Cattle, goats	Thyroglobulin
Henny feathering	Chickens	Aromatase
Leucocyte adhesion deficiency (LAD)	Cattle, dogs	β-2 Integrin (CD18)
Myotonia congenita	Dogs, goats and horses	Chloride channel
Malignant hyperthermia	Pigs	Ryanodine receptor
X-linked muscular dystrophy	Cats and dogs	Dystrophin

Table 24.2 Some genetically-based diseases or conditions in humans with single gene aetiology, displaying dominant or recessive inheritance patterns.

Disease or condition	Pattern of inheritance
Albinism	Recessive
Ataxia telangiectasia	Recessive
Brachydactyly	Dominant
Colour blindness	Recessive
Duchenne muscular dystrophy	Dominant
Haemophilia	Recessive
Huntington's chorea	Dominant
Phenylketonuria	Recessive
Pseudo-achondroplastic dwarfism	Dominant
Sickle cell anaemia	Recessive

at gene loci occur with a certain frequency per generation, known as the spontaneous mutation rate. This is typically one per million. Based on the underlying mechanisms which result in genetic change, mutations can be divided into two broad categories, spontaneous and induced. Spontaneous mutations result from errors in DNA replication and repair as well as errors which occur during recombination or movement of transposable elements. Induced mutation is a consequence of accidental or deliberate exposure to chemical or physical agents or mutagens which cause heritable alterations to DNA. Radiation can induce a variety of non-specific chromosomal and DNA aberrations. Following exposure to chemical mutagens, agents which induce mutation, DNA replication is affected in a manner which increases the rate of mutation above background level.

The simplest genetic models are exemplified by traits encoded by single genes which conform to classic Mendelian principles (Table 24.1). Single genes can exist in a number of alternate states, termed alleles, which can be described as dominant, recessive, co-dominant or partially dominant (Table 24.2). A recessive allele is one whose phenotypic effect is not expressed in the heterozygote. The phenotypic effect of a recessive allele is expressed only in animals homozygous for that allele. Animals homozygous for a non-functional tyrosinase gene exhibit the disease trait, albinism. Tyrosinase is required for the production of melanin from tyrosine. Dominant alleles are phenotypically expressed in animals heterozygous for that allele. Mutations in genes which are essential for survival are described as lethal mutations. Such mutations invariably result in premature death and consequently are not passed on to subsequent generations. Gangliosidosis is an example of a recessive lethal gene resulting from an inherited deficiency in β-galactosidase. This condition is not lethal in the heterozygous state. Some mutations in regions encoding for a gene product may not affect the animal's viability. They may, however, ultimately affect the animal's performance. Classically, animal breeders select animals for specific characteristics. Negative aspects of selective breeding include reduced variation, reduction in genetic fitness, increased homozygosity and potential for expression of undesirable characteristics, within a given population.

Chromosomal abnormalities

Deletions or aberrations which occur at a chromosomal level can sometimes be observed cytologically. Aberrations which have a deleterious effect on the developing animal frequently result in embryonic death. When the chromosome complement of a cell is altered by the addition or loss of a chromosome, this condition is termed aneuploidy. If a pair of chromosomes loses one of its number, the condition is referred to as monosomy, while the addition of a chromosome to a pair of chromosomes is referred to as trisomy. A number of conditions resulting from monosomy and trisomy have been characterised in humans (Table 24.3).

A chromosome can undergo changes whereby part of its structure is either relocated within the same chromosome

Table 24.3 Important autosomal and sex-linked conditions in humans due to chromosomal abnormalities.

Condition	Chromosomal abnormality
Cri du chat syndrome	Partial monosomy, chromosome 5
Down syndrome	Trisomy, chromosome 21
Patau syndrome	Trisomy, chromosome 13
Edward's syndrome	Trisomy, chromosome 18
Klinefelter syndrome	Additional X chromosome
Turner syndrome	One X chromosome absent

or transferred to another chromosome. Reciprocal translocations result when two non-homologous chromosomes break into two segments and reciprocal exchange of the segments between the two chromosomes occurs. Animals possessing a reciprocal translocation within their genomes have a normal phenotype but display a significant reduction in fertility. The phenotype remains unchanged as the animal has a full complement of genetic material, albeit with an altered arrangement. During meiosis this altered arrangement leads to an unequal distribution of genetic material within a significant number of gametes.

Tandem translocations occur when part of an arm of one chromosome breaks and joins to the end of another chromosome. This type of aberration is rarer than reciprocal translocation.

Centric fusion occurs when two acrocentric chromosomes fuse forming one metacentric chromosome. An animal carrying this aberration has a normal phenotype as it possesses a complete genome, despite the fact that the animal's karyotype is atypical. An increased frequency of monosomy or trisomy occurs in the offspring of cattle with centric fusion.

Occasionally a metacentric chromosome can split forming two acrocentric chromosomes. As a consequence of this, the animal appears to have an extra chromosome without the acquisition of additional genetic material. This aberration, termed centric fission, has been reported in donkeys.

Deletion and inversion of sections of a chromosome can result from breakages at two points in a chromosome. Deletion results in the loss of genetic information and inversion results in the realignment of genetic information within the chromosome. These aberrations are rarely reported.

Teratogens

A teratogen is an agent which can cause a permanent alteration to the structure or function of an embryo or foetus. Teratogens acting at vulnerable periods of embryogenesis or foetal development can cause serious non-inherited malformations. A number of malformations caused by teratogens are linked to alterations in the function or expression of genes instrumental in the developmental process. The ultimate effect of exposure to teratogens depends on the gestational age of the embryo or foetus at the time of exposure and the nature and mode of action of the damaging factor. The modes of action of agents which can cause congenital defects conform to basic rules. These include the stage of gestation at which they exert their effects, the dose or degree of exposure required to induce change and the manner in which these agents are metabolised. Drugs or chemicals must cross the placental barrier in order to exert deleterious effects on the developing embryo. Species differences account for much of the variation in the effects of drugs and chemicals on developing embryos. Species susceptibility is especially important for viral teratogens as these infectious agents usually exhibit species specificity.

Although the embryo is shielded from mechanical injury by the foetal membranes and from the adverse affects of toxic or infectious agents by the placental barrier, a number of drugs, chemicals and infectious agents can cause serious damage to the developing embryo. The effect of exposure of a pregnant animal or human to teratogens usually follows a toxicological dose-response curve. There is a threshold below which no effect is observed, but as the dose of teratogen is increased, both the severity of the alterations in the embryo or foetus and the frequency at which they occur in a given species increases. The zygote is inherently susceptible to genetic mutations and chromosomal abnormalities but is usually resistant to teratogens. Although the developing embryo is highly susceptible to the damaging influence of environmental teratogens, this susceptibility declines as the embryo undergoes progressive development. The foetus becomes increasingly resistant to teratogens as it matures. However, late-differentiating structures such as the cerebellum, the palate and portions of the urinary and reproductive systems remain susceptible to many teratogens until late in gestation. Agents, imbalances and factors implicated in the disruption of embryonic or foetal development through their teratogenic effects are summarised in Table 24.4.

Therapeutic drugs and chemicals

At defined exposure levels, therapeutic drugs can be potentially teratogenic. The effects of some drugs on the

Table 24.4 Chemicals, environmental pollutants, infectious agents, metabolic imbalances, mycotoxins, physical factors, poisonous plants and therapeutic drugs implicated in the disruption of normal embryonic or foetal development through their teratogenic effects.

Agent, imbalance or factor	Susceptible species	Comments
Addictive chemicals/drugs		
Cocaine	Humans	The effects of cocaine on *in utero* development include foetal death, growth retardation, microcephaly, cerebral infarctions, urogenital anomalies and post-natal neuro-behavioural disturbances. Because poor nutrition and multiple drug abuse may be a feature of some pregnancies, the precise teratogenic effects of cocaine are not clearly established.
Ethyl alcohol	Humans	Foetal alcohol syndrome occurs in babies born to women with severe alcoholism during pregnancy. Because it can readily cross the placental barrier, ethyl alcohol is exceptionally dangerous for the developing foetus. Features of the condition include growth deficiency, mental retardation, altered facial appearance and congenital heart defects. Children with foetal alcohol syndrome are both developmentally and mentally retarded and exhibit behavioural disturbances. Studies using pregnant mice indicate that ethyl alcohol interferes with neural crest cell migration. It can also cause apoptosis of neurons in the developing forebrain and interfere with the activity of cell adhesion molecules. In the chick embryo, ethyl alcohol disrupts development by causing apoptosis of neural crest cells and by interfering with the formation of the fronto-nasal prominence. These developmental defects correlate with the loss of *Sonic Hedgehog* gene expression in the pharyngeal arches.
Toluene and other organic solvents	Humans	Repetitive deliberate inhalation of organic solvents such as toluene during pregnancy increases the risk of teratogenesis and abortion. Foetal changes include growth retardation, cranio-facial anomalies and microcephaly. Neurotoxicity, which affects adults who abuse toluene, also occurs in the foetus.
Environmental pollutants		
DDT (dichlorodiphenyl-trichloroethane)	Humans and wildlife species	The damaging effect of pesticides such as DDT on wildlife species was reported in the early 1960s. However, it took more than a decade to implement a ban on DDT. Birds of prey such as peregrine falcons and bald eagles became endangered species because of their position at the top of the food chain. The fragility of egg shells of birds of prey was linked to residues of DDT in prey which, when consumed, was concentrated in the tissues of falcons and eagles. Although banned as a pesticide in the early 1970s, in regions where it was used extensively, DDT remains at appreciable concentrations in soil as this chemical has a half-life of approximately 15 years. A metabolic by-product of DDT, DDE (1,1-dichloro-2,2 bis (p-chlorophenyl) ethylene), is reported to exert its effect either by mimicking oestrogen activity or by inhibiting the effectiveness of androgens. Feminisation of fish in Lake Superior, a decline in human sperm counts and an increased frequency of breast cancer worldwide have been attributed to environmental pollution by DDT and DDE. Due to its persistence in the environment, its potential to accumulate in the tissues of animals and its toxicity for humans, DDE has been listed as a pollutant of particular concern. Developmental effects of oral feeding of DDT in animals include toxicity for the embryo and foetus.
Dioxin	Humans, monkeys, rats, mice, fish	This halogenated hydrocarbon is a contaminant of many industrial processes. When used as a herbicide, dioxin has been linked to congenital anomalies in the human population, especially where it was used as a defoliant. The male offspring of female rats exposed to this toxic molecule had reduced sperm counts, decreased testicular size and altered sexual behaviour. Fish embryos are reported to be particularly susceptible to the toxic effects of dioxin. The offspring of rhesus monkeys exposed to less than I ng/kg/day before pregnancy had measurable behavioural changes. Exposure of pregnant mice to dioxin induces cleft palate, kidney, brain and other defects in their offspring. Using *in vitro* culture of palate cells from mouse, rat and human embryos, it was shown that dioxin treatment altered proliferation and differentiation of epithelial cells and that palate epithelial cells had a high-affinity receptor for dioxin. It has been suggested that the teratogenic effect of dioxin is due to its interference with epidermal growth factor or transforming growth factor.
Lead	Humans and animals	Due to environmental pollution, high levels of lead in drinking water, in vegetables and in the air can lead to toxicity. Lead crosses the placenta and can accumulate in foetal tissues. Reports indicate that children born to mothers who were exposed to sub-clinical levels of lead had behavioural changes and psychomotor disturbances. Lead toxicity may damage the developing human central nervous system leading to decreased IQ and functional deficits.
Mercury	Humans	Ingestion of food contaminated with methyl mercury during pregnancy resulted in damage to the foetal central nervous system. Cerebral palsy, microcephaly, blindness, cerebral atrophy and mental retardation are the principal developmental defects attributed to the teratogenic activity of organic mercury. Selective absorption by regions of the cerebral cortex has been reported.

Table 24.4 (continued)

Agent, imbalance or factor	Susceptible species	Comments
Polychlorinated biphenyls	Humans and wildlife	Polychlorinated biphenyls (PCBs) are mixtures of synthetic organic chemicals with the same basic chemical structure and similar physical properties. Due to their chemical stability, non-flammability, high boiling point and electrical insulating properties, PCBs were widely used commercially for more than half a century. Concern over their toxicity and persistence in the environment led to prohibition of their manufacture in the United States of America in 1976. There is substantial evidence that halogenated aromatic hydrocarbons including PCBs are carcinogenic, teratogenic, neurotoxic and immunosuppressive. From the late 1920s until the late 1970s, PCBs were extensively used for commercial purposes and these toxic substances are still present in the food chain. They have been blamed for the decline in the reproductive capabilities of otters, seals, mink and fish. Some polychlorinated biphenyls structurally resemble diethylstilboestrol and it is postulated that they can act as environmental oestrogens. If ingested in large amounts by pregnant women, these teratogens can cause reduced foetal growth rate and abnormal skull calcification. These compounds can also cause hypoplastic deformed nails and hyperpigmentation of gums, nails and other tissues. It is reported that body residues of PCBs in exposed women can affect pigmentation in their babies born up to four years after exposure. In addition to their oestrogenic activity, polychlorinated biphenyls structurally resemble thyroid hormones. Hydroxylated polychlorinated biphenyls have a high affinity for transthyretin, a serum protein involved in thyroid hormone transport, and can lead to excretion of thyroid hormones. As thyroid hormones are critical for development of the cochlea, the offspring of pregnant rats exposed to polychlorinated biphenyls had deficient cochlear development and were deaf.

Infectious agents

Bacteria

Treponema pallidum subspecies *pallidum*	Humans	*In utero* infection with *T. pallidum* subspecies *pallidum* can lead to serious foetal disease referred to as congenital syphilis. Infection acquired during pregnancy, primary maternal infection, invariably leads to serious foetal infection resulting in foetal death or congenital anomalies. When infection is acquired before pregnancy, foetal infection and congenital anomalies are unlikely. Congenital infection may result in maculopapular rash, central nervous system defects including deafness, hydrocephalus and mental retardation, destructive lesions of the palate and nasal septum and deformed teeth, bones and nails. Syphilis increases the risk of abortion.

Protozoa

Toxoplasma gondii	Humans, sheep, goats, pigs, cats	In both humans and animals, a primary infection with *T. gondii* during pregnancy can lead to congenital infection. When human or animal infection with *T. gondii* occurs before pregnancy, no congenital infection follows. In humans, primary infection during early pregnancy can lead to foetal death and abortion, stillbirth, chorioretinitis, brain damage with intracerebral calcification, hydrocephalus, microcephaly, rash and hepatosplenomegaly. Psychomotor or mental retardation are features of severe congenital toxoplasmosis. Infection late in gestation can result in mild or subclinical foetal disease with delayed manifestations. In sheep, goats and pigs, abortion late in gestation and perinatal deaths are common findings. Encephalitis is often associated with congenital infections in animals.

Viruses

Cytomegalovirus (Family *Herpesviridae*, subfamily *Betaherpesvirinae*)	Humans	Infection with cytomegalovirus (human herpesvirus 5) is one of the most common viral causes of congenital defects in humans. Up to 2% of newborn babies may have cytomegalovirus infection and approximately one-tenth of these infected *in utero* have signs of severe generalised infection. The outcome of severe intra-uterine infection may be foetal death or congenital defects. *In utero* infection, which is a consequence of primary maternal infection, can result in hepatosplenomegaly, chorioretinitis, microcephaly, intracerebral calcification and mental retardation.
Herpes simplex virus type 1 and herpes simplex virus type 2 (Family *Herpesviridae*, subfamily *Alphaherpesvirinae*)	Humans	Although rarely described, both herpes simplex virus type 1 and herpes simplex virus type 2 can cause congenital infections. Infection with herpes simplex virus type 2 can be acquired at the time of birth as the baby passes through the genital tract. Congenital malformations attributed to infection with these herpes viruses which occurs in late pregnancy include vesicular rash, ocular defects, hepatitis, microcephaly and mental retardation.
Parvovirus B19 (Family *Parvoviridae*, genus *Parvovirus*)	Humans	*In utero* infection with this virus in early pregnancy can cause anaemia in approximately 10% of infected foetuses. As the virus replicates in erythroid precursor cells, it can cause severe anaemia leading to congenital heart failure, hydrops foetalis and foetal death.

Table 24.4 (*continued*)

Agent, imbalance or factor	Susceptible species	Comments
Rubella virus (Family *Togaviridae*, genus *Rubivirus*)	Humans	Up to 90% of babies born to women who were first infected with rubella virus (German measles) during the first 3 months of pregnancy are at risk of developing severe congenital defects. Infection during the early embryonic period produces stage-specific malformations which can result in intrauterine death, spontaneous abortion or congenital malformations of major organs. Prominent congenital anomalies include deafness, cataracts and other ocular defects, cardiovascular malformations, microcephaly and mental retardation. The term congenital rubella syndrome is applied to the severe malformations arising from *in utero* infection with rubella virus. The risk of severe congenital defects declines as the foetus matures, and infections after the 20th week of gestation rarely results in serious defects. Maternal immunity following infection with the virus, or resulting from vaccination, prevents congenital infection.
Varicella-zoster virus (Family *Herpesviridae* subfamily *Alphaherpesvirinae*)	Humans	Infection with varicella-zoster virus (human herpesvirus 3), the cause of chickenpox, early in pregnancy may be associated with congenital anomalies which include skin and muscle defects, limb hypoplasia, ocular defects, microcephaly and mental retardation. As the foetus matures, the risk of congenital defects declines and infection after the 20th week of gestation is unlikely to cause serious defects.
Human immunodeficiency virus (Family *Retroviridae*, genus *Lentivirus*)	Humans	A high percentage of babies born to infected mothers are congenitally infected and subsequently develop the acquired immunodeficiency syndrome. Currently, there is uncertainty about the outcome of *in utero* infection with human immunodeficiency viruses on the developing foetus. Some reports suggest that congenital infection with these retroviruses may cause foetal growth retardation, cranio-facial defects and microcephaly.
Akabane virus (Family *Bunyaviridae*, genus *Bunyavirus*)	Cattle, sheep and goats	*In utero* infection of calves results in congenital defects which are related to foetal age at time of infection. Arthrogryposis, hydranencephaly, abortion and foetal death are possible sequelae to *in utero* infection. Infection between 70 and 100 days of gestation frequently results in hydranencephaly. When infection occurs between 100 and 170 days of gestation, the principal deformities are associated with arthrogryposis. Abortion and foetal death may also occur. Infection late in pregnancy may result in encephalomyelitis. The congenital defects present in the offspring of pregnant sheep and goats include hydranencephaly, arthrogryposis, scoliosis, porencephaly and microcephaly.
Bluetongue virus (Family *Reoviridae*, genus *Orbivirus*)	Sheep; cattle and goats are also susceptible	Some bluetongue virus strains, especially those in attenuated virus vaccines, can cause embryonic death, cerebral abnormalities and other defects. If pregnant ewes become infected early in gestation, embryonic death is likely. When infection occurs from approximately 40 to 100 days of gestation, congenital malformations may include hydranencephaly, porencephaly, blindness and ataxia. Rarely, congenital deformities can occur in calves following *in utero* infection. Unlike foetal infections with pestiviruses, bluetongue viruses are unlikely to induce immunotolerance in developing foetuses.
Border disease virus (Family *Flaviviridae*, genus *Pestivirus*)	Sheep; goats are also susceptible	Infection of pregnant ewes can result in a wide range of embryonic or foetal changes which include embryonic death and resorption, central nervous system defects, skeletal growth retardation, fleece abnormalities and ocular defects. The age of the foetus at time of infection determines the outcome. Embryonic death and resorption may follow infection of the developing embryo. Infections which occur during organogenesis result in skeletal growth retardation, hypomyelinogenesis, cerebellar dysplasia and enlarged primary hair follicles with reduction in the number of secondary hair follicles. Foetuses which survive *in utero* infection become immunotolerant to the virus and remain persistently infected. Characteristic signs of infection in newborn lambs include altered body conformation, changes in fleece quality and tremors. Projecting hairs along the neck and back extend above the wool and impart a halo effect which is most noticeable in fine-coated breeds.
Bovine viral diarrhoea virus (Family *Flaviviridae*, genus *Pestivirus*)	Cattle	Infection of a non-immune pregnant cow with this pestivirus can result in transplacental transmission with the outcome dependent on the age of the embryo or foetus at time of infection and the strain of the infecting virus. During the first 30 days of gestation, infection may result in embryonic death and resorption with return of the cow to oestrus. The effects of intra-uterine infection between 30 and 90 days of gestation include abortion, mummification, congenital abnormalities of the central nervous system and ocular abnormalities. Cerebellar hypoplasia, microphthalmia, retinal dysplasia and alopecia due to hypoplasia of infected hair follicles may occur. Foetuses which become infected before 120 days of gestation are immunologically incompetent and consequently develop immunotolerance to the virus, with persistent infection for the lifetime of the animal. Although such foetuses may survive, a range of congenital defects may be present. Because the bovine foetus acquires immunocompetence close to 120 days of gestation, infections after that time are less severe than in an immunologically incompetent foetus or signs of disease may be absent, as the foetus can produce neutralising antibodies which lead to the elimination of the virus.

Table 24.4 *(continued)*

Agent, imbalance or factor	Susceptible species	Comments
Classical swine fever virus (Family *Flaviviridae*, genus *Pestivirus*)	Pigs	Infection of pregnant sows results in a range of embryonic and foetal changes which include early embryonic death, abortions, stillbirths, mummification and the birth of persistently infected piglets. The age of the embryo or foetus determines the outcome of *in utero* infection. If infection occurs during the first 3 weeks of gestation, embryonic death with resorption is likely. When infection occurs during organogenesis, growth retardation, mummification, abortion, stillbirths and congenital malformations of the central nervous system may occur. Neural defects include cerebellar and spinal hypoplasia and congenital tremors. If infection occurs before the development of immunological competence, such animals remain persistently infected and excrete virus continuously. Foetal infections late in gestation are often characterised by post-natal changes which include growth retardation, depressed immune responsiveness and other evidence of tissue damage which frequently leads to death weeks or months later.
Feline panleukopenia virus (Family *Parvoviridae*, genus *Parvovirus*)	Cats	The effects of transplacental infection with this parvovirus on foetal development relate to the stage of gestation at time of infection and range from cerebellar hypoplasia and retinal dysplasia to foetal death. Infection early in gestation may result in resorption or abortion. Stillbirths, early neonatal deaths and teratogenic changes such as cerebellar hypoplasia and retinal dysplasia may occur in the litters of queens infected in late pregnancy. *In utero* infection during the last 2 weeks of pregnancy or early neonatal infection results in selective destruction of the external granular layer of the cerebellum. The subsequent cerebellar hypoplasia, which is evident when kittens become active, is characterised by ataxia, hypermetria and incoordination. These neurological signs persist for life.
Japanese encephalitis virus (Family *Flaviviridae*, genus *Flavivirus*)	Pigs; sometimes horses and other species	Infection of sows towards mid-pregnancy can cause abortion and foetal changes ranging from mummification and stillborn foetuses to weak piglets with neurological signs but also clinically normal piglets. Experimental infection of pregnant sows produces congenital defects which include hydrocephalus, cerebellar hypoplasia and hypomyelinogenesis.
Porcine herpesvirus 1 (Family *Herpesviridae*, genus *Varicellovirus*)	Pigs	In pigs, this virus causes Aujeszky's disease or pseudorabies. Up to 50% of pregnant sows may abort when the virus is introduced into a non-immune herd. Following *in utero* infection, foetal death may occur at any stage of gestation. Infection of sows in early pregnancy usually results in resorption of embryos and return to oestrus. Later in pregnancy, infection affecting all or part of the litter may result in abortion, or in stillborn, mummified, weak or normal piglets. Porcine herpesvirus 1 is one of a number of viruses implicated in the SMEDI syndrome.
Porcine parvovirus (Family *Parvoviridae*, genus *Parvovirus*)	Pigs	When infection occurs during the first 4 weeks of gestation, embryonic death and resorption usually occur. Foetal death and mummification are likely when infection occurs between 30 and 70 days of gestation. With the development of immunological competence at approximately 70 days, foetal damage is less marked; some stillbirths may occur and litter sizes may be smaller than normal. If the number of viable foetuses is reduced below four, the entire litter is usually lost. Infection with porcine parvovirus is a major cause of SMEDI.
Porcine respiratory and reproductive syndrome virus (Family *Arteriviridae*, genus *Arterivirus*)	Pigs	Infection with this arterivirus causes reproductive failure in sows, characterised by abortions late in gestation, stillbirths, mummified foetuses, weak neonatal piglets and a high rate of return to oestrus. Foetal and placental abnormalities are not consistently present. Reproductive problems may persist for up to 5 months following an initial outbreak of disease. As the virus seems to be capable of crossing the placenta only late in gestation, late-term abortions or premature farrowings are a feature of congenital infections caused by this infectious agent.
Rift Valley fever virus (Family *Bunyaviridae*, genus *Phlebovirus*)	Sheep, cattle and goats	Following primary infection with Rift Valley fever virus, a high percentage of pregnant sheep, goats and cattle abort. The virus replicates in the placentomes producing placentitis and abortion. A live attenuated vaccine, which is widely used in endemic areas and during outbreaks of disease, can cause congenital defects or abortion. Changes induced by this live vaccine include arthrogryposis, hydranencephaly, cerebellar hypoplasia and microcephaly.

Metabolic disturbances

Chemicals or drugs which affect thyroid functioning or development	Humans, animals	Iodides such as potassium iodide readily cross the placenta and can interfere with foetal thyroxine production. Radioactive iodine may cause congenital goitre. Maternal iodine deficiency may cause congenital cretinism, characterised by arrested physical and mental development and bone dystrophy. Administration of anti-thyroid drugs, such as propylthiouracil, to pregnant women may interfere with foetal synthesis of thyroxine and may cause congenital goitre. Because of their structural similarity to thyroid hormones, polychlorinated biphenyls, which are environmental pollutants, can affect the functioning of these hormones.

Table 24.4 (*continued*)

Agent, imbalance or factor	Susceptible species	Comments
Iodine deficiency	Horses, cattle, sheep and pigs	Increased neonatal mortality and goitre are features of iodine deficiency in domestic animals. Iodine deficiency may be due to a deficient intake of this element. It can also occur as a consequence of a high intake of calcium and diets with a high content of *Brassica* species. The condition is characterised by stillbirths and weak newborn animals, by partial or complete alopecia and by palpable enlargement of the thyroid gland.
Copper deficiency	Sheep and cattle	Copper deficiency may be primary, when the dietary supply is inadequate, or secondary, when the dietary intake is sufficient but copper uptake is impeded by a high dietary intake of inorganic sulphate in combination with molybdenum. A deficiency of copper interferes with myelin formation in the developing embryo. In pregnant ewes on a copper-deficient diet, defective foetal myelination is evident close to mid-pregnancy. As a consequence of defective myelination first affecting the cerebrum and later the spinal cord, hind limb incoordination and other neurological signs are evident at birth (swayback).
Diabetes	Humans	Because vascular lesions in long-standing diabetes may produce placental dysfunction, foetal growth retardation can occur in the babies of insulin-dependent diabetic mothers. Other malformations include congenital heart disease, caudal dysplasia and proximal femoral hypoplasia. Risk of congenital defects are greatest in patients with untreated or poorly controlled diabetes.
Folic acid deficiency	Humans	Evidence gained from studies of neural tube anomalies in the human population suggests a decreased risk of neural tube defects in babies born to mothers who had received folic acid supplementation before and during pregnancy.
Maternal phenylketonuria	Humans	The children of women with phenylketonuria are at risk of being exposed to high levels of phenylalanine during pregnancy, particularly if such women are not treated during pregnancy. High levels of phenylalanine interfere with embryonic cell metabolism and may lead to mental retardation, microcephaly and intra-uterine growth retardation.
Vitamin A		
(a) Deficiency	Pigs and cattle	Ocular agenesis has been reported in piglets born to sows on a vitamin A-deficient diet. A vitamin A-deficient diet has been associated with congenital blindness in calves due to pressure on the optic nerve as a result of defective bone growth.
(b) Excess	Humans, dogs, pigs, monkeys and chickens	If ingested in high concentrations, vitamin A and its analogues act as teratogens. The term vitamin A denotes specific chemical compounds such as retinol or its esters. Retinoic acid has many of the biological activities of retinol and a large number of analogues such as isotretinoin and etretinate have been synthesised. Retinoic acid has an important role in the formation of the cranio-caudal axis of mammalian embryos and also in limb formation. If present in high concentrations in the diet of pregnant women at the late gastrulation – early neurulation stage of development, retinoic acid and the synthetic retinoids isotretinoin and etretinate have teratogenic activity. This activity is apparently related to their ability to alter expression of *Hox* genes involved in specifying the cranio-caudal axis and to inhibit neural crest cell migration. Pregnant women who took a retinoic acid formulation for the treatment of acne had babies with a range of congenital anomalies including central nervous system defects, cleft palates, thymic aplasia and abnormalities of the heart and aortic arch.

Mycotoxins

Aflatoxins	Animals, sometimes humans	Mycotoxins are secondary metabolites of certain fungal species. Ingestion of aflatoxins produced by *Aspergillus flavus* and some other *Aspergillus* species can result in immunosuppression, neoplasia, mutagenesis and teratogenesis.
Patulin	Animals; may affect humans	Patulin, produced by *Penicillium expansum*, is reported to be mutagenic, carcinogenic and teratogenic.
Zearalenone	Animals; may affect humans	When fed to pregnant sows, zearalenone, a mycotoxin with oestrogenic activity produced by *Fusarium graminearum* and other *Fusarium* species, can cause reduced litter size, stillbirths, foetal malformations, mummification, neonatal mortality and splay-leg in piglets.

Physical factors

Hyperthermia	Rats, mice, guinea-pigs, hamsters, sheep, monkeys, chickens	Experimentally, it has been shown that offspring of pregnant animals subjected to hyperthermia can have congenital malformations. The spectrum of congenital malformations induced by experimental hyperthermia is reported to be characteristic for a given species. Lambs born to pregnant ewes exposed to hyperthermia between the 18th and 25th days of pregnancy had central nervous system abnormalities; hyperthermia between the 30th and 80th day of gestation resulted in foetal growth retardation. In monkeys subjected to hyperthermia, congenital defects included midfacial hypoplasia, anophthalmia and tetralogy of Fallot. The most common manifestation of heat-induced damage in guinea-pigs was microcephaly. In rodents subjected to hyperthermia, congenital malformations included tooth, cranial and vertebral defects. Sustained elevated body temperature in pregnant women due to fever or high environmental temperatures is a suspected cause of developmental defects in some babies.

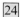

Table 24.4 *(continued)*

Agent, imbalance or factor	Susceptible species	Comments
Ionising radiation	Humans and animals	Exposure to high levels of ionising radiation following atomic explosions or accidents involving nuclear reactors causes a high incidence of foetal malformations in human and animal populations. Teratogenic risk depends on dose and stage of exposure. For the human foetus, the period of greatest susceptibility is from the eighth to the 16th week of gestation. *In utero* exposure to ionising radiation can lead to microcephaly, eye anomalies, growth retardation and mental retardation. X-rays, in large doses, can also interfere with normal *in utero* development. Ingestion of radioactive isotopes in food or water can delay mitotic activity and produce cell death. The effect of radioactive isotopes on the developing foetus is dependent on dose, distribution, metabolism and localisation. Administration of radioactive iodine to pregnant women after the 8th week of gestation can cause foetal thyroid hypoplasia.

Poisonous plants

Acorns, alleged toxicity	Cattle	A feed-related condition of cattle, referred to as acorn calves, was formerly attributed to ingestion of acorns by pregnant cows in the western United States of America, Canada and Australia. This disease, which has been given the name congenital joint laxity and dwarfism, has been associated with feeding grass or legume silage during pregnancy. Because Timothy grass, fed as silage, produced the disease which was prevented by adding hay or grain to the silage ration, it seems probable that the condition was due not to toxicity but rather to a consequence of a deficiency state. Affected calves have shortened long bones, overdistension of distal joints and slight doming of the cranium. Calves with this condition survive but do not thrive.
Astragalus species, *Oxytropis* species	Sheep, cattle, horses	When pregnant ewes consume the locoweeds *Astragalus* species and *Oxytropis* species, congenital anomalies in their lambs include brachygnathia, contractures or over-extension of joints, limb rotations, osteoporosis and bone fragility. Foetal death and abortion may also occur when these toxic plants are consumed by pregnant ewes. Calves born to cows which have consumed locoweeds have developmental anomalies which include permanent flexure of the carpal joints and contracted tendons. Limb deformities in a foal born to a mare which had consumed locoweeds have been reported.
Conium maculatum	Cattle, pigs, horses, sheep	Congenital skeletal malformations caused by *Conium maculatum* have been recorded in cattle and pigs. The toxic affects of this plant, also referred to as poison hemlock, are less evident in horses and sheep. In grazing animals, hemlock alkaloids cause paralysis of motor nerve endings and over-stimulation, followed by depression of the central nervous system. There are at least five piperidine alkaloids in *Conium maculatum*, of which coniine and γ-coniceine are considered to be teratogenic. Limb deformities, cleft palate and muscular tremors have been reported in piglets born to sows which had eaten hemlock. The piperidine alkaloids cause arthrogryposis and spinal deformities in the offspring of sows fed these toxic factors between days 43 and 53 of gestation; similar deformities occur in calves born to cows fed these alkaloids between the 55th and 75th days of gestation. Cleft palates occur in piglets exposed to these teratogens between the 30th and 45th days of pregnancy.
Lupinus species	Cattle	When pregnant cows consume certain wild lupins, malformations of the limbs, especially the forelimbs, occur in their calves. There are more than 100 species of lupins, and among these, some are toxic and teratogenic. Based on feeding trials and epidemiological data, *Lupinus laxiflorus*, *Lupinus caudatus*, *Lupinus sericeus* and *Lupinus formosus* have been implicated in 'crooked calf disease'. The quinolizidine alkaloid, anagyrine, is considered to be the teratogenic agent present in many lupin species. However, *Lupinus formosus* contains only trace amounts of anagyrine and high concentrations of the piperidine alkaloid ammodendrine, the latter also teratogenic in pregnant cattle. Limb abnormalities consist of flexion contracture and arthrogryposis associated with disordered growth of joints and shortening and rotation of the bones. Lack of foetal movement caused by the sedative or anaesthetic effect of lupin alkaloids may be responsible for skeletal deformities observed. Cleft palate is also a feature of this disease.
Nicotiana tabacum	Pigs, cattle, sheep	Ingestion of *Nicotiana tabacum* by pregnant sows between the 22nd and 53rd day of gestation causes arthrogryposis and sometimes brachygnathia and kyphosis in their piglets. The teratogen present in this variety of burley tobacco is the piperidine alkaloid, anabasine. Cleft palate and arthrogryposis has also been produced experimentally in the foetuses of cattle and sheep fed *Nicotiana glauca* (wild tree tobacco) during pregnancy. As this plant is not palatable, it is unlikely to be a cause of natural disease in cattle and sheep.

Table 24.4 (*continued*)

Agent, imbalance or factor	Susceptible species	Comments
Veratrum californicum	Sheep, cattle, goats	When fed to dams in early pregnancy, *Veratrum californicum* (skunk cabbage or false hellebore) causes severe congenital deformities of the head and defects affecting other structures in offspring. If ewes are fed this toxic plant at specific times in their pregnancies, congenital cyclopean deformities of the head, absence or displacement of the pituitary gland, cleft palate, limb deformities and tracheal stenosis occur. Foetal death and resorption can also occur. Ingestion of *Veratrum californicum* by pregnant cows may result in cleft palate, syndactylia and other limb deformities. Although sheep, cattle and goats are susceptible to the teratogens in this toxic plant, field cases are reported only in sheep. A prolonged gestation period occurs in pregnant ewes fed *Veratrum californicum*. Of the more than 50 steroid alkaloids present in *Veratrum californicum*, cyclopamine, cycloposine and jervine are the teratogenic components which cause disturbances in embryological development during formation of the neural tube. These toxic alkaloids are known to interfere with Sonic Hedgehog signalling. Their mode of action relates to interference with components within the Sonic Hedgehog signalling pathway, possibly as a result of interaction with the transmembrane protein, smoothened. The effects on bone development are attributed to interference with cartilage metabolism.

Therapeutic drugs

Angiotensin-converting enzyme inhibitors	Humans	Exposure to these anti-hypertensive drugs is not associated with embryonic damage during the first trimester. During the second or third trimester, these drugs can cause oligohydramnios, pulmonary hypoplasia, intra-uterine growth retardation, skull hypoplasia and renal dysfunction. Foetal and neonatal death can result from severe foetal hypotension due to the action of these drugs.
Benzodiazepines	Humans	A range of psycho-active drugs including diazepam, chlordiazepoxide and oxazepam, which are commonly used as sedatives, readily cross the placental barrier. Use of these drugs during the first trimester of pregnancy has been associated with cranio-facial anomalies and transient withdrawal symptoms.
Benzimidazole compounds	Sheep	Benzimidazole compounds are widely used as anthelmintics in domestic animals. When administered to pregnant ewes between the 14th and 24th days of pregnancy, some benzimidazole compounds produce skeletal, renal and vascular anomalies in ovine embryos.
Carbamazepine	Humans	This drug, used for the control of epilepsy, may cause a range of malformations including cranio-facial defects, fingernail hypoplasia and delayed intra-uterine development. There may be an increased risk of neural tube defects in babies born to women taking this drug during the first trimester of pregnancy. Formation of epoxide intermediates during the metabolism of carbamazepine has been implicated in the induction of foetal malformation.
Coumarin derivatives	Humans	These anticoagulants, which cross the placental barrier, can cause nasal hypoplasia, bone stippling, intra-uterine growth retardation and anomalies of the eyes, hands, neck and central nervous system. The foetus is particularly susceptible to exposure from the 6th to the 14th week of gestation. Although bleeding is unlikely to cause defects during the first trimester, central nervous system defects, which may occur at any time after the first trimester, may be related to foetal haemorrhage. Neonatal haemorrhage may also occur.
Diethylstilboestrol	Humans, mice	This synthetic oestrogen was used for almost 30 years, from the 1940s to the 1970s, for the prevention of threatened miscarriage and other complications of pregnancy in humans. Because this compound stimulates oestrogen-receptor-containing tissue, it may cause both structural and functional defects in developing male and female reproductive organs. In mice, prenatal exposure to diethylstilboestrol causes structural abnormalities of the uterus and uterine tubes in females and testicular and epididymal defects in males. Female offspring of women treated with diethylstilboestrol during early pregnancy had an increased risk of morphological abnormalities of the reproductive tract and adenocarcinoma of the vagina and cervix. Male children of women treated early in pregnancy with this synthetic oestrogen had a higher incidence of genital tract anomalies, including epididymal cysts and hypoplastic testes, than occurs in the normal population. Experimentally, it has been shown in pregnant mice that diethylstilboestrol represses expression of *Hox a-10* in the paramesonephric (Müllerian) duct. Wnt proteins, in association with Hox gene expression, influence uterine development. Diethylstilboestrol, acting through the oestrogen receptor, represses the *Wnt 7a* gene and this repression prevents the maintenance of Hox gene expression. Absence of Hox gene expression prevents the activation of *Wnt 5a* which encodes a protein required for cellular proliferation in the developing uterus.
Griseofulvin	Dogs, cats, horses; humans are also susceptible	This anti-fungal compound is used orally for the treatment of fungal infections of the skin. Toxic effects include bone marrow suppression and teratogenicity.

Table 24.4 (continued)

Agent, imbalance or factor	Susceptible species	Comments
Lithium carbonate	Humans	Lithium therapy is widely used as an antidepressant for patients with manic depressive illness. Treatment of women with lithium carbonate during pregnancy has been associated with an increased frequency of congenital anomalies, mainly of the heart and great vessels.
Methadone	Humans	Methadone, which is used for the treatment of heroin addiction, is considered to be a 'behavioural teratogen'. Babies born to mothers on methadone therapy had lower birth weights than non-exposed babies and also had central nervous system defects. The effects of methadone are not clearly established, as other drugs, including alcohol, are frequently used by narcotic-dependent women.
Methallibure	Pigs	This drug, which is an inhibitor of pituitary gonadotrophin, is used to control oestrus in sows. When fed to sows early in pregnancy, methallibure causes cranial and limb deformities in piglets.
Phenytoin	Humans	This drug, used for the control of epilepsy, is associated with a range of congenital defects. Babies born to mothers treated with phenytoin or hydantoin in the first trimester of pregnancy have patterns of anomalies which include microcephaly, mental retardation, cleft palate, hypoplastic nails and distal phalangeal hypoplasia. The formation of epoxide intermediates during the metabolism of phenytoin has been implicated in the induction of foetal malformations.
Streptomycin	Humans	Prolonged treatment of mothers with streptomycin during pregnancy is associated with hearing deficiency in their babies. The ototoxic activity of streptomycin relates to its deleterious effects on the eighth cranial nerve.
Tetracycline	Humans	Bone and tooth staining can occur in children if tetracycline is used at therapeutic levels during pregnancy. Used at high dosage levels, this antibiotic can induce hypoplastic tooth enamel. Because tetracycline interacts with calcified tissue, its staining effects are observed only if exposure occurs late in the first trimester or after that time.
Trimethadione	Humans	This drug, used for the control of epilepsy, has been superseded by other drugs in recent years. It is sometimes used in patients whose clinical condition is inadequately controlled by conventional therapy. When administered to pregnant women, this drug causes the foetal trimethadione syndrome characterised by pre-natal and post-natal growth retardation, V-shaped eyebrows, low-set ears, cleft lip or palate, irregular teeth and cardiac and central nervous system defects. This drug affects cell membrane permeability but the mechanism whereby it exerts its teratogenic effects has not been determined.
Valproic acid	Humans, rodents and non-human primates	Valproic acid, a widely prescribed anticonvulsant drug, has been linked to malformation in human and murine embryos and also in non-human primates. In utero exposure in humans has been associated with neural, cranio-facial, cardiovascular and skeletal defects. The embryos of laboratory mice show a pattern of susceptibility to this drug similar to human embryos. Spina bifida was recognised as a consequence of in utero exposure to valproic acid and subsequently it was found that this drug induced other malformations.
Fluoroquinolones	Humans	Because of their potential teratogenic effects on foetal cartilage and bone, fluoroquinolones are contraindicated in pregnant women.
Sulphonamides	Humans	Sulphonamide administration is contraindicated in the third trimester of pregnancy because these antimicrobial drugs may lead to displacement of bilirubin from plasma albumin and predispose to neonatal hyperbilirubinaemia. In newborn babies, free bilirubin can become deposited in the basal ganglia and sub-thalamic nuclei of the brain, causing an encephalopathy called kernicterus.
Thalidomide	Humans. Non-human primates and rabbits are also susceptible	From the late 1950s to the early 1960s, more than 10,000 babies whose mothers had taken the mild sedative thalidomide during pregnancy were born with serious birth defects. Thalidomide exerts its teratogenic effect from approximately 20 to 36 days of gestation. Phocomelia, a condition in which long bones of the limbs are deficient or absent, oesophageal and duodenal atresia, ventricular septal defects, ocular and otic defects and renal agenesis were the anomalies most frequently reported in affected babies. The teratogenic activity of thalidomide is attributed to the drug's ability to interfere with the production of angiogenesis factors in the developing limb buds and elsewhere by binding to sites which cause down-regulation of the transcription of two target genes.

Drugs used in cancer chemotherapy

Alkylating agents

| Busulfan Cyclophosphamide | Humans | These cytotoxic drugs, which are widely used in cancer chemotherapy, act by damaging DNA, thereby interfering with cell replication. Growth retardation, vascular anomalies, syndactyly and other minor anomalies are reported following treatment with these drugs. The risk of teratogenesis is usually related to the gestation age of the embryo or foetus and is also dose related. |

Table 24.4 (*continued*)

Agent, imbalance or factor	Susceptible species	Comments
Anti-metabolites		
Methotrexate Mercaptopurine	Humans	Methotrexate is a folic acid antagonist which inhibits dihydrofolate reductase, essential for the synthesis of purines and pyrimidines. Mercaptopurine is a purine analogue. These drugs exert their teratogenic effects by inhibiting cell proliferation. Intra-uterine growth retardation, microcephaly, hydrocephalus, cleft palate and post-natal growth retardation and mental retardation are consequences of exposure to these drugs.
Natural products		
Mitomycin	Humans, mice	This cytotoxic drug, which is classified as an antibiotic, arrests cell division. A single treatment of murine embryos with mitomycin at the primitive streak stage of development results in extensive cell death so that at the neural plate stage, cell numbers are greatly depleted. Most embryos survive and at the end of organogenesis appear normal. Less than 10% of embryos show gross malformation, with microphthalmia the most common defect. Despite their appearance of normality, newborn animals have severe neurological defects and few survive to weaning.

developing embryo are well characterised and the mechanisms by which they exert their effects are understood. Retinoids at defined concentrations and at a particular stage in pregnancy cause congenital defects in humans. These compounds may alter the expression of some genes central to normal development such as the Hox genes and *Sonic Hedgehog* (*Shh*). There is increasing concern that many newly-synthesised chemical compounds, which either accidentally or deliberately become incorporated into food for human consumption or into animal feed, may have potentially harmful effects on the developing embryo or foetus. It is estimated that several thousand new compounds or by-products of manufacturing industrial processes enter the environment annually. Monitoring the effects of these compounds on the developing human embryo or foetus presents many challenges as the effects of a chemical compound or therapeutic drug cannot be predicted reliably from the type of chemical or drug, or from data relating to its structure, pharmacology or toxicology. Studies using laboratory animals are limited by their inability to predict teratogenesis in humans because of the wide variation in species susceptibility. Thalidomide, which is highly teratogenic in humans, some non-human primates and rabbits, does not exert teratogenic effects in many laboratory animals. Because preclinical drug trials must of necessity exclude women who might be pregnant, the teratogenic effect of newly developed drugs on the human population cannot be determined from such trials. Commonly used therapeutic drugs with known teratogenic activity, used in food-producing animals may sometimes be present in milk or meat products. In view of the known teratogenicity of some anthelmintics such as members of the benzimidazole group in some domestic animals, producers should adhere strictly to withdrawal periods because of the possible risks to consumers associated with anthelmintic tissue residues.

Cytotoxic drugs used for treating neoplastic diseases

By their nature cytotoxic agents act at specific phases of the cell cycle and, accordingly, have activity only against dividing cells. In the treatment of neoplastic disease, cytotoxic drugs which are administered to halt the proliferation of neoplastic cells interfere either directly or indirectly with DNA replication. As a consequence of their interference with cell division, exposure of the embryo or foetus to cytotoxic drugs leads to serious developmental disruption ranging from intrauterine death to severe malformation. Because many chemotherapeutic drugs used for treating neoplastic disease are actually or potentially teratogenic, they should not be prescribed for pregnant women, especially during the first trimester of pregnancy. Cytotoxic drugs can be arbitrarily classified according to their modes of action or their source. Major categories include alkylating agents, antimetabolites, natural products, hormones and their antagonists, and a miscellaneous group comprising compounds with diverse activity. Treatment with many cytotoxic drugs during pregnancy leads either to death of the embryo or to phase-specific damage to the developing organ primordia at the time of exposure. Low dose exposure to cytotoxic drugs can cause an increase in the mutation rate of proliferating cells.

Poisonous plants

Many poisonous plants have been implicated in congenital defects in animals and a number of the toxic factors responsible for teratogenesis have been identified (Table 24.4). Considerable species variation to plant teratogens is recognised. At precise times during gestation, the embryo or foetus is particularly susceptible to plant teratogens. An example of this susceptibility is the ability of *Veratrum californicum* to induce congenital cyclopean deformities if consumed by pregnant ewes at the 14th day of pregnancy. The alkaloids produced by this plant, jervine and cyclopamine, selectively block Hedgehog signal transduction. The congenital malformations induced by consumption of poisonous plants range from skeletal deformities to cleft palate and tracheal stenosis. Some toxic alkaloids in particular plants interfere with the normal pattern of migration of embryonic cells while other plant teratogens may exert their effects through their sedative or anaesthetic effects on the developing foetus.

Infectious agents

A number of infectious agents, which can either damage the placenta or cross the placental barrier and infect the developing embryo or foetus, are important causes of congenital defects in humans and domestic animals. These infectious agents include pathogenic bacteria, fungi, protozoa and viruses (Table 24.4). Some of these agents can also cause foetal death and abortion. Because the embryo is particularly susceptible to infectious agents early in gestation, a number of these pathogens can produce serious congenital defects following a primary maternal infection early in pregnancy. The lesions which infectious agents produce and the times during pregnancy at which they exert their maximum pathogenic effects are often distinguishing characteristics of particular pathogens which cause congenital defects. When replicating in embryonic or foetal tissue, viruses can interfere with cellular proliferation, differentiation or maturation. Placentitis and foetal tissue necrosis are two obvious consequences of viral replication in the placenta or in developing foetal organs. The ability of a virus to produce teratogenic effects is related to the susceptibility of undifferentiated and differentiated cells to attachment and penetration of a given virus and to its replication within the cell. Strain differences of some viruses may account in part for their teratogenic effects. The pathogenicity of a virus, its effects on embryonic or foetal tissue, the stage of gestation at which infection occurs and the degree of immunological competence of the foetus may determine the outcome of *in utero* viral infection (Fig. 24.1). In humans, infection with rubella virus causes stage-specific malformations which can result in intra-uterine death, abortion or congenital malformations of major organs. Infection of pregnant cattle, sheep and goats with Akabane virus results in congenital defects which are related to foetal age at time of infection. Arthrogryposis, hydranencephaly, abortion or foetal death are possible sequelae to *in utero* infection in these species. While most viral pathogens tend to cause more serious damage if infection occurs early in gestation, infection of sheep or goats with the

protozoan parasite *Toxoplasma gondii* tends to cause abortion late in gestation.

In humans, the period of greatest susceptibility to teratogens is during organogenesis, from approximately the 18th to the 40th days of gestation. Exposure to teratogens after the 40th day of gestation may result in malformation of the reproductive tract, urinary system, the palate or the brain. Although the gestation periods of domestic animals range from 63 days in cats to approximately 330 days in horses, the period of greatest embryonic susceptibility in all of these species is during organogenesis. The specificity of particular pathogens often limits their host range. As a consequence of this specificity, many viruses associated with congenital defects in animals cause disease only in one or a limited number of species. This specificity is clearly illustrated by the teratogenicity of feline panleukopenia virus which is confined to cats. In contrast, bacteria and protozoa tend to be less specific in their host preferences. The protozoan pathogen, *Toxoplasma gondii*, can cause congenital disease in humans, sheep, goats and pigs. Most of the infectious agents associated with congenital defects in humans and domestic animals cause malformations by crossing the placental barrier and destroying existing embryonic or foetal tissue, or by interfering with cellular growth, differentiation or migration. The majority of infectious diseases associated with congenital defects in humans and animals are caused by viruses which have an affinity for the placenta or for tissue in the embryo or foetus. When viral replication in the foetus is rapid, foetal death and abortion are likely even if infection occurs late in gestation. The deleterious influences of teratogenic viruses on the developing embryo or foetus can extend from embryonic death and resorption, mummification, abortion and stillbirth to gross and microscopically identifiable malformations. The acronym SMEDI describes porcine reproductive failure in which **s**tillbirths, **m**ummification, **e**mbryonic **d**eath and **i**nfertility occur (Table 24.4). Depending on the tissue or organ damaged by the infectious agent and the stage of gestation at which infection occurs, clinical signs can range from severe defects to barely discernible changes in post-natal neurological behaviour. If the foetus is immunologically competent at time of infection with a particular virus, its immune response may be able to contain the viral infection with minimal foetal damage evident post-natally.

A limited number of bacteria and protozoa cause developmental defects in human and animal populations. A wide range of bacterial pathogens, however, are implicated in abortions in domestic animals (Tables 24.5 to 24.10). Among these, *Brucella* species, *Leptospira interrogans* serovars and *Salmonella* serotypes feature prominently in ruminant and porcine abortions.

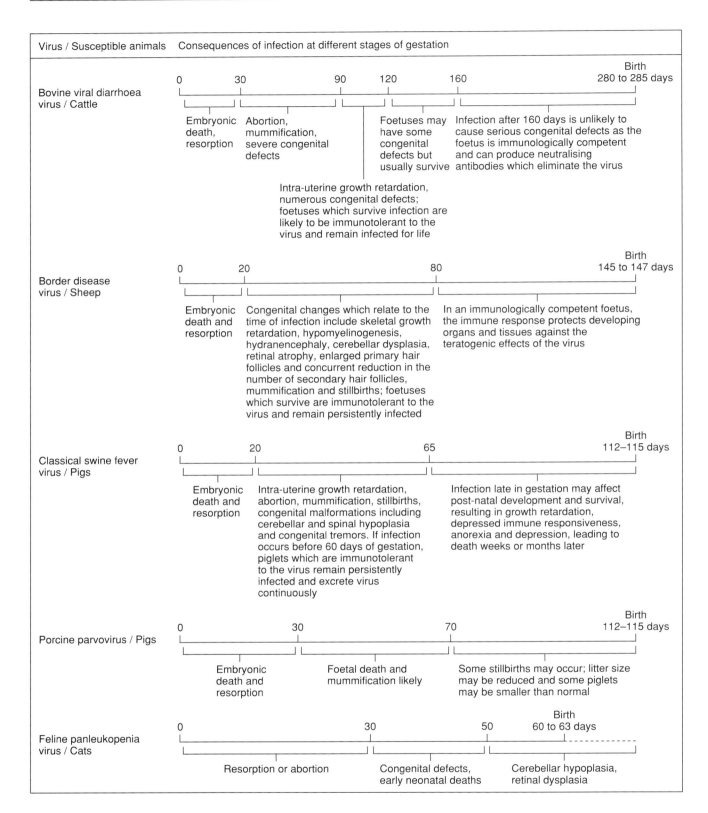

Figure 24.1 The consequences of *in utero* infection with teratogenic viruses in domestic animals at different stages of gestation.

Table 24.5 Infectious agents implicated in bovine abortion.

Agent	Comments
Bacteria	
Bacillus licheniformis	Causes sporadic abortions
Brucella abortus	Major cause of abortion in many countries
Brucella melitensis	Causes sporadic abortions
Campylobacter fetus subspecies *venerealis*	Occasional cause of abortion
Chlamydophila abortus	Causes sporadic abortions late in gestation
Anaplasma phagocytophila	Abortion may occur late in gestation
Leptospira interrogans serovars	Abortions tend to occur after 6 months of gestation
Listeria monocytogenes	Causes sporadic abortions late in gestation
Salmonella Dublin and other serotypes	Causes sporadic or epidemic abortions in some herds
Ureaplasma diversum	Causes sporadic abortions late in gestation
Fungi	
Aspergillus fumigatus	Causes sporadic abortions late in gestation
Mortierella wolfii	Causes sporadic abortions late in gestation
Protozoa	
Neospora caninum	May be an important cause of bovine abortion in some countries
Trichomonas foetus	Infection usually results in early embryonic death; occasionally abortion may occur in the first half of pregnancy
Viruses	
Akabane virus	May cause foetal death, abortion, stillbirth; major cause of congenital defects
Bovine viral diarrhoea virus	May cause foetal death, abortion or congenital defects
Infectious bovine rhinotracheitis virus	May cause foetal death, abortion after the 5th month of gestation
Rift Valley fever virus	May cause foetal death and abortion

Table 24.6 Infectious agents implicated in ovine abortion.

Agent	Comments
Bacteria	
Bacillus licheniformis	Causes sporadic abortions
Brucella melitensis	Major cause of abortion in many countries. Placentitis is a feature of this disease
Brucella ovis	Sporadic abortions may occur; mummification and autolysis of the foetus sometimes observed
Campylobacter fetus subspecies *fetus*	Abortion, which usually occurs late in gestation, is a consequence of placentitis
Campylobacter jejuni	Abortion tends to occur late in gestation
Chlamydophila abortus	Causes a disease referred to as enzootic abortion of ewes. Abortion usually occurs in the last month of pregnancy as a consequence of placentitis
Coxiella burnetii	A rare cause of abortion late in gestation
Anaplasma phagocytophila	Abortion may occur late in gestation
Listeria monocytogenes	Sporadic abortion late in gestation following placentitis
Salmonella serotypes	A number of *Salmonella* serotypes cause abortion late in gestation. *Salmonella* Dublin and *Salmonella* Typhimurium can produce both systemic disease and abortion
Protozoa	
Toxoplasma gondii	Major cause of abortion in sheep. Abortion late in gestation and perinatal death are common findings in sheep
Viruses	
Akabane virus	Abortion may occur when foetuses are infected late in pregnancy
Bluetongue virus	Some bluetongue virus strains may cause abortion together with congenital abnormalities
Cache Valley virus	Occasionally associated with congenital defects and abortion
Rift Valley fever virus	Causes high mortality rates in neonatal lambs and abortion in pregnant ewes

Table 24.7 Infectious agents implicated in porcine abortion.

Agent	Comments
Bacteria	
Brucella suis	Abortion may occur in the second half of pregnancy
Erysipelothrix rhusiopathiae	Abortion may occur in association with systemic disease
Leptospira interrogans serovars	Abortions late in gestation
Viruses	
African swine fever virus	Abortion often occurs in association with systemic disease
Classical swine fever virus	Associated with severe infection in sows, abortion is common; the SMEDI syndrome is a feature of infection with this virus
Japanese encephalitis virus	Abortions and stillbirths may occur
Porcine enteroviruses	The SMEDI syndrome and sporadic abortions may occur
Porcine herpesvirus 1 (Aujeszky's disease virus)	Abortion is usually secondary to fever and systemic disease; the SMEDI syndrome may occur
Porcine parvovirus	The SMEDI syndrome is a feature of infection with this virus
Porcine respiratory and reproductive virus	Late-term abortions may follow infection with this virus; SMEDI syndrome occurs in affected herds

Table 24.8 Infectious agents implicated in equine abortion.

Agent	Comments
Bacteria	
Ehrlichia risticii	May cause abortion in the second half of gestation
Leptospira interrogans serovars	Abortion may be a consequence of acute leptospirosis
Fungi	
Aspergillus fumigatus	May cause abortion late in gestation, a consequence of mycotic placentitis
Viruses	
Equine herpesvirus 1	This is the most common viral cause of abortion which occurs after the 8th month of gestation; equine herpesvirus 4 causes sporadic abortion in mares
Equine viral arteritis virus	Infection may result in a high rate of abortion; stillbirths are also a feature of infection with this virus

Table 24.9 Infectious agents implicated in canine abortion.

Agent	Comments
Bacteria	
Brucella canis	Decreased fertility and abortions are features of infection with this pathogen
Protozoa	
Neospora caninum	May be a rare cause of abortion in bitches
Viruses	
Canine herpesvirus 1	Primary infection of pregnant bitches may result in abortion or stillbirths

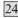

Table 24.10 Infectious agents implicated in feline abortion or early embryonic death.

Agent	Comments
Viruses	
Feline leukaemia virus	Reduced reproductive performance occurs in a high percentage of infected queens; early embryonic death and abortion midway through pregnancy may occur
Feline panleukopenia virus	Early intra-uterine infection with this parvovirus may result in resorption or abortion; infection during late pregnancy results in cerebellar hypoplasia

Table 24.11 Features of congenital diseases of animals which can be used to determine whether they are due to genetic or chromosomal factors or caused by teratogenic agents.

Feature of condition	Of genetic or chromosomal aetiology	Resulting from exposure to teratogens
Nature of defect	Phenotypical expression well characterised and relatively constant in affected animals	Usually variable; developmental defects relate to gestational age of embryo or foetus at time of exposure
Distribution pattern of defect in animals	Occurs more frequently in defined populations or breeds	Defects not related to breed of animal
Numbers of animals affected	Usually sporadic over a long time period	May involve many animals on one farm or in one breeding unit
Geographical distribution	Distribution often confined to a particular breed in a defined area	Disease may be confined to a particular species of animal, independent of breed, and may affect discrete groups of susceptible animals
Mechanism of disease production	Defect usually specific for a defined tissue, body system or protein molecule	Tissue changes or developmental defects often affect more than one body system
Role of environmental factors in disease production	Usually independent of environmental factors. Clinical manifestations of the condition can be induced by environmental influences	Typically, congenital defects are associated with exposure to environmental pollutants or damaging physical factors, consumption of poisonous plants, treatment with specific therapeutic drugs or infection with pathogenic microorganisms

Assessing the aetiology of congenital disease

Careful evaluation of field data combined with laboratory findings from affected foetuses is required to determine whether congenital disease was due to genetic or chromosomal factors, or caused by teratogenic agents (Table 24.11). When groups of pregnant animals are affected, flock or herd histories may provide a useful insight into the possible causes of the congenital defects. The species affected, the number of animals involved and the nature of the congenital malformations observed along with laboratory findings should provide sufficient information to determine the probable aetiology of the congenital defects observed.

Laboratory tests which may be used to confirm the genetic or chromosomal nature of a congenital disease include karyotyping, pedigree analysis and genotyping. Karyotyping can be used to detect obvious chromosomal aberrations. Pedigree analysis provides information relating to the genetic history of a given animal population or breed. Genotyping can be used to identify alleles or markers associated with a genetic trait. Confirmation of the possible role of chemicals, drugs, environmental pollutants, metabolic imbalances or poisonous plants in the aetiology of congenital disease requires pathological, toxicological or other appropriate laboratory tests. When dealing with infectious agents, the presence of antibodies in foetal serum for a specific pathogen is consistent with *in utero* infection. Isolation of an infectious agent from foetal tissue confirms the involvement of such an agent in the aetiology of congenital disease.

Further reading

Brent, R.L. and Beckman, D.A. (1999) Teratogens. In *Encyclopedia of Reproduction*, Vol. 4. Eds. E. Knobil and J.D. Neill. Academic Press, San Diego, pp. 735–749.

Cheeke, P.R. (1998) *Natural Toxicants in Feeds, Forages and Poisonous Plants*, 2nd edn. Interstate Publishers, Danville, IL.

Finnell, R.H., Gellineau-Van Waes, J., Eudy, J.D. and Rosenquist, T.H. (2002) Molecular basis of environmentally induced birth defects. *Annual Review of Pharmacology and Toxicology* **42**, 181–208.

Gilbert, S.F. (2003) *Developmental Biology*, 7th edn. Sinauer Associates, Sunderland, Mass.

James, L.F., Panter, K.E., Gaffield, W. and Molyneux R.J. (2004) Biomedical applications of poisonous plant research. *Journal of Agricultural Food Chemistry* **52**, 3211–3230.

Moore, K.L. and Persaud, T.V.N. (1998) *Before We Are Born*, 5th edn. W.B. Saunders, Philadelphia, PA.

Murphy, F.A., Gibbs, E.P.J., Horzinek, M. and Studdert, M.J. (1999) *Veterinary Virology*, 3rd edn. Academic Press, San Diego.

Navarro, M., Cristofol, C., Carretero, A., Arboix, M. and Ruberte, J. (1998) Anthelmintic induced congenital malformations in sheep embryos using netobimin. *Veterinary Record* **142**, 86–90.

Nicholas F.W. (1996) *Introduction to Veterinary Genetics.* Oxford University Press, Oxford.

Oberst, R.D. (1993) Viruses as teratogens. *Veterinary Clinics of North America: Food Animal Practice* **9**, 23–31.

Quinn, P.J., Markey, B.K., Carter, M.E., Donnelly, W.J. and Leonard, F.C. (2002) *Veterinary Microbiology and Microbial Disease*. Blackwell Science, Oxford.

Szabo, K.T. (1989) *Congenital Malformations in Laboratory and Farm Animals*. Academic Press, San Diego.

Thorogood, P. (1997) *Embryos, Genes and Birth Defects.* John Wiley, Chichester.

WHO (1977) Non-Mendelian developmental defects: animal models and implications for research into human disease. *Bulletin of the World Health Organisation* **55**, 475–487.

Glossary

Abortion premature expulsion of the products of conception, either an embryo or a non-viable foetus, from the uterus

Achondroplasia failure of growth of cartilage in endochondral ossification leading to dwarfism

Acrocentric chromosome a chromosome which has a terminally-placed centromere

Acrosomal reaction the release of enzymes and other proteins from the acrosomal vesicle of a spermatozoon which occurs after the spermatozoon binds to the zona pellucida

Agammaglobulinaemia absence of gamma globulins in the blood

Agenesis failure of development

Alar plate dorsal region of grey matter in the developing neural tube

Albinism an autosomal recessive condition resulting in the absence of pigmentation from the hair, skin and eyes

Allantois endodermal diverticulum extending from hindgut. It forms one of the extra-embryonic membranes; it provides vascularity to the chorion and acts as an extra-embryonic bladder

Alleles One of two or more alternative forms of a particular gene at a defined locus

Alopecia absence or deficiency of hair or wool coat

Amelia congenital absence of the limbs

Amniogenesis development of amnion by folding (domestic animals) or by cavitation (primates)

Amnion the innermost extra-embryonic membrane which encloses the developing foetus

Amniotic fluid an aqueous fluid which fills the amniotic sac

Anal membrane dorsal division of cloacal membrane

Anastomosis a natural communication between two blood vessels or two tubular organs

Anencephaly congenital absence or severe reduction in size of the cerebral hemispheres

Aneuploidy a condition where the chromosome number of cells of an individual is not the diploid number characteristic for that species

Angioblast precursor cell of capillary endothelium

Angiogenesis the process whereby existing blood vessels lengthen or branch by sprouting

Ankylosis abnormal fixation of a joint

Antibodies serum proteins produced in response to infection or immunisation by an antigenic agent; these proteins, referred to as immunoglobulins, are found in the gamma globulin fraction of serum

Antrum cavity of Graafian follicle which is filled with follicular fluid

Aortic sac expanded distal end of truncus arteriosus from which the aortic arch arteries arise during cardiac development

Apical ectodermal ridge ectodermal thickening at tip of limb bud which secretes factors required for embryonic limb development and growth

Aplasia incomplete or defective development of a tissue or organ

Apoptosis a form of programmed cell death caused by activation of endogenous caspases leading to degeneration of DNA by DNase

Arthrogryposis persistent flexion of a joint

Artiodactyla a division of the ungulate or hoofed animals, having an even number of toes, two or four

Athelia congenital absence of teats

Atresia congenital absence or closure of a normal body opening

Atrophy decrease in the normal size of a tissue, which can result from lack of use, decreased blood supply or from nutritional deficiencies

Autocrine a mode of extracellular signalling where the target cell is the same cell or cell type as that which secreted the signalling factor originally

Autosomes chromosomes other than the sex chromosomes

Barr body the condensed single de-activated X chromosome observed in the nuclei of female mammalian somatic cells

Basal plate ventral region of grey matter in the developing neural tube

Bilaminar embryonic disc disc-shaped embryo comprising ectoderm and endoderm

Blastocyst a stage of development in a mammalian embryo which follows the morula stage. It typically consists of a hollow sphere of trophoblastic cells, a central fluid-filled cavity called the blastocoele and a cluster of cells on the interior called the inner cell mass

Blastomeres cells produced by cleavage of a fertilised ovum

Blood islands clusters of angiogenic mesenchymal cells on the surface of the yolk sac

Brachydactyly abnormal shortness of the digits

Brachygnathia abnormal shortness of the lower jaw

Capacitation the physiological changes spermatozoa must undergo in the female genital tract or *in vitro* before being capable of fertilising ova

Carcinogenic describes a substance which can cause cancer

Cardiogenic plate mesoderm which gives rise to the cardiac tubes

CD cluster of differentiation; term given to cell surface molecules identifiable by monoclonal antibodies. Clusters of differentiation are used to characterise blood and tissue cells such as lymphocytes and macrophages

Cell-mediated immunity immune responses mediated by T lymphocytes, in contrast to humoral immunity, which is mediated by antibodies

Centriole a self-reproducing cellular organelle, which consists of short cylinders containing nine groups of microtubules, generally arranged as triplets

Centromere a region of the chromosome where kinetochore microtubules attach during mitosis and meiosis

Centrosome a dense cytoplasmic region surrounding a pair of centrioles which is devoid of a membrane

Chimera an organism composed of genetically different cell populations derived from genetically different zygotes

Chorion the outermost of the foetal membranes composed of trophoblast lined with somatic mesoderm

Chromatids the daughter strands of a duplicated chromosome, which are joined at the centromeres

Chromatin a complex of nucleic acids, histones and non-histone proteins which make up chromosomes

Cleavage the phase of repeated mitotic cell division without an increase in cell size that transforms the zygote into a morula

Cloaca dilated caudal end of embryonic hindgut in mammals; common opening of the urinary, digestive and reproductive tracts in some lower vertebrates

Cloacal bursa a dorsal outpouching of the cloaca in birds which is the site of B lymphocyte development, also referred to as the bursa of Fabricius

Codominant designation given to genes when both alleles are fully expressed in the heterozygous state

Coelom cavity between splanchnic and somatic mesoderm

Competence the ability of a cell to receive and respond to inductive signals produced by another cell

Conceptus the product of conception including the embryo and foetal membranes

Congenital defects abnormalities of the structure or function of cells, tissues or organs which are present at birth

Corona radiata a layer of radially elongated cells derived from the cumulus oophorus, which surround the zona pellucida of an oocyte

Corpus albicans fibrous remnant of corpus luteum

Corpus luteum a yellow-coloured transient endocrine structure in the ovary formed from the ruptured Graafian follicle and the surrounding thecal cells after ovulation

Cortical reaction the release of the contents of the oocyte cortical granules into the perivitelline space after contact with the fertilising spermatozoon; the cortical reaction is a method of preventing polyspermy in some species

Cotyledons villi of the chorioallantoic membrane which interdigitate with crypts of caruncles in ruminants forming placentomes

Cyclin-dependent kinase (Cdk) a protein kinase which is active when it forms a complex with a cyclin protein. Particular Cdk–cyclin complexes trigger different steps of the cell cycle through the phosphorylation of target proteins

Cyclins proteins which play a role in the progression of the cell cycle through the activation of kinases

Cyclopia complete or partial fusion of the orbits and eyes

Cytokines soluble biological messenger proteins which can mediate cellular interactions and regulate cell growth and secretion

Cytokinesis process of cytoplasmic division, which usually follows nuclear division

Cytoneme actin-based extracellular cytoplasmic projections believed to mediate long-range cell-to-cell communication in *Drosophila*

Cytotrophoblast cellular layer of trophoblast

Dendritic cells macrophage-like cells with dendritic morphology which function as antigen-presenting cells for T lymphocytes

Dental lamina ectodermal precursor of tooth buds

Dental sac condensed mesenchyme surrounding enamel organ

Dermatome subdivision of the somite which contributes to the formation of the dermis

Dermomyotome the dorso-lateral section of the somite which consists of the dermatome and myotome

Determination a process by which the potential for differentiation of cells or tissues becomes limited to a particular lineage

Diencephalon the caudal part of the forebrain comprising epithalamus, thalamus and hypothalamus

Differentiation structural and biochemical changes within a cell or cell group leading to the production of cell types with defined specialised functions

Dominant referring to alleles that are fully expressed in the heterozygous state

Drosophila a genus of flies containing about 900 described species; *Drosophila melanogaster* is the most extensively studied species in this genus from the standpoint of genetics and cytology

Ductus arteriosus shunt connecting the left pulmonary artery to the aortic arch

Ductus venosus shunt through the liver connecting the left umbilical vein to the caudal vena cava

Dyad the product of tetrad separation or disjunction at the first meiotic prophase, consisting of two sister chromatids joined at the centromere

Dysgenesis defective development or malformation

Dysplasia developmental abnormality leading to alteration in shape, size or development of tissues or cells

Ectoderm outer germ layer that gives rise to the nervous system, the epidermis of the skin, the outer lining of the chorion and inner lining of the amnion

Ectopia abnormal location of an organ or tissue

Embryonic disc large cells of the early embryo arranged in a disc-shaped structure

Embryonic period the period of development from the completion of implantation to the formation of organ primordia

Embryotrophe nourishing material which an embryo may absorb and utilise

Enamel organ ectodermal precursor of tooth enamel

Endoderm the inner germ layer which forms the epithelial lining of the embryonic alimentary and respiratory tracts

Enhancer sequences of nucleotides which potentiate the transcriptional activity of physically-linked genes

Epiblast outer layer of the inner cell mass

Epimere dorsal portion of a myotome

Epispadias congenital defect where the urethral opening is located on the dorsal surface of the penis

Erythropoietin a hormone produced by kidney cells which acts on stem cells in the bone marrow, stimulating erythrocyte production

Exon region of a gene containing DNA which codes for a protein

Fate map a diagram that illustrates the origin and fate of cells in the embryo

Foetal membranes membranes which provide prolection, nutrition and respiration for the developing embryo; they include the yolk sac, amnion, chorion and allantois

Foetal period the period of development from the formation of organ primordia to the end of gestation

Foregut (embryonic) the formation of the gut extending from the oro-pharyngeal membrane to the level of the hepatic diverticulum

Freemartin a mammalian intersex sterile animal, phenotypically female, born co-twin with a male sibling

G_0 phase state of withdrawal from the eukaryotic cell cycle by entry into a quiescent G_1 phase

G_1 phase a period of the cell cycle between the end of cytokinesis and commencement of DNA synthesis

G_2 phase a period of the cell cycle between the end of DNA synthesis and the beginning of mitosis

Gamete mature haploid germ cell from a male or female animal; the union of a gamete from a male animal, a spermatozoon, with a gamete from a female animal, an ovum, initiates the development of a new individual

Gametogenesis development of male and female gametes

Gastrulation   a process of cell migration that gives rise to the germ layers ectoderm, mesoderm and endoderm

Gene   a fundamental physical unit of heredity, which occupies a specific location on a chromosome

Germ cells   descendants of primordial cells which originate in the yolk sac endoderm and migrate to the gonadal ridges of the embryo where they give rise to either spermatozoa or ova; the term is also used to describe spermatozoa or ova

Germ layers   the ectoderm, mesoderm and endoderm

Graafian follicle   a large follicle found in mammalian ovaries which contains an ovum; after ovulation, it forms the corpus luteum

Gubernaculum   a column of mesenchyme that extends from the caudal pole of the gonad to the inguinal region. It is associated with descent of the testis

Gut-associated lymphoid tissue   lymphoid tissue, located in the gastrointestinal mucosa and submucosa, which constitutes the gastrointestinal immune system

Haematopoiesis   the production of blood cells

Haemotrophe   nutrient source for embryo or foetus from maternal blood or its breakdown products

Haploid   describes a cell which has a single set of unpaired chromosomes, half the number of a typical somatic cell, given the notation 'n'

Head fold   the rostral body fold

Hedgehog proteins   the Hedgehog (Hh) family of proteins originally identified in *Drosophila* has three mammalian homologues: Sonic Hedgehog (Shh), Desert Hedgehog (Dhh) and Indian Hedgehog (Ihh).

Hindgut   the portion of the gut extending from the caudal end of the midgut loop to the cloacal membrane

Hippomane   calculus found in the allantoic fluid of mares

Histogenesis   development of a tissue

Histotrophe   nutrient source for embryo or foetus derived from maternal tissue other than blood

Humoral immunity   immune responses which involve antibodies

Hydranencephaly   absence of the cerebral hemispheres, with their normal site filled with cerebrospinal fluid

Hydrocephalus   abnormal accumulation of cerebrospinal fluid within the cerebral ventricular system

Hyoid arch   second pharyngeal arch

Hyperplasia   excessive growth of tissues due to an increase in cell numbers

Hypoblast   a cuboidal layer of cells on the ventral surface of the inner cell mass

Hypomere   ventral–lateral subdivision of a myotome, which gives rise to the hypaxial muscles of the lateral and ventral body wall

Hypoplasia   incomplete development or underdevelopment of an organ or tissue

Hypotrichosis   the presence of less hair than normal

Ichthyosis   skin condition marked by dryness, roughness and scaliness due to hypertrophy of the epidermis or defective keratinisation

Ig   abbreviation for immunoglobulin; examples of immunoglobulins are IgM, IgG and IgA

Immunodeficiency   a failure in non-specific immunity or specific immunity which may be either primary or secondary in origin

Implantation   attachment of the blastocyst to the epithelial lining of the uterus; in some species the blastocyst becomes embedded in the endometrium

In vitro   outside of the living body or in an artificial environment

In vivo   in the living body

Induction   the developmental process in which the fate of a group of cells is determined by interactions with another group of cells

Integrins   a family of cell-surface adhesion molecules found on leukocyte membranes; they have an important role in the adhesion of antigen-presenting cells and lymphocytes and also in leukocyte migration into tissues

Intermediate mesoderm   subdivision of the mesoderm between paraxial and lateral plate mesoderm

Intron   untranslated intervening sequences which are interspersed between coding sequences of a particular gene and which are removed from the primary RNA transcript to yield mRNA

Iso-   prefix signifying equal or alike

Isolecithal   denoting a uniform distribution of yolk within an egg

Karyotype   the chromosomal complement of a cell, individual or species; the karyotype is often illustrated with a photomicrograph showing the size, shape and number of chromosomes present

Kinetochore   complex protein structure which forms on the centromeres of mitotic and meiotic chromosomes to which microtubules attach

Kyphosis   an abnormal dorsal curvature of the thoracic region of the vertebral column as viewed from the side

Labio-gingival sulcus   groove between lip and gum

Labio-scrotal folds   paired folds which form the scrotum (male) or labia (female)

Langerhans cells   dendritic cells found in the skin which belong to the monocyte family; function as effective antigen-presenting cells for T-lymphocytes

Lens placode   surface ectodermal structure from which the lens vesicle develops

Lens vesicle   invagination of lens placode which forms the lens

Limb bud   mesodermal outgrowth from which a limb develops; each limb bud consists of an outer ectodermal cap and an inner mesodermal core

Lineage   line of descent from a progenitor cell

Linguo-gingival sulcus   groove between tongue and gum

Liquor folliculi   fluid in the cavity of a Graafian follicle

Lordosis   abnormal ventral curvature of the thoraco-lumbar region of the vertebral column

Male pronucleus   the haploid nuclear material of the head of a spermatozoon after it has entered the ovum and acquired a pronuclear membrane

Mandibular arch   the first pharyngeal arch

Maxillary process   dorsal division of the first pharyngeal arch

Meiosis   a special type of cell division which occurs only during the formation of gametes; in this form of cell division, the number of chromosomes is halved from diploid to haploid

Mendelian principles   the principles of inheritance proposed by Gregor Mendel. (1) Genetic characters are controlled in unit factors which exist in pairs in individual organisms. (2) When alleles control a single trait, one allele is dominant over the other which is said to be recessive. (3) During the formation of gametes, the paired unit factors separate or segregate randomly

Meningomyelocoele   protrusion of the spinal cord and meninges through a defect in the vertebral column

Meromelia   congenital absence of part of a limb

Mesencephalon   the midbrain vesicle, one of the three primary brain vesicles

Mesenchyme   loose connective tissue of mesodermal or neural crest origin

Mesoderm   the middle of the three primary germ layers of the embryo, located between the ectoderm and endoderm

Mesonephric duct   duct of the mesonephros; in males, first functions in excretion of urine and subsequently contributes to the formation of the male duct system; degenerates in females

Mesonephros   temporary middle foetal kidney formed from intermediate mesoderm. In males, a number of its tubules give rise to efferent ductules of the testis

Metacentric chromosome   a chromosome with a centrally-placed centromere

Metanephros   the definitive kidney

Metencephalon   rostral part of hind-brain from which the pons and cerebellum form

Microcephaly   decreased head size relative to the rest of the body

Microphthalmos   abnormal reduction in the size of one or both eyes

Microtubule   hollow cylinders with a diameter of about 25 nm, composed of long chains of the proteins α-tubulin and β-tubulin. They function as part of the cytoskeleton, maintaining cell shape and aiding in intra-cellular transport; they play a central role in cell division. Microtubules are dynamic; they grow and shrink depending on the needs of the cell

Midgut   region of the developing gut which extends from point of entry of bile duct to the hindgut

Mitogen   an extra-cellular substance which induces mitosis

Mitosis   division of the nucleus during cell division resulting in the formation of two daughter cells having the same diploid complement of chromosomes as the original cell

Morula   solid sphere of cells produced by cleavage of the fertilised ovum

Mummification   conversion of a foetus to a dehydrated state with a leathery appearance

Mutagen   a substance which induces DNA mutations at a rate above that normally observed for a given gene

Mutation   the process by which a gene undergoes structural change

Mycotoxin   toxic substance produced by a fungus

Myelencephalon   caudal part of hindbrain; forms the medulla oblongata

Myotome   that portion of a somite which gives rise to striated muscle

Neural crest   population of cells which arise from the edge of the neural plate and migrate to different regions of the body, giving rise to many tissues

Neural folds   folds formed during neurulation

Neural plate   thickened plate of neural ectoderm from which neural tube and neural crest develop

Neural tube   ectodermal tube formed by union of neural folds; develops into the central nervous system

Neuroblast   neuroepithelial embryonic cell which gives rise to neurons

Neuroectoderm   neural epithelium which arises from ectoderm within the neural plate

Neuropores   transient openings at each end of the neural tube

Neurulation   the process of folding of the neural plate, leading to formation of the neural tube

NK cells   natural killer cells; large granular lymphocytes without antigenic specificity which can destroy tumour cells and virus-infected cells without prior stimulation by immunisation

Non-disjunction   failure of homologous chromosomes to separate properly and move to opposite poles during mitosis or meiosis

Notochord   rod-like rostral extension of primitive node which extends from the cranial to the caudal region ventral to the developing neural tube

Oligohydramnios   deficiency in the amount of amniotic fluid in the amnion

Ontogeny   developmental history of an individual

Oocyte   immature ovum

Oogenesis   the process of ovum formation

Oogonia   primordial cells of the female germ line

Organogenesis   the formation of organs during embryological development

Oro-pharyngeal membrane   a membrane of ectoderm and endoderm which separates the stomodeum from the foregut

Osteopetrosis   a hereditary disease characterised by abnormally dense bones which are prone to fracture

Otic placode   ectodermal precursor of the otocyst

Otocyst   precursor of the inner ear; the auditory vesicle of the embryo

Ovulation   the process whereby a mature ovum is released from the Graafian follicle

Ovum   the mature female gamete or egg

Paracrine   a form of cell-to-cell communication which depends on a secreted substance acting over a short distance without entering the circulation

Paramesonephric (Müllerian) duct   duct formed by an invagination of the coelomic epithelium lateral to the mesonephric duct; forms the uterine tubes and uterus

Paraxial mesoderm   embryonic mesoderm lateral to the neural tube which undergoes segmentation, forming somites

Parenchyma   the functional elements of an organ as distinct from its connective tissue framework

Parthenogenesis   development without fertilisation; cleavage of an unfertilised ovum

Partial dominance   referring to the partial phenotypic expression of an allele in the heterozygous state

Parturition   birth

Pathogenic microorganisms   Bacteria, fungi and viruses which can cause disease in animals and humans

Perivitelline space   the space between the oocyte (ovum) cell membrane and the zona pellucida

Phagocytes   cells such as macrophages and neutrophils with the ability to engulf foreign particles, especially bacteria

Pharyngeal arches   paired structures in mammals which correspond to branchial arches in fish

Phenotype   the appearance of an animal as determined by its genotype and environmental influences

Phosphorylation   the chemical addition of a phosphate group (phosphate and oxygen) into an organic molecule

Placenta   the organ of physiological exchange between endometrium and foetal membranes in the uterus of pregnant mammals, composed of maternal and foetal tissue

Placental barrier   the tissues which separate the maternal and foetal circulations

Placentitis   inflammation of the placenta

Polar bodies   haploid cells containing a nucleus but little cytoplasm, extruded from the oocyte during meiosis

Polyploidy   the presence of more than two haploid sets of chromosomes in a cell; having more than two sets of homologous chromosomes

Polythelia   the presence of supernumerary teats

Prechordal plate   mass of mesoderm which forms cranial to the notochord

Primary palate   the structure which separates the oral cavity from the developing nasal cavities

Primary villus   villus composed only of trophoblast

Primitive streak   a linear region of cell migration from the ectoderm (epiblast) which forms the embryonic endoderm and mesoderm. The primitive streak defines the cranial–caudal axis of the embryo

Primitive (Hensen's) node expanded ectoderm at the rostral end of the primitive streak

Primordial germ cell the earliest precursor of the gamete

Primordium bud, or early rudiment; an aggregation of cells in the embryo which indicates the first stage in the development of an organ or structure

Proctodeum depression of ectoderm external to the cloacal membrane

Pronephros initial excretory organ present in vertebrate embryos which persists in some fish

Pronucleus the haploid nucleus of a gamete; the nucleus of the spermatozoon or ovum prior to fusion

Prosencephalon fore-brain vesicle; the most rostral of the three early divisions of the brain

Proteoglycans glycoproteins formed primarily in connective tissue; composed of glycosaminoglycans linked to a protein core

Proto-oncogene a gene involved in the regulation of cell proliferation which can cause cancer if it mutates or is expressed abnormally

Rachischisis congenital fissure of the vertebral column

Random assortment the random distribution of paternally-derived and maternally-derived chromosomes during gamete formation

Rathke's pouch a dorsal evagination of the stomodeum from which the adenohypophysis develops

Recessive gene a gene which is expressed in the homozygous state but not in the presence of a dominant allelle

Reduction division the first meiotic division, which reduces the chromosome number of gametes from 2n to n

Resorption breakdown and assimilation of a structure such as an embryo

Rhombencephalon hind-brain vesicle

Rhombic lips thickenings of alar laminae of rhombencephalon; form the cerebellar primordia

RNA polymerase II an enzyme which catalyses the synthesis of mRNA from DNA

S phase stage in the eukaryotic cell cycle during which DNA synthesis takes place

Sclerotome ventro-medial sub-division of a somite which contributes to the formation of a vertebra

Scoliosis an abnormal, exaggerated lateral curvature of the vertebral column

Secondary palate portion of palate formed from fused lateral palatal processes

Septum transversum transverse mesodermal partition between the pericardium and the developing foregut which gives rise to the tendinous centre of the diaphragm

Sinus venosus caudal chamber of the embryonic heart which receives blood from the vitelline, umbilical and cardinal veins prior to remodelling of the heart

Small interfering RNA short (or small) interfering RNA (siRNA); this is a short 21–23 nt RNA duplex involved in inducing the RNA interference response in mammalian cells. The siRNA stimulates the cleavage of other single-stranded RNA with the same sequence as the siRNA

SMEDI acronym which describes porcine reproductive failure characterised by **s**tillbirths, **m**ummification, **e**mbryonic **d**eath and **i**nfertility

Somatic mesoderm portion of lateral plate external to the embryonic coelom

Somatopleure the embryonic layer formed by the union of the somatic layer of mesoderm with ectoderm

Somite period the period during which the somites are observed in an embryo; the number of pairs may be used to estimate the age of the embryo

Somites segmented blocks of mesoderm formed from paraxial mesoderm

Spermatogenesis the production of spermatozoa

Spermiogenesis maturation of spermatids to spermatozoa

Splanchnic mesoderm portion of lateral plate medial to embryonic coelom

Splanchnopleure the embryonic layer composed of splanchnic mesoderm and endoderm

Spontaneous mutation rate the natural rate of mutation for a given gene locus. Mutation rate is expressed as the number of mutation events per gene per unit time

Stem cells cells with self-renewing capabilities which can differentiate into multiple cell lineages

Stomodeum the ectodermal depression at the rostral end of the embryo which becomes the rostral portion of the mouth

Stratum granulosum the layer of cells derived from follicular cells lining the antrum of a maturing ovarian follicle

Stroma the connective tissue forming the framework of an organ as distinct from its functional cells, referred to as parenchyma

Sulcus limitans groove between alar and basal plates of the neural tube

Survival factors factors which inhibit apoptosis and promote survival of a cell or cell populations

Symplasma multinucleate syncytium-like mass of degenerating uterine tissue produced as a reaction to invading trophoblastic villi

Synaptic signalling signalling relating to a synapse; the minute gap between adjacent neurons across which nerve impulses pass. As an impulse reaches a synapse, a neurotransmitter is released which diffuses across this gap and stimulates an electrical impulse in the post-ganglionic neuron

Syncytiotrophoblast the outer syncytial layer of the trophoblast formed from the inner cytotrophoblast

Syncytium multinucleate cellular mass resulting from mitosis without cell boundaries

Syndactyly incomplete separation of digits; fusion of claws or digits

Tail fold caudal body fold

TATA box a DNA sequence, thymine–adenine–thymine–adenine, to which RNA polymerase binds; present in many promoter regions

Telencephalon the cerebral vesicles; secondary paired brain vesicles which arise from the prosencephalon

Teratogen an agent which can cause a permanent alteration to the structure or function of an embryo or foetus

Teratology the study of abnormal development and congenital malformations

Teratoma tumour containing derivatives of two or three germ layers which arise from primordial germ cells

Tetrad four homologous chromatids (two pairs of sister chromatids) synapsed during first meiotic prophase and metaphase

Thrombopoietin a hormone produced by the liver which acts on megakaryocytes, regulating platelet production

Thymus primary lymphoid organ for T lymphocyte differentiation and maturation

Transcription the synthesis of RNA copy from genomic template of DNA by RNA polymerase

Transforming growth factor family a large family of structurally-related, secreted proteins which act as mediators, controlling a wide range of functions during foetal development and post-natally. Members of this protein family include the TGF-β, bone morphogenic proteins and activins

Translation the synthesis of a polypeptide using the instruction carried by an mRNA strand

Transposable elements a class of DNA sequences which have the capability of moving from one chromosomal site to another; movement is mediated by the enzymes transposase and resolvase

Trilaminar embryonic disc disc-shaped embryo comprising ectoderm, mesoderm and endoderm

Trophoblast the cells of the blastocyst, excluding those which form the embryo; the cells of the trophoblast attach the fertilised ovum to the endometrium and contribute to the formation of the foetal membranes and placenta

Truncus arteriosus cranial dilation of the cardiac tube

Tubal pregnancy implantation and development occurring in the uterine tube

Tuberculum impar medial swelling which contributes to the rostral third of the tongue

Tumour suppressor gene gene which appears to prevent neoplastic cell formation

Umbilical cord the structure which connects the embryo or foetus with the placenta, containing loose mesenchymal tissue, blood vessels, the urachus and vestige of the yolk sac

Urogenital folds elevations flanking the urogenital groove which enclose the urethra in the body of the penis in the male embryo and form the labia in the female embryo

Urogenital groove midline depression between urogenital folds

Urogenital membrane ventral subdivision of cloacal membrane

Urogenital sinus ventral sub-division of the cloaca

Urorectal septum mesodermal septum which divides the cloaca into the dorsal rectum and ventral primitive urogenital sinus

Vaginal plate endodermal proliferation from the urogenital sinus; when canalised it contributes to the formation of the vagina

Variation the divergence among individuals of a group, which are not due to differences in age or sex

Vitelline membrane the cell membrane of the ovum

Viviparity giving birth to living young which develop within the maternal body

Wharton's jelly the mucoid matrix of the umbilical cord

Yolk sac an extra-embryonic foetal membrane made up of an inner endodermal layer and an outer splanchnic mesodermal layer which communicates with the embryonic midgut through the vitello-intestinal duct

Zona pellucida transparent, non-cellular layer surrounding the oocyte

Zona reaction alteration of the zona pellucida induced by the action of the cortical granules when the head of a spermatozoon comes in contact with the surface of an oocyte; this reaction prevents adhesion to and penetration of the zona pellucida by additional spermatozoa

Zygote the diploid cell resulting from the fusion of the male and female gametes; the fertilised ovum

Index

All numbers refer to page numbers. Numbers in **bold** refer to major entries.